Imaging of Disorders Spanning the Spectrum from Childhood into Adulthood

Editor

EDWARD Y. LEE

RADIOLOGIC CLINICS OF NORTH AMERICA

www.radiologic.theclinics.com

Consulting Editor
FRANK H. MILLER

May 2020 • Volume 58 • Number 3

ELSEVIER

1600 John F. Kennedy Boulevard • Suite 1800 • Philadelphia, Pennsylvania, 19103-2899

http://www.theclinics.com

RADIOLOGIC CLINICS OF NORTH AMERICA Volume 58, Number 3
May 2020 ISSN 0033-8389, ISBN 13: 978-0-323-71116-6

Editor: John Vassallo (j.vassallo@elsevier.com)
Developmental Editor: Donald Mumford

Radiologic Clinics of North America (ISSN 0033-8389) is published bimonthly by Elsevier Inc., 360 Park Avenue South, New York, NY 10010-1710. Months of issue are January, March, May, July, September, and November. Periodicals postage paid at New York, NY and additional mailing offices. Subscription prices are USD 513 per year for US individuals, USD 980 per year for US institutions, USD 100 per year for US students and residents, USD 594 per year for Canadian individuals, USD 1253 per year for Canadian institutions, USD 703 per year for international individuals, USD 1253 per year for international institutions, USD 100 per year for Canadian students/residents, and USD 315 per year for international students/residents. To receive student and resident rate, orders must be accompanied by name of affiliated institution, date of term and the signature of program/residency coordinatior on institution letterhead. Orders will be billed at individual rate until proof of status is received. Foreign air speed delivery is included in all *Clinics* subscription prices. All prices are subject to change without notice. **POSTMASTER:** Send address changes to *Radiologic Clinics of North America*, Elsevier Health Sciences Division, Subscription Customer Service, 3251 Riverport Lane, Maryland Heights, MO63043. **Customer Service: Telephone: 1-800-654-2452** (U.S. and Canada); **1-314-447-8871** (outside U.S. and Canada). **Fax: 1-314-447-8029. E-mail: journalscustomerservice-usa@elsevier.com (for print support); journalsonlinesupport-usa@elsevier.com (for online support)**.

Reprints. For copies of 100 or more of articles in this publication, please contact the Commercial Reprints Department, Elsevier Inc., 360 Park Avenue South, New York, New York 10010-1710. Tel.: +1-212-633-3874; Fax: +1-212-633-3820; E-mail: reprints@elsevier.com.

Radiologic Clinics of North America also published in Greek Paschalidis Medical Publications, Athens, Greece.

Radiologic Clinics of North America is covered in *MEDLINE/PubMed (Index Medicus), EMBASE/Excerpta Medica, Current Contents/Life Sciences, Current Contents/Clinical Medicine, RSNA Index to Imaging Literature, BIOSIS, Science Citation Index,* and *ISI/BIOMED*.

Contributors

CONSULTING EDITOR

FRANK H. MILLER, MD, FACR
Lee F. Rogers MD Professor of Medical
Education, Chief, Body Imaging Section and
Fellowship Program, Medical Director, MRI,
Department of Radiology, Northwestern
Memorial Hospital, Northwestern University
Feinberg School of Medicine, Chicago, Illinois,
USA

EDITOR

EDWARD Y. LEE, MD, MPH
Associate Professor and Chief, Division of
Thoracic Imaging, Department of Radiology,
President, International Society of Pediatric
Thoracic Imaging, Boston Children's Hospital,
Harvard Medical School, Boston,
Massachusetts, USA

AUTHORS

APEKSHA CHATURVEDI, MD
Associate Professor, Division of Pediatric
Radiology, Department of Imaging Sciences,
University of Rochester Medical Center, Strong
Memorial Hospital, Rochester, New York,
USA

JUNGWHAN JOHN CHOI, MD
Instructor, Department of Radiology, Boston
Children's Hospital, Harvard Medical School,
Boston, Massachusetts, USA

NATHAN DAVID P. CONCEPCION, MD
Head, Section of Pediatric Radiology, Institute
of Radiology, St. Luke's Medical Center-Global
City, Taguig City, Philippines; Clinical Assistant
Professor, St. Luke's Medical Center College
of Medicine-William H. Quasha Memorial,
Quezon City, Philippines; Vice President,
Philippine Society for Pediatric Radiology

CARLO N. DE CECCO, MD, PhD
Division of Cardiothoracic Imaging,
Department of Radiology and Imaging
Sciences, Emory University Hospital, Atlanta,
Georgia, USA

PETER D. FILEV, MD
Division of Cardiothoracic Imaging,
Department of Radiology and Imaging
Sciences, Emory University Hospital, Atlanta,
Georgia, USA

MICHAEL S. FURMAN, MD
Clinical Assistant Professor, Diagnostic
Imaging, Warren Alpert Medical School of
Brown University, Providence, Rhode Island,
USA; Department of Diagnostic Imaging,
Rhode Island Hospital, Providence, Rhode
Island, USA

VARUNA K. GADIYARAM, MD
Division of Cardiothoracic Imaging,
Department of Radiology and Imaging
Sciences, Emory University Hospital, Atlanta,
Georgia, USA

JARED R. GREEN, MD
Division Head, Pediatric Interventional
Radiology, Assistant Professor of Radiology,
Department of Medical Imaging, Ann and
Robert H. Lurie Children's Hospital, Chicago,
Illinois, USA

BRADFORD HASTINGS, MD, MPH
Radiology Resident and Clinical Fellow,
Department of Radiology, Beth Israel
Deaconess Medical Center, Harvard Medical
School, Boston, Massachusetts,
USA

PARTHA HOTA, DO
Division of Thoracic Imaging, Department of
Radiology, Brigham and Women's Hospital,
Boston, Massachusetts, USA; Atlantic Medical
Imaging, Galloway, New Jersey, USA

BERNARD F. LAYA, MD, DO
Professor, St. Luke's Medical Center College
of Medicine-William H. Quasha Memorial,
Head, Section of Pediatric Radiology, Institute
of Radiology, St. Luke's Medical
Center-Quezon City, Quezon City,
Philippines; President, Philippine
Society for Pediatric Radiology

EDWARD Y. LEE, MD, MPH
Associate Professor and Chief, Division of
Thoracic Imaging, Department of Radiology,
President, International Society of Pediatric
Thoracic Imaging, Boston Children's Hospital,
Harvard Medical School, Boston,
Massachusetts, USA

TERESA I-HAN LIANG, MD, FRCPC
Department of Radiology, University of Alberta,
Stollery Children's Hospital, Edmonton,
Alberta, Canada

RACHNA MADAN, MD
Assistant Professor of Radiology, Harvard
Medical School, Associate Staff Radiologist,
Division of Thoracic Imaging, Department of
Radiology, Brigham and Women's Hospital,
Boston, Massachusetts, USA

ROBERT P. MAS, BAS
Ross University School of Medicine, St
Michael, Barbados, West Indies

CATERINA B. MONTI, MD
Department of Biomedical Sciences for Health,
Università degli Studi di Milano, Milano,
Italy

KOENRAAD MORTELE, MD
Dover, Massachusetts, USA

GIUSEPPE MUSCOGIURI, MD
Centro Cardiologico Monzino, IRCCS, Milano,
Italy

LISET PELAEZ, MD
Department of Pathology, Nicklaus Children's
Hospital, Nicklaus, Florida, USA

RACHEL PEVSNER, DO
Department of Pediatric Radiology, Chief of
Ultrasound Division, Nicklaus Children's
Hospital, Miami, Florida, USA

GRACE S. PHILLIPS, MD
Associate Professor, Division Chief, Computed
Tomography, Department of Radiology,
Seattle Children's Hospital, University of
Washington School of Medicine, Seattle,
Washington, USA

DOMEN PLUT, MD, PhD
Department of Pediatric Radiology, Clinical
Radiology Institute, University Medical Centre
Ljubljana, Ljubljana, Slovenia

SCOTT A. RESNICK, MD
Professor of Radiology and Surgery, Division of
Vascular and Interventional Radiology,
Northwestern University Feinberg School of
Medicine, Chicago, Illinois, USA

RICARDO RESTREPO, MD
Chief, Division of Interventional Pediatric
Radiology and Body Imaging, Professor,
Department of Radiology, Nicklaus Children's
Hospital, Miami, Florida, USA

ERIN K. ROMBERG, MD
Acting Assistant Professor, Department of
Radiology, Seattle Children's Hospital,
University of Washington School of Medicine,
Seattle, Washington, USA

ANURAG SAHU, MD
Cardiac Intensive Care Unit, Emory University
Hospital, Atlanta, Georgia, USA

FRANCESCO SARDANELLI, MD
Department of Biomedical Sciences for Health,
Università degli Studi di Milano, Department of
Radiology, IRCCS Policlinico San Donato,
Milan, Italy

SCOTT SCHIFFMAN, MD
Assistant Professor, Division of
Musculoskeletal Radiology, Department of
Imaging Sciences, University of Rochester
Medical Center, Strong Memorial Hospital,
Rochester, New York, USA

JEDIDIAH SCHLUNG, MD
Department of Imaging Sciences, Strong
Memorial Hospital, Rochester, New York, USA

GARY R. SCHOOLER, MD
Assistant Professor, Department of Radiology,
Duke University Medical Center, Durham,
North Carolina, USA

FRANCESCO SECCHI, MD, PhD
Department of Biomedical Sciences for Health,
Università degli Studi di Milano, Department of
Radiology, IRCCS Policlinico San Donato,
Milan, Italy

BINDU N. SETTY, MD
Assistant Professor, Department of Radiology,
Boston Medical Center, Boston,
Massachusetts, USA

ARTHUR E. STILLMAN, MD, PhD
Division of Cardiothoracic Imaging,
Department of Radiology and Imaging
Sciences, Emory University Hospital, Atlanta,
Georgia, USA

Contents

Congenital brain malformations comprise a spectrum of disorders that result from a variety of causes, including genetic abnormalities, ischemia, infections, and toxic exposures. Although most cases are discovered in infancy or childhood, clinically occult abnormalities may prove to be confounding, especially if first encountered later in life on imaging examinations obtained for other indications or in the context of superimposed pathology. This review article provides an overview of congenital brain malformations because they may be encountered at all ages for general radiologists.

Advanced pulmonary disease continues to remain the leading cause of morbidity and mortality in patients with cystic fibrosis (CF), with pulmonary imaging playing a crucial role in early detection, longitudinal monitoring, as well as prelung and post-lung transplant evaluation. This article reviews the specific imaging features of CF using conventional imaging modalities (chest radiographs and high-resolution computed tomography [HRCT]) as well as emerging imaging technologies (digital chest tomosynthesis and MR imaging). In addition, the authors review the CF-specific HRCT imaging findings that are essential in the evaluation of these patients in the pre–lung transplant and post–lung transplant settings.

Childhood interstitial lung disease (chILD) in children, teenagers, and young adults presents a challenge to the clinicians and radiologist, given its rarity, diverse imaging manifestations, and often nonspecific clinical examination findings. This article discusses the utility of available imaging techniques and associated characteristic imaging findings, and reviews the 2015 chILD classification scheme, with clinical examples highlighting the imaging features to help the radiologist aid in an efficient and accurate multidisciplinary diagnosis of chILD.

Because of a recent increase in survival rates and life expectancy of patients with congenital heart disease (CHD), radiologists are facing new challenges when imaging the peculiar anatomy of individuals with repaired CHD. Cardiac computed tomography and magnetic resonance are paramount noninvasive imaging tools that are useful in assessing patients with repaired CHD, and both techniques are increasingly performed in centers where CHD is not the main specialization. This review provides general radiologists with insight into the main issues of imaging patients with repaired CHD, and the most common findings and complications of each individual pathology and its repair.

Inflammatory bowel disease (IBD) has a rising prevalence in children and an increasing number of adults living with IBD were diagnosed in childhood. This chronic disorder requires frequent cross-sectional imaging for evaluating disease progression. Radiologists must be vigilant to detect and understand imaging manifestations of acute and chronic, alimentary, and extraintestinal findings of IBD. This article discusses the role of imaging in evaluation of IBD transitioning from pediatric to adult patients. Imaging modalities and techniques used for evaluating IBD are reviewed. Characteristic acute and chronic imaging findings of IBD are discussed with emphasis on what radiologists need to clearly understand.

Congenital, developmental, and acquired conditions of the pediatric hip frequently present with sequelae in the adult. There is substantial overlap in the end-stage results of these pathologic conditions, including osseous changes, chondral/labral injuries, and premature osteoarthritis. This review discusses the top 10 etiopathogeneses of pediatric hip conditions and presents associated dysmorphisms in the adult on an illustrative, multimodality, case-based template. Quantitative imaging metrics and the role of advanced imaging techniques are reviewed. The ultimate goal is enhanced understanding of the expected evolution of childhood hip pathologic conditions and their associated complications for general radiologists.

End-stage organ failure is commonly treated with transplantation of the respective failing organ. Although outcomes have progressively improved over the decades, early and late complications do occur, and are often diagnosed by imaging. Given the increasing survival rates of transplant patients, the general radiologist may encounter these patients in the outpatient setting. Awareness of the normal radiologic findings after transplantation, and imaging findings of the more common complications, is therefore important. We review and illustrate the imaging assessment of complications from lung, liver, and renal transplantation, highlighting the key similarities and differences between pediatric and adult patients.

and screening recommendations for a selected group of clinically relevant genetic syndromes affecting both pediatric and adult populations.

Congenital entities sharing imaging characteristics with true pathologies occasionally are discovered incidentally in adults. These may occur in the neck, chest, abdomen/pelvis, or musculoskeletal systems. Although these incidental findings share imaging features with true pathologic processes, up-to-date knowledge and assessment with the most appropriate imaging modalities generally allow a distinction between congenital entities that may be safely dismissed and pathologic processes requiring further assessment and treatment. This article reviews several of the most common congenital processes that may present incidentally in adult patients mimicking disease. Emphasis is on findings that can be used to distinguish congenital process from true disease processes.

PROGRAM OBJECTIVE

The objective of the *Radiologic Clinics of North America* is to keep practicing radiologists and radiology residents up to date with current clinical practice in radiology by providing timely articles reviewing the state of the art in patient care.

TARGET AUDIENCE

Practicing radiologists, radiology residents, and other healthcare professionals who provide patient care utilizing radiologic findings.

LEARNING OBJECTIVES

Upon completion of this activity, participants will be able to:

1. Review imaging for congenital brain malformations, repaired congenital heart disease (CHD), complications from lung, liver, and renal transplantation (pediatric and adult), and the expected evolution of childhood hip pathologies.
2. Discuss emerging imaging modalities for cystic fibrosis, childhood interstitial lung disease (chILD), and a select group of clinically relevant genetic syndromes (pediatric and adult),
3. Recognize the spectrum of characteristic acute and chronic imaging findings of IBD, vascular malformations and vascular tumors, differences between intramuscular venous malformations (IMVM), intramuscular capillary type hemangioma (ICTH), and Fibroadipose vascular anomaly (FAVA), and distinctions between incidental congenital entities that may be safely dismissed versus those requiring further assessment and treatment.

ACCREDITATION

The Elsevier Office of Continuing Medical Education (EOCME) is accredited by the Accreditation Council for Continuing Medical Education (ACCME) to provide continuing medical education for physicians.

The EOCME designates this journal-based CME activity for a maximum of 12 *AMA PRA Category 1 Credit*(s)™. Physicians should claim only the credit commensurate with the extent of their participation in the activity.

All other healthcare professionals requesting continuing education credit for this enduring material will be issued a certificate of participation.

DISCLOSURE OF CONFLICTS OF INTEREST

The EOCME assesses conflict of interest with its instructors, faculty, planners, and other individuals who are in a position to control the content of CME activities. All relevant conflicts of interest that are identified are thoroughly vetted by EOCME for fair balance, scientific objectivity, and patient care recommendations. EOCME is committed to providing its learners with CME activities that promote improvements or quality in healthcare and not a specific proprietary business or a commercial interest.

The planning committee, staff, authors and editors listed below have identified no financial relationships or relationships to products or devices they or their spouse/life partner have with commercial interest related to the content of this CME activity:

Apeksha Chaturvedi, MD; Jungwhan John Choi, MD; Nathan David P. Concepcion, MD; Peter D. Filev, MD; Michael S. Furman, MD; Varuna K. Gadiyaram, MD; Jared R. Green, MD; Bradford Hastings, MD, MPH; Partha Hota, DO; John Vassallo; Marilu Kelly, MSN, RN, CNE, CHCP; Pradeep Kuttysankaran; Bernard F. Laya, MD, DO; Edward Y. Lee, MD, MPH; Teresa I-Han Liang, MD, FRCPC; Rachna Madan, MD; Robert P. Mas, MD; Caterina B. Monti, MD; Koenraad Mortele, MD; Giuseppe Muscogiuri, MD; Liset Pelaez, MD, FRCPC; Rachel Pevsner, DO; Grace S. Phillips, MD; Domen Plut, MD, PhD; Scott A. Resnick, MD; Ricardo Restrepo, MD; Erin K. Romberg, MD; Anurag Sahu, MD; Scott Schiffman, MD; Jedidiah Schlung, MD; Gary R. Schooler, MD; Francesco Secchi, MD, PhD, Bindu N. Setty, MD; Arthur E. Stillman, MD, PhD.

The planning committee, staff, authors and editors listed below have identified financial relationships or relationships to products or devices they or their spouse/life partner have with commercial interest related to the content of this CME activity:

Carlo N. De Cecco, MD, PhD: research support and a speaker for Bayer AG and Siemens.

Francesco Sardanelli, MD: research support and a speaker for Bracco, Bayer AG, and General Electric.

UNAPPROVED/OFF-LABEL USE DISCLOSURE

The EOCME requires CME faculty to disclose to the participants:

1. When products or procedures being discussed are off-label, unlabelled, experimental, and/or investigational (not US Food and Drug Administration [FDA] approved); and
2. Any limitations on the information presented, such as data that are preliminary or that represent ongoing research, interim analyses, and/or unsupported opinions. Faculty may discuss information about pharmaceutical agents that is outside of FDA-approved labelling. This information is intended solely for CME and is not intended to promote off-label use of these medications. If you have any questions, contact the medical affairs department of the manufacturer for the most recent prescribing information.

TO ENROLL

To enroll in the *Radiologic Clinics of North America* Continuing Medical Education program, call customer service at 1-800-654-2452 or sign up online at http://www.theclinics.com/home/cme. The CME program is available to subscribers for an additional annual fee of USD 330.00.

METHOD OF PARTICIPATION

In order to claim credit, participants must complete the following:

1. Complete enrolment as indicated above.
2. Read the activity.
3. Complete the CME Test and Evaluation. Participants must achieve a score of 70% on the test. All CME Tests and Evaluations must be completed online.

CME INQUIRIES/SPECIAL NEEDS

For all CME inquiries or special needs, please contact elsevierCME@elsevier.com.

RADIOLOGIC CLINICS OF NORTH AMERICA

RELATED SERIES

Magnetic Resonance Imaging Clinics
Neuroimaging Clinics
PET Clinics

THE CLINICS ARE AVAILABLE ONLINE!
Access your subscription at:
www.theclinics.com

Preface

Imaging of Disorders Spanning the Spectrum from Childhood to Adulthood

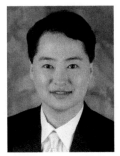

Edward Y. Lee, MD, MPH
Editor

Due to recent rapid advances in surgical and nonsurgical management of congenital and acquired pediatric disorders, many pediatric patients are now living longer and reaching adulthood. Increasing survival rates and life expectancy has presented radiologists with new challenges when interpreting imaging studies for long-term survivors of pediatric diseases. In addition, congenital entities sharing similar imaging characteristics with true pathologic conditions can be incidentally discovered in adults, potentially resulting in confusion, delayed diagnosis, or even misdiagnosis.

Therefore, the aim of the articles in this issue of *Radiologic Clinics of North America* is to provide general radiologists with insight into the imaging findings of disorders that now span from childhood to adulthood. In addition, this issue also addresses imaging findings that can be used to distinguish the congenital processes that occur beyond childhood from true disease processes in need of additional evaluation and treatment.

As the editor for this issue, I have selected topics that are considered to be of current importance with widespread clinical relevance in the imaging management of disorders that now bridge from childhood to adulthood. A clear understanding of the up-to-date imaging techniques combined with characteristic imaging findings of these disorders, which were previously exclusively seen in pediatric patients, is essential for optimal patient care.

I had the great privilege and pleasure of working with highly experienced and talented contributing authors, all of whom are experts in the field of medical imaging. Their invaluable efforts and extraordinary expertise have helped create a resource of information that should facilitate the better understanding of this unique group of congenital and acquired pediatric disorders that span from childhood to adulthood. I would also like to thank Dr Frank H. Miller, consulting editor of the *Radiologic Clinics of North America*, for his insightful guidance; John G. Vassallo, Donald Mumford, and their colleagues at Elsevier, for their superb administrative and editorial assistance; and my family, for their constant encouragement and invaluable support.

Edward Y. Lee, MD, MPH
Division of Thoracic Imaging
Department of Radiology
Boston Children's Hospital
Harvard Medical School
300 Longwood Avenue
Boston, MA 02115, USA

E-mail address:
Edward.Lee@childrens.harvard.edu

Radiol Clin N Am 58 (2020) xv
https://doi.org/10.1016/j.rcl.2020.02.004
0033-8389/20/© 2020 Published by Elsevier Inc.

Brain Malformations at All Ages
From Aunt Minnie to Zebras for General Radiologists

Jungwhan John Choi, MD[a], Bindu N. Setty, MD[b], Edward Y. Lee, MD, MPH[a],*

KEYWORDS

- Congenital brain malformations • Pediatric brain • Congenital brain

KEY POINTS

- Congenital brain malformations often manifest in an imaging spectrum of mild to severe forms with clinical phenotype often corresponding with the imaging findings.
- In milder manifestations of brain malformations, affected patients may present as adults with first time seizure, developmental delay, or for other unrelated causes.
- Surgery for brain malformations is often directed toward the management of secondary findings, such as hydrocephalus or seizures.
- In a patient with history of shunted hydrocephalus or epilepsy surgery, one should look for possible underlying congenital malformations.

INTRODUCTION

Congenital brain malformations can be encountered in both pediatric and adult patients and with the improving resolution of fetal MR imaging, they are increasingly being diagnosed in the prenatal period as well.[1] Although most malformations are discovered in infancy or childhood, milder phenotypes may manifest clinically later in life or remain clinically silent until discovered incidentally on imaging obtained for other indications. These malformations may prove to be confounding to a general radiologist, particularly if encountered in the context of superimposed pathology or in the setting of surgical complications.

The etiologies for congenital brain malformations are varied and can result from genetic abnormalities, ischemia, infections, and toxic exposures. Recently, the Zika virus epidemic brought much public attention to the effect of congenital infections on the developing brain and importance of early screening and detection.[2] Although the scope of congenital brain malformations are as varied as the causes, identifying the pattern of malformation may suggest the underlying cause or genetic abnormality. This review article provides an overview of brain malformations because they may be encountered at all ages for general radiologists.

IMAGING TECHNIQUES
Plain Radiography

Skull radiography is still commonly obtained in the setting of suspected nonaccidental trauma in the pediatric population. However, it is no longer considered standard of care for most clinical indications in either children or adults owing to its lack of sensitivity and specificity at the cost of radiation dose, which is not insignificant when multiple views are obtained.

[a] Department of Radiology, Boston Children's Hospital, Harvard Medical School, 300 Longwood Avenue, Main Building, 2nd Floor, Boston, MA 02115, USA; [b] Department of Radiology, Boston Medical Center, FGH Building, 3rd Floor, Boston, MA 02118, USA
* Corresponding author.
E-mail address: Edward.lee@childrens.harvard.edu

Radiol Clin N Am 58 (2020) 463–474
https://doi.org/10.1016/j.rcl.2019.12.002
0033-8389/20/© 2020 Elsevier Inc. All rights reserved.

Ultrasound Imaging

Ultrasound examination is the primary modality for imaging the fetal and neonatal brain until approximately 9 to 12 months of age, at which time the closing anterior fontanelle provides a limited acoustic window. In infants and neonates, ultrasound examination can be used to screen for intracranial hemorrhage, hydrocephalus, periventricular leukomalacia, and congenital anomalies.

Ultrasound examination is typically performed via the open anterior as well as mastoid fontanelles through which a series of sagittal, parasagittal, and coronal grayscale images are obtained. The mastoid fontanelle offers an optimal window for evaluation of the fourth ventricle and posterior fossa. Color and spectral Doppler can be performed to evaluate the circle of Willis, superficial cortical veins, venous sinuses, and vascular anomalies, such as vein of Galen malformations.

Advantages of ultrasound examination include real-time diagnostic information; portability with the ability to image infants who may be too unstable to travel to computed tomography scanning/MR imaging, and its low cost, allowing for serial screening examinations. Disadvantages include limited sensitivity for detecting early ischemic changes and limited views of structures located deep or peripheral to the field of view provided by the anterior and mastoid fontanelle acoustic windows, such as the lateral temporal lobes or periphery of the posterior fossa structures, an important site of hemorrhage detection in patients on extracorporeal membrane oxygenation.[3]

Computed Tomography Scans

Multidetector computed tomography scanning offers the advantages of rapid acquisition times; the ability to recreate isotropic, multiplanar, reformatted images, and 3-dimensional reconstructions in various algorithms; and fine osseous detail over MR imaging. These advantages should be heavily weighed against the risks associated with the use of ionizing radiation, particularly in children with chronic conditions, who may undergo multiple diagnostic imaging investigations throughout their lifetime. For both children and adults, dose reduction should be optimized via appropriate collimation of the area of interest; indication-appropriate kilovoltage and milliampere-second parameters; and iterative reconstruction techniques, if available, to further decrease the radiation dose.

MR Imaging

In most circumstances in which imaging of the brain are required, MR imaging is the imaging modality of choice. MR imaging offers excellent soft tissue resolution, spatial resolution, and ability for multiplanar imaging acquisition, all with lack of ionizing radiation. Disadvantages include longer image acquisition times and susceptibility to motion, which may be problematic in the pediatric population, particularly between the ages of 6 months and 4 years of age. For children who may be unable to remain still for MR imaging, sedation may be required.

Individual sequences chosen for an MR imaging protocol vary depending on the clinical indication with standard protocols including sagittal T1-weighted imaging; axial and coronal T2-weighted imaging; axial T2 fluid attenuation inversion recovery (FLAIR) imaging; and axial diffusion-weighted imaging. Pediatric patients at the authors' institution with suspected structural brain abnormalities are imaged with isotropic T1-weighted FLAIR and magnetization prepared T1-weighted MR imaging at isotropic resolution, which accentuate subtle cortical and white matter abnormalities and beautifully depict gray–white matter interfaces.[4] Gadolinium contrast may be administered to better assess primary and metastatic brain tumors, leptomeningeal disease, intracranial infections, demyelination, and neurocutaneous disorders. However, evaluation of brain malformations typically does not require gadolinium contrast.

SPECTRUM OF BRAIN MALFORMATIONS
Malformations of Cortical Development

Disorders of neuronal proliferation
Hemimegalencephaly Hemimegalencephaly refers to hamartomatous overgrowth of all or part of a cerebral hemisphere. Often, additional abnormalities such as polymicrogyria, lissencephaly, or gray matter heterotopias are present and may involve the contralateral hemisphere. Clinically, affected patients often present within the first year of life with seizure disorder, macrocephaly, hemiplegia, and profound developmental delay. The incidence of hemimegalencephaly is rare, accounting for 0.2% of children with epilepsy and among those 1% to 14% have malformations of cortical development.[5] If no contralateral malformations are present, seizures are managed with anatomic or functional hemispherectomy, which often requires shunting of the surgical cavity. Surgical shunt malfunctions are common and may present in the adult emergency setting (**Fig. 1**).

Focal cortical dysplasias
Focal cortical dysplasias are areas of cortical disorganization and abnormal laminar architecture (**Fig. 2**). They often present in

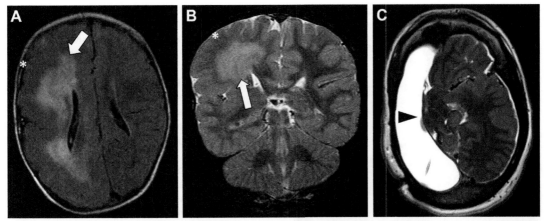

Fig. 1. A 1-year-old boy with intractable epilepsy in the setting of hemimegalencephaly who underwent right hemispherectomy and placement of a shunt into a hemicranial cerebrospinal fluid (CSF) cavity presents to the emergency department as a 19-year-old man with increased lethargy. (*A*) Axial nonenhanced FLAIR MR image of the brain shows an abnormally large right cerebral hemisphere with diffuse cortical malformation (*asterisk*) and diffuse right-sided white matter signal abnormality (*arrow*), characteristic of hemimegalencephaly. (*B*) Coronal nonenhanced T2-weighted MR image shows asymmetry of the right cerebral hemisphere with diffuse cortical malformation (*asterisk*) and diffuse right sided white matter signal abnormality (*arrow*). (*C*) Axial nonenhanced T2-weighted MR image shows postoperative changes related to right hemispherectomy and occipital approach shunt placement with shift of the left cerebral hemisphere across midline into the resection cavity (*arrowhead*). This appearance represents the patient's baseline after hemispherectomy, not substantially changed over many years.

childhood in the setting of intractable epilepsy and are recognized as the most common cause of neocortical pharmacoresistant epilepsy.[6] However, in some instances, focal cortical dysplasias can be clinically occult and are discovered later in life on MR imaging examinations performed for indications other than seizure.

In the setting of medically refractory seizures, a multidisciplinary and multimodality evaluation with MR imaging, nuclear imaging, and subdural localization by electroencephalogram can guide focal resection for treatment with favorable long-term seizure outcomes observed in up to 80% of patients undergoing surgery. Factors associated with recurrent seizures following surgery include operation after 18 years of age, long duration of epilepsy before surgery and the presence of multilobar focal cortical dysplasia.[7]

Disorders of neuronal migration

Lissencephaly Lissencephaly (literally, smooth brain) is characterized by reduced gyral and sulcal development with patterns of both pachygyria and agyria. There are a variety of gene alterations resulting in lissencephaly, which have classically been grouped into 2 major subtypes: type 1 (classic) and type 2 (cobblestone) lissencephaly or cobblestone malformation.

Classic lissencephaly arises from disruption of neuronal migration between the 10th and 14th

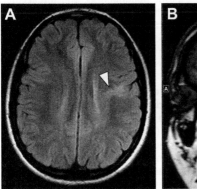
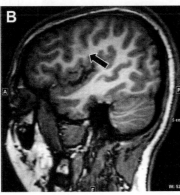

Fig. 2. A 14-year-old girl who presented with an acute episode of psychosis. (*A*) Axial nonenhanced FLAIR MR image of the brain shows linear signal abnormality in the white matter extending from the ventricular margin and widening at the cortex (*arrowhead*), an example of the transmantle sign of focal cortical dysplasia. (*B*) Sagittal nonenhanced T1-weighted MR image shows hazy, indistinct appearance of the gray–white matter junction, suggestive of focal cortical dysplasia (*arrow*).

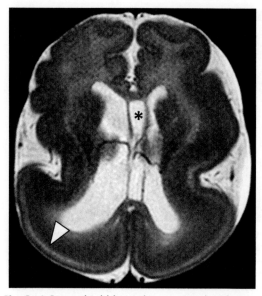

Fig. 3. A 3-month-old boy who presented with new-onset seizures. An axial nonenhanced T2-weighted MR image of the brain shows a simplified gyral pattern with smooth parieto-occipital cortex and thin T2 hyperintense layer known as the cell sparse zone (*arrowhead*), suggestive of classic lissencephaly. Also seen is a cavum septum pellucidum (*asterisk*).

weeks of gestation. Imaging findings of lissencephaly range from the classic hourglass or figure of 8 shape, reflecting diffusely thickened and abnormally smooth cerebral cortex in its more severe form (Fig. 3), to milder forms of subtle band heterotopias. More severe forms are manifested in infancy with hypotonia, seizures and developmental delay. Milder forms with only subcortical band heterotopia are more commonly observed in heterozygous female carriers of the X-linked DCX gene mutation and may be minimally symptomatic with mild seizures and present later in childhood or in the adult setting.[8]

Cobblestone malformation (once known as type II lissencephaly) results from an overmigration of neurons through the pia and into the subarachnoid space. The best known cause results from a mutation involving the dystroglycan complex, which anchors the neuronal cytoskeleton to the extracellular matrix. This mutation results in a heterogeneous group of disorders, affecting the brain, muscles, and eyes, including Fukuyama muscular dystrophy, muscle-eye-brain disease, and Walker-Warburg syndrome. The imaging appearance ranges from mild pachygyria to a cobblestone multinodular appearance of the cortex, most pronounced anteriorly (Fig. 4).

Clinical presentation typically varies based on the underlying syndrome with varying phenotypes of developmental delay, hypotonia, and visual problems. Muscle-eye-brain disease has the least severe phenotype and may present later in life with mean age of 9 ± 5.5 years (range, 2-19 years) with varying degrees of spasticity and additional imaging findings of periventricular white matter abnormalities, ventriculomegaly, pontocerebellar hypoplasia, and cerebellar cysts.[9]

Gray matter heterotopia Heterotopic gray matter refers to focal collections of gray matter arising from interruptions in normal neuronal migration. They are subdivided into 3 subgroups, which describe their location and include periventricular/subependymal, focal subcortical, and leptomeningeal (double cortex or band heterotopia). The most common presentation is with seizures, with onset and severity depending on the location and degree of heterotopia. Patients with subependymal heterotopias have relatively late onset of clinical symptoms manifesting as simple partial seizures and/or developmental delay (Fig. 5).[10] In cases

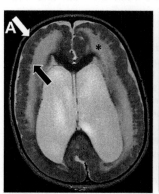
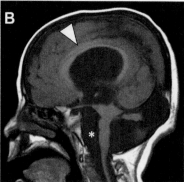

Fig. 4. A 5-year-old boy with epilepsy, spastic quadriparesis, and intellectual disability. (*A*) Axial nonenhanced T2-weighted MR image of the brain shows a smoothly undulating outer cortex contour (*white arrow*) with cobblestone appearance of the inner cortical layer (*black arrow*), characteristic of cobblestone malformation. There is also diffuse signal abnormality in the white matter, indicating dysmyelination (*asterisk*) and ventriculomegaly. (*B*) Sagittal nonenhanced T1-weighted MR image shows pontocerebellar hypoplasia (*asterisk*) and thinning of the corpus callosum (*arrowhead*).

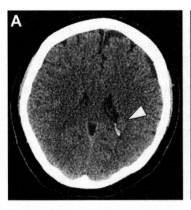
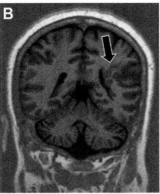

Fig. 5. A 37-year-old woman with seizures. (A) Axial nonenhanced soft tissue window setting CT scan of the brain shows nodularity along the left ventricular margin (*arrowhead*). (B) Axial nonenhanced coronal inversion recovery MR image of the brain shows heterotopic gray matter extending from the ventricle to the cortex suggestive of periventricular and subcortical heterotopia (*arrow*).

of intractable seizures, which is more common with the leptomeningeal subtype, palliative surgery may be performed.

Disorders of neuronal organization

Polymicrogyria Polymicrogyria refers to malformation of the deep cortex with formation of small and convoluted gyri arising from late disruption of neuronal migration and cortical organization. Polymicrogyria can be unilateral, bilateral, focal, or diffuse with the perisylvian region most commonly involved (**Fig. 6**). Affected patients can present with developmental delay, focal neurologic symptoms, or seizures depending on the cortical area involved. Treatment can be pursued via focal resection in cases of medically refractory epilepsy or corpus callosotomy in cases of diffuse or bilateral, unresectable lesions.

Schizencephaly Schizencephaly refers to a gray matter–lined cleft in the cerebral hemisphere extending from the ependymal surface to the pia mater overlying the cerebral cortex. It arises from a congenital disorder of neuronal organization as opposed to porencephaly, which results

from an encephaloclastic insult in late gestation, resulting in a white matter–lined cystic cleft. Affected patients may be asymptomatic; present with seizures and motor deficits from unilateral lesions; or have severe developmental delay, paresis, and spasticity with bilateral lesions (**Fig. 7**). Treatment is usually for management of seizures and may involve lesionectomy or hemispherectomy, depending on disease severity.

Abnormalities of ventral induction

Holoprosencephaly Holoprosencephaly (HPE) is characterized by incomplete cleavage of the forebrain with absence of the interhemispheric falx and fusion of the central gray nuclei. There are a few variants reflecting a spectrum of severity ranging from (1) a milder variant of lobar HPE with hypoplasia of the frontal poles and agenesis of the septum pellucidum (**Fig. 8**); (2) a semilobar HPE with hypoplastic globus pallidi and fusion of the caudate nuclei and thalami (**Fig. 9**), and (3) the most severe variant of alobar HPE with complete fusion of the cerebral hemisphere, absence of the falx, corpus callosum, and septum

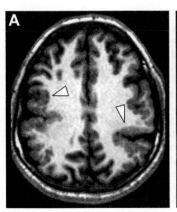
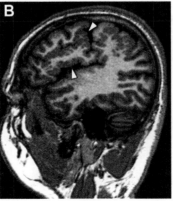

Fig. 6. A 25-year-old woman with seizures. (A) Axial nonenhanced 3-dimensional T1-weighted MR image of the brain shows thickened cortex with an irregular bumpy contour along the perisylvian regions (*arrowheads*) consistent with bilateral perisylvian polymicrogyria. (B) Sagittal nonenhanced 3-dimensional T1-weighted MR image shows extensive perisylvian polymicrogyria (*arrowhead*).

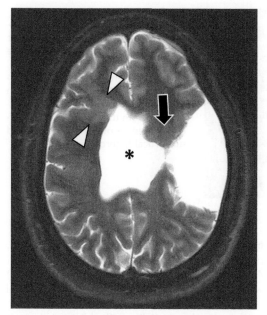

Fig. 7. A 41-year-old man with long-standing history of seizures and new-onset right hemiparesis. An axial nonenhanced T2-weighted MR image of the brain shows a large gray matter lined cerebrospinal fluid (CSF) cleft extending from the ventricle on the left, suggestive of an open lip schizencephaly (*arrow*). Additionally, there is a thin gray matter–lined cleft extending from the frontal horn of the right lateral ventricle, suggestive of a closed lip schizencephaly (*arrowhead*). The septum pellucidum is absent (*asterisk*).

pellucidum and a rudimentary monoventricle (**Fig. 10**). HPE is associated with midline facial anomalies with commonly taught adage that the face predicts the brain, indicating that HPE severity correlates with facial anomalies, which can include hypotelorism, central megaincisor, cebocephaly, ethmocephaly, and cyclopia.

HPE is the most common malformation of the brain and face with prevalence of 1.3 in 10,000

live births.[11] Affected patients often present in infancy or early childhood with facial malformations, seizures (50%), developmental delay, hypothalamic/pituitary dysfunction (most commonly diabetes insipidus seen in up to 70% of patients), dystonia, and hypotonia with clinical severity and a life expectancy that depends on degree of variant cleavage.[12] Treatment is often directed toward the management of seizures and hormone replacement therapy.

Septo-optic dysplasia Septo-optic dysplasia refers to any combination of optic nerve hypoplasia, pituitary hypoplasia, and midline ventral cerebral abnormalities and is considered a mild variant of HPE. Cortical abnormalities include schizencephaly, polymicrogyria, and gray matter heterotopias.[13] Septo-optic dysplasia is often detected in infancy or early childhood, with hypoglycemic seizures, apnea, hypotonia, endocrine dysfunction, or short stature (**Fig. 11**). Visual impairments include normal and/or color blindness, nystagmus, or strabismus. Treatment is directed toward hormone replacement therapy.

Corpus callosum anomalies Agenesis and hypogenesis of the corpus callosum are relatively common accounting for 3% of central nervous system malformations.[14] Hypogenesis of the corpus callosum commonly manifests as an abnormally short corpus callosum with preservation of the splenium and dorsal body and absence of the inferior genu and rostrum, resulting from an interruption of normal callosal development during the 12th and 20th weeks of gestation. Complete callosal agenesis is characterized by absence of the corpus callosum and cingulate gyrus with parallel orientation of the trigones and occipital horns (colpocephaly) and longitudinally oriented Probst bundles observed along the medial aspect of the lateral ventricles, formed by axons, which failed to cross the midline (**Fig. 12**).

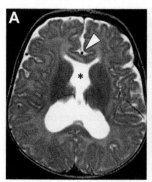 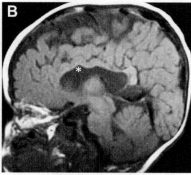

Fig. 8. A 5-day-old girl with multiple congenital anomalies, microcephaly, and cleft palate. (*A*) Axial nonenhanced T2-weighted MR image of the brain shows complete separation of the interhemispheric fissure and thalami with hypoplasia of the frontal lobes, compatible with lobar HPE. Note the absent septum pellucidum (*asterisk*) and azygous anterior cerebral artery (*arrowhead*). (*B*) Sagittal nonenhanced T1-weighted MR image shows an incompletely formed corpus callosum (*asterisk*).

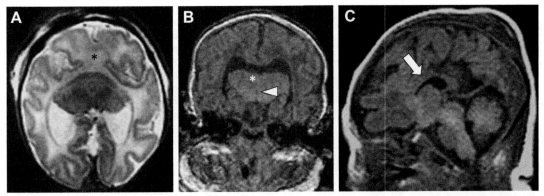

Fig. 9. A 5-day-old girl with multiple congenital anomalies. (A) Axial nonenhanced T2-weighted MR image of the brain shows fusion of the frontal lobes (asterisk) and deep nuclei with partial formation of the occipitotemporal lobes and interhemispheric fissure posteriorly, characteristic findings of semilobar HPE. (B) Coronal nonenhanced 3-dimensional T1-weighted MR image shows the deep nuclei are fused into a single midline mass (asterisk) with a rudimentary third ventricle (arrowhead). (C) Sagittal nonenhanced 3-dimensional T1-weighted MR image shows an incompletely formed corpus callosum (arrow).

Although callosal malformations can be seen in isolation, they are often seen in association with other chromosomal abnormalities (17.3%) and central nervous system malformations (49.5%), such as Chiari II malformation or aqueductal stenosis.[15] In isolated cases, affected patients may be normal to near normal with subtle cognitive defects presenting later in life. In more severe cases associated with other malformations, clinical prognosis can be poor with treatment directed toward the management of hydrocephalus and seizures.

Malformations of the cerebellar vermis
Dandy–Walker spectrum The Dandy–Walker spectrum represents a broad continuum of cystic posterior fossa malformations. The classic Dandy–Walker malformation consists of an enlarged posterior fossa with elevated torcula, severe hypoplasia or agenesis of the cerebellar vermis, and a dilated, cystic appearing fourth ventricle (**Fig. 13**). The Dandy–Walker spectrum

encompasses a number of anomalies in addition to the classic Dandy–Walker malformation, including the Dandy–Walker variant (less dilation of the fourth ventricle and less enlargement of the posterior fossa), retrocerebellar arachnoid cysts, Blake pouch cysts (ballooning of the superior medullary velum into the cisterna magna), and mega cisterna magna.

The clinical presentation varies depending on the severity of the abnormality. The Dandy–Walker spectrum is seen in approximately 1 in 30,000 live births with a number of genes as well as different modes of inheritance implicated.[16,17] Up to 80% of patients with classic Dandy–Walker malformation present in the first year of life with symptoms secondary to hydrocephalus. Less severe forms of retrocerebellar arachnoid cysts and mega cisterna magna may be found incidentally on imaging performed for other indications. If required, treatment is directed toward management of hydrocephalus with cerebrospinal fluid

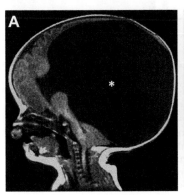

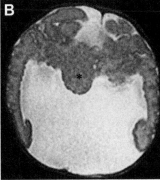

Fig. 10. A 2-day-old boy with abnormal facial features and macrocephaly. (A) Sagittal nonenhanced T1-weighted MR image of the brain shows a large dorsal cyst (asterisk) with resultant mass effect on the posterior fossa structures, which are otherwise intact. (B) Axial nonenhanced T2-weighted MR image shows the thalami are fused into a single midline mass (asterisk) indenting the inferior aspect of the dorsal cyst resulting in the characteristic horse-shoe–shaped monoventricle of alobar HPE.

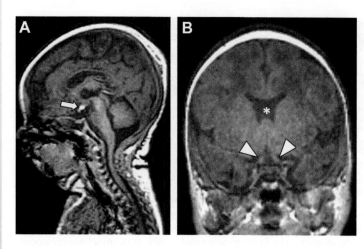

Fig. 11. A 5-year-old girl with short stature. (*A*) Sagittal nonenhanced 3-dimensional T1-weighted MR image of the brain shows an ectopic posterior pituitary bright spot (*arrow*). (*B*) Coronal nonenhanced 3-dimensional T-weighted MR image shows absent septum pellucidum (*asterisk*) and hypoplastic optic nerves (*arrowhead*).

(CSF) diversion and in some cases cyst and shunt marsupialization.

Joubert syndrome Joubert syndrome is an autosomal-recessive disorder resulting in impaired ciliary function. On imaging of the brain, there is underdevelopment of the cerebellar vermis with thickened superior cerebellar peduncles and elongated configuration of the fourth ventricle, resulting in a characteristic molar tooth configuration of the hindbrain (**Fig. 14**). Prevalence is approximately 1 in 100,000 in the United States, with an increased prevalence among isolated populations, such as the Ashkenazi Jews or the Hutterites owing to founder effects.[18] Uniquely, clinical phenotype is independent of the severity of imaging findings with most patients surviving infancy and reaching adulthood. Affected children have a spectrum of abnormalities, including

developmental delay, oculomotor apraxia and speech dyspraxia, hypotonia, and seizure disorders with treatment directed toward the management of seizures.

Rhomboencephalosynapsis
Rhomboencephalosynapsis is a rare, but increasingly recognized malformation, in which there is hypogenesis or complete agenesis of the cerebellar vermis with fusion of the cerebellar hemispheres (**Fig. 15**). It is often associated with other abnormalities, including hydrocephalus, callosal anomalies, and HPE. Clinical presentation varies with prenatal hydrocephalus reflecting poor outcomes and most cases presenting with cognitive impairment. Although the prognosis is often poor, there are survivors to early adulthood as well as a case report of newly diagnosed rhombencephalosynapsis at 55 years of age in

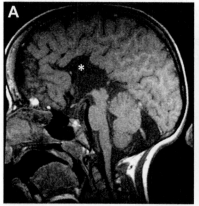
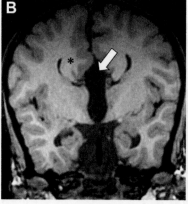
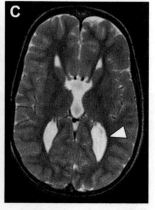

Fig. 12. A 15-year-old girl with developmental delay. (*A*) Sagittal nonenhanced T1-weighted MR image of the brain shows absence of the corpus callosum (*asterisk*). (*B*) Coronal nonenhanced 3-dimensional T1-weighted MR image shows steer horn shape of the lateral ventricles caused by white matter tracts (Probst bundles), which parallel the interhemispheric fissure (*asterisk*). Note the additional finding of a high-riding third ventricle (*arrow*). (*C*) Axial nonenhanced T2-weighted MR image shows parallel orientation of the lateral ventricles and colpocephaly (*arrowhead*).

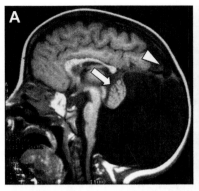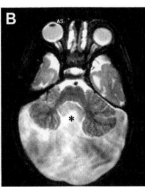

Fig. 13. A 3-year-old boy with developmental delay. (*A*) Sagittal nonenhanced T1-weighted MR image of the brain shows an enlarged posterior fossa with elevation of the torcula herophili (*arrowhead*), hypoplastic vermis (*arrow*), and a large posterior fossa cyst, characteristic findings of the classic Dandy–Walker malformation. (*B*) Axial nonenhanced T2-weighted MR image shows communication of the fourth ventricle with the large posterior fossa cyst (*asterisk*).

an employed male with a normal IQ.[19] If necessary, treatment is directed toward the management of hydrocephalus, often with shunt placement.

Abnormalities of dorsal induction

Chiari I malformations Chiari I malformations are defined as caudal extension of the cerebellar tonsils below the level of the foramen magnum, related to a congenitally small, bony posterior fossa. On imaging, the tonsils extend to a variable degree (typically ≥5 mm), have a pointed configuration, and, as a result, obstruct the flow of CSF at the foramen magnum (**Fig. 16**). This finding is in contradiction to milder tonsillar ectopia, which is thought to be an incidental, clinically silent finding, with rounded configuration of the tonsils and no substantial impediment to CSF flow. Hydromyelia of the cervical cord is present in 23% of affected patients with variable caudal extension into the thoracic cord.[20]

Many patients with Chiari I malformation are asymptomatic with degree of tonsillar ectopia (>12 mm), narrow CSF space posterior to the cerebellar tonsils, and molded morphology of the cerebellar tonsils often correlating with clinical severity. Clinically, affected patients may present with various signs and symptoms, including suboccipital headaches, cranial nerve palsies, ocular disturbances, otoneurologic dysfunction, cord motor or sensory abnormalities, scoliosis, gait disturbance, neuropathic joints, or rarely sudden death.[21]

Treatment for asymptomatic patients remains controversial. For symptomatic patients, posterior fossa decompression and resection of the posterior arch of C1 with cerebellar tonsil resection is performed. Children respond better to treatment than adults, with reported improvement of up to 81% of brainstem signs after surgery.[22]

Chiari II malformations The Chiari II malformation is a complex malformation of the hindbrain and skull that occurs in association with an open neural tube defect, most commonly a myelomeningocele. During fetal development, the malformation is thought to occur from chronic leakage of CSF through the neural tube defect, resulting

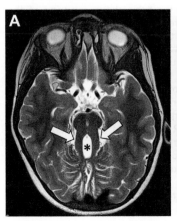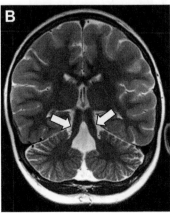

Fig. 14. A 6-year-old girl who presented with a first-time seizure. (*A*) Axial nonenhanced T2-weighted MR image of the brain shows thickened and elongated superior cerebellar peduncles in a molar tooth configuration (*arrows*) and elongation of the fourth ventricle (*asterisk*), characteristic of Joubert syndrome. (*B*) Coronal nonenhanced T2-weighted MR image shows thickened and elongated superior cerebellar peduncles (*arrows*) and absence of the cerebellar vermis.

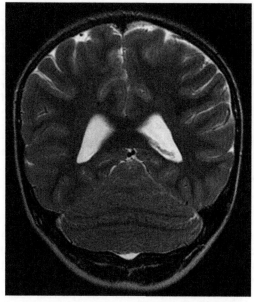

Fig. 15. A 10-year-old boy with developmental delay. A coronal nonenhanced T2-weighted MR image of the brain shows fusion of the cerebellar hemispheres with absence of the cerebellar vermis, characteristic of rhomboencephalosynapsis.

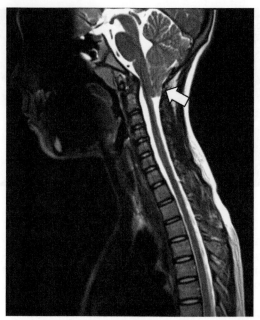

Fig. 16. An 11-year-old girl presenting with headaches and problems with proprioception. A sagittal nonenhanced T2-weighted MR image of the cervical and upper thoracic spine shows descent of the cerebellar tonsils more than 5 mm below the foramen magnum (white arrow), compatible with a diagnosis of Chari I malformation. Note the pointed configuration of the cerebellar tonsils and narrowing of the CSF space posterior to the cerebellar tonsils.

in incomplete expansion of the rhombencephalic vesicle leading to abnormal growth of the skull base and a resultant small posterior fossa. Features commonly seen in Chiari II include hydrocephalus, dysplastic tentorium, small bony posterior fossa, inferior displacement and elongation of the brainstem, kinking at the cervicomedullary junction, enlarged massa intermedia, tectal beaking, callosal hypogenesis, stenogyria, and subependymal heterotopia (Fig. 17).

Chiari II malformations are relatively common with an incidence of approximately 1 in 1000 live births.[23] Diagnosis is often made prenatally with elevated maternal alpha-fetoprotein or the characteristic lemon sign (indentation of the frontal bones) and banana sign (cerebellar crowding and

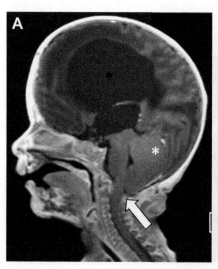

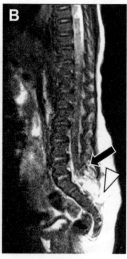

Fig. 17. A 60-day-old boy with known open spinal dysraphism. (A) Sagittal nonenhanced T1-weighted MR image of the brain shows towering of the cerebellum (white asterisk), kinking at the cervicomedullary junction (arrow), inferior displacement and elongation of the brainstem, hypoplasia of the corpus callosum, and hydrocephalus (black asterisk) in this patient with Chiari II malformation. (B) Sagittal nonenhanced T2-weighted MR image of the thoracic and lumbar spine shows the neural placode resting at the L5 level (arrow) and postoperative changes related to prior myelomeningocele repair (arrowhead).

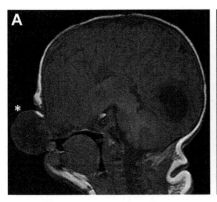
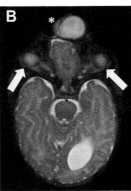

Fig. 18. A 39-day-old boy referred for evaluation of a midline facial mass. (*A*) Sagittal nonenhanced T1-weighted MR image of the brain shows herniation of CSF and brain tissue into a midline facial defect (*asterisk*), compatible with a meningoencephalocele through a Tessier facial cleft. (*B*) Axial nonenhanced T2-weighted MR image shows the midline herniation of CSF and brain tissue (*asterisk*) and hypertelorism (*white arrows*) in this patient with midline facial cleft and meningoencephalocele.

wrapping around the brainstem) observed on prenatal ultrasound examination or fetal MR imaging.

Standard management has been early neonatal repair of the myelomeningocele and shunting of hydrocephalus with a recent trend toward prenatal surgical repair of the myelomeningocele at select fetal centers. Although there are no established long-term data on prenatal surgical repair, evolving literature has reported reduced hydrocephalus, reduced requirement for postnatal ventriculoperitoneal shunt placement, and improved motor outcomes at 30 months of age.[24–26] It is conceivable that, with improving prenatal surgical dexterity and postnatal outcomes, more patients will be imaged as young adults.

Cephalocele Cephalocele refers to herniation of central nervous system tissue through a defect in the skull. They are further classified according to their contents as meningoceles (containing CSF-lined meninges), meningoencephaloceles (containing CSF and brain tissue) (**Fig. 18**), and meningoencephalocystoceles (containing CSF, brain, and ventricle).

Presentation may vary depending on the size and location, with most discovered at birth. Nasopharyngeal cephaloceles may present later, near the end of the first decade of life. Treatment entails resection of the dysplastic herniated brain tissue to prevent CSF leakage and meningitis. More recently, 3-dimensional printing has been applied in modeling cranial vaults in preparation for repair with reincorporation of brain tissue in select cases.

SUMMARY

Congenital brain malformations are not uncommon and may be encountered in both the pediatric and adult practice settings. Milder forms of brain malformations may be first diagnosed in the adult practice setting on an imaging evaluation obtained for a first-time seizure, developmental delay, or for unrelated indications such as trauma or headache. Alternatively, children with known malformations may be encountered in the adult practice setting for routine imaging follow-up for shunted hydrocephalus or seizures. Therefore, it is important for the general radiologist to have an understanding of the patterns and types of congenital brain malformations because they may be encountered in their daily practice.

DISCLOSURE

The authors have nothing to disclose.

REFERENCES

1. Kline-Fath BM, Calvo-Garcia MA. Prenatal imaging of congenital malformations of the brain. Semin Ultrasound CT MR 2011;32(3):167–88.
2. Trevathan E. Editorial brain malformation surveillance in the Zika era. Birth Defects Res A Clin Mol Teratol 2016;106(11):869–74.
3. Bulas DI, Taylor GA, Fitz CR, et al. Posterior fossa intracranial hemorrhage in infants treated with extracorporeal membrane oxygenation: sonographic findings. AJR Am J Roentgenol 1991;156(3):571–5.
4. Yang E, Chu WC, Lee EY. A practical approach to supratentorial brain malformations. Radiol Clin North Am 2017;55(4):609–27.
5. Massimi L, Rocco CD. Hemimegalencephaly. In: Rocco CD, Pang D, Rutka JT, editors. Textbook of Pediatric Neurosurgery. Springer International Publishing; 2018. p. 1–43.
6. Shorvon SD, Andermann F, Guerrini R. The causes of epilepsy common and uncommon causes in adults and children. Cambridge: Cambridge University Press; 2011.
7. Fauser S, Schulze-Bonhage A. In response: long-term seizure outcome in 211 patients with focal cortical dysplasia. Epilepsia 2015;56(7):1177–8.
8. Moffat JJ, Ka M, Jung E-M, et al. Genes and brain malformations associated with abnormal neuron

positioning. Mol Brain 2015;8(1). https://doi.org/10.1186/s13041-015-0164-4.

9. Yiş U, Uyanık G, Rosendahl D, et al. Clinical, radiological, and genetic survey of patients with muscle–eye–brain disease caused by mutations in POMGNT1. Neuromuscul Disord 2016;26. https://doi.org/10.1016/j.nmd.2016.06.288.

10. Donkol RH. Assessment of gray matter heterotopia by magnetic resonance imaging. World J Radiol 2012;4(3):90.

11. Orioli IM, Castilla EE. Epidemiology of holoprosencephaly: prevalence and risk factors. Am J Med Genet C Semin Med Genet 2010;154C(1):13–21.

12. Levey EB, Stashinko E, Clegg NJ, et al. Management of children with holoprosencephaly. Am J Med Genet Part C Semin Med Genet 2010;154C(1):183–90.

13. Alt C, Shevell MI, Poulin C, et al. Clinical and radiologic spectrum of septo-optic dysplasia: review of 17 cases. J Child Neurol 2017;32(9):797–803.

14. Morris JK, Wellesley DG, Barisic I, et al. Epidemiology of congenital cerebral anomalies in Europe: a multicentre, population-based EUROCAT study. Arch Dis Child 2019. https://doi.org/10.1136/archdischild-2018-316733.

15. Glass HC, Shaw GM, Ma C, et al. Agenesis of the corpus callosum in California 1983-2003: a population-based study. Am J Med Genet A 2008;146A(19):2495–500.

16. Correa GG, Amaral LF, Vedolin LM. Neuroimaging of dandy-walker malformation. Top Magn Reson Imaging 2011;22(6):303–12.

17. Bosemani T, Orman G, Boltshauser E, et al. Congenital abnormalities of the posterior fossa. Radiographics 2015;35(1):200–20.

18. Hevner RF, Dobyns WB, Valente EM. Joubert Syndrome. In: Adle-Biassette H, Harding BN, Golden JA, editors. Developmental Neuropathology. Hoboken (NJ): Wiley Blackwell; 2018. p. 151–7.

19. Bell B, Stanko H, Levine R. Normal IQ in a 55-year-old with newly diagnosed rhombencephalosynapsis. Arch Clin Neuropsychol 2005;20(5):613–21.

20. Strahle J, Muraszko KM, Kapurch J, et al. Chiari malformation Type I and syrinx in children undergoing magnetic resonance imaging. J Neurosurg Pediatr 2011;8(2):205–13.

21. Heiss JD. Epidemiology of the Chiari I Malformation. In: Tubbs RS, Oakes WJ, editors. The Chiari Malformations. New York: Springer; 2013. p. 83–92.

22. Arnautovic A, Splavski B, Boop FA, et al. Pediatric and adult Chiari malformation Type I surgical series 1965–2013: a review of demographics, operative treatment, and outcomes. J Neurosurg Pediatr 2015;15(2):161–77.

23. Burn S. Spina Bifida: management and outcome. JAMA 2009;301(4):439.

24. Adzick NS. Fetal myelomeningocele: natural history, pathophysiology, and in-utero intervention. Semin Fetal Neonatal Med 2010;15(1):9–14.

25. Houtrow AJ, Burrows PK, Thom EA. Comparing neurodevelopmental outcomes at 30 months by presence of hydrocephalus and shunt status among children enrolled in the MOMS trial. J Pediatr Rehabil Med 2018;11(4):227–35.

26. Farmer DL, Thom EA, Brock JW, et al. The Management of Myelomeningocele Study: full cohort 30-month pediatric outcomes. Am J Obstet Gynecol 2018;218(2). https://doi.org/10.1016/j.ajog.2017.12.001.

Cystic Fibrosis from Childhood to Adulthood
What Is New in Imaging Assessment?

Partha Hota, DO[a,b], Rachna Madan, MD[a,*]

KEYWORDS

- Cystic fibrosis - Pulmonary disease - Lung transplantation - High-resolution computed tomography

KEY POINTS

- Radiographs and high-resolution computed tomography (HRCT) continue to be the primary imaging modalities in the initial assessment and longitudinal monitoring of cystic fibrosis (CF).
- Recently, emerging imaging modalities, including digital chest tomosynthesis and magnetic resonance imaging, have shown promise in the evaluation of CF with their exact roles yet to be defined.
- With an increasing number of patients with CF receiving lung transplantations, it is crucial for the radiologist to be aware of the CF-specific pre-transplant and post-transplant HRCT findings when assessing these patients.

INTRODUCTION

Cystic fibrosis (CF) is the most common lethally inherited disease in Caucasians with approximately 30,000 affected individuals in the United States alone, as of 2017.[1,2] Characterized by mutations resulting in dysfunctional chloride channel ion transporters, CF is a multisystem disorder with pulmonary, pancreatic, hepatobiliary, gastrointestinal, reproductive, osseous, and infectious manifestations.[1] Of these complications, advanced pulmonary disease dominates the clinical landscape and results from abnormal mucociliary clearance with subsequent episodes of chronic bronchopulmonary infection, mucus obstruction, and eventual bronchiectasis.[1] The resultant morbidity and mortality rates from pulmonary disease approach 95%; with lung transplantation remaining the only definitive cure for CF. Therefore, pulmonary imaging plays a vital role in the early detection, longitudinal monitoring, and pre-transplant and post-transplant evaluation of patients with CF.[3–5]

This article has the two following purposes: (1) to review the specific imaging features of CF with conventionally used imaging modalities (chest radiographs and high-resolution computed tomography [HRCT]) as well as with emerging imaging technologies (digital chest tomosynthesis, hyperpolarized gas magnetic resonance (MR) imaging, and noncontrast MR imaging); and (2) to review the HRCT imaging findings that are essential in the evaluation of these patients in the pre–lung transplant and post–lung transplant settings.

IMAGING TECHNIQUES
Conventional Imaging Techniques

Chest radiographs
Chest radiographs are the most commonly used and often the initial imaging modality when evaluating patients with CF in both pediatric and adult populations. Although less sensitive than HRCT, chest radiographs continue to be used because of the low radiation dose, low cost, and widespread availability. Early in the disease process, chest radiographs may appear entirely normal.

[a] Division of Thoracic Imaging, Department of Radiology, Brigham and Women's Hospital, 75 Francis Street, Boston, MA 02115, USA; [b] Atlantic Medical Imaging, Galloway, NJ, USA
* Corresponding author.
E-mail address: rmadan@bwh.harvard.edu

Radiol Clin N Am 58 (2020) 475–486
https://doi.org/10.1016/j.rcl.2019.12.003
0033-8389/20/© 2019 Elsevier Inc. All rights reserved.

The earliest radiographic findings include hyperinflation secondary to distal airway mucus obstruction or cylindrical bronchiectasis (with tram track opacities).[1,6] By the time patients with classic CF reach adulthood, chronic episodes of mucus obstruction and bronchopulmonary infection result in classic chest radiograph findings, including central and upper lung predominant varicoid and cystic bronchiectasis, bronchial wall thickening, peribronchial cuffing, increased interstitial markings, and scattered nodular opacities (Fig. 1).[1,6] Pneumothoraces are frequently seen and can be recurrent.[1,6,7] Patients with nonclassic CF tend to be adults with fewer clinical symptoms and can have chest radiographs demonstrating mild to very subtle or absent radiographic changes when compared with those of patients with classic CF.[1]

Superimposed bacterial infection (such as with *Pseudomonas aeruginosa* or *Burkholderia* species) often results in mucoid impaction or areas of consolidation (Fig. 2). Mucus-impacted central bronchiectasis in a so-called finger-in-glove appearance is classically observed in the setting of allergic bronchopulmonary aspergillosis (ABPA) and develops in up to 20% of patients with CF.[6,8]

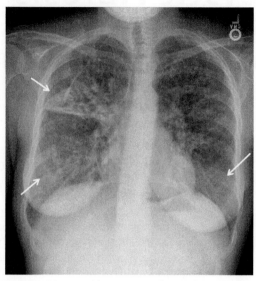

Fig. 2. A 30-year-old woman with CF who presented with fever. Frontal chest radiograph demonstrates patchy bilateral parenchymal opacities (*arrows*) in keeping with pneumonia superimposed on classic findings of CF, including diffuse bronchiectasis, increased interstitial markings, and bronchial wall thickening.

Several chest radiograph scoring systems for CF exist, including the Brasfield, Chrispin-Norman, and Wisconsin systems. Most of these involve scoring of air trapping, bronchiectasis, disease extent, and severity, and all of these have been demonstrated to have good correlation with lung function.[9] Ultimately, choosing which scoring system to evaluate patients with CF for longitudinal monitoring is the responsibility of the reader or institution. Recently developed machine learning models using deep convolution neural networks have been used in the scoring of chest radiographs with one study reporting similar accuracy of a machine learning algorithm to a pediatric radiologist in predicting the Brasfield score.[10] Although promising, these models remain in infancy, and their exact clinical role has yet to be determined.

High-resolution computed tomography
HRCT remains the current gold standard in the evaluation of CF with several studies demonstrating superior accuracy when compared with incentive spirometry and chest radiography alone.[11–13] HRCT findings of classic CF include central and upper lung predominant varicoid and cystic bronchiectasis, bronchial wall thickening, endobronchial mucoid impaction, hyperinflation with air trapping, distal atelectasis, and sacculations (Fig. 3).

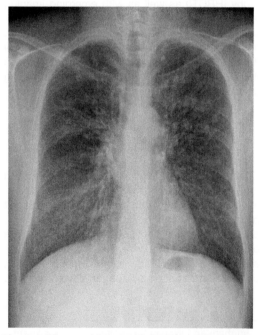

Fig. 1. A 38-year-old man with CF. Frontal chest radiograph demonstrates classic findings of CF, including diffuse bronchiectasis, increased interstitial markings, bronchial wall thickening, and scattered nodular opacities.

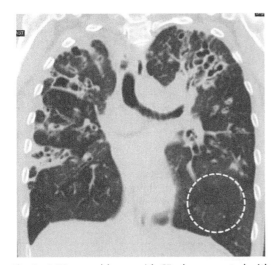

Fig. 3. A 38-year-old man with CF who presented with shortness of breath and hemoptysis. Coronal lung window setting CT image demonstrates mid and upper lung predominant bilateral varicoid bronchiectasis with bronchial wall thickening and endobronchial mucoid impaction. There is mild mosaicism in keeping with air trapping (*dashed circle*).

Superimposed infection can have a variety of imaging manifestations. In the setting of bacterial infection (commonly *Pseudomonas*), lobar and multifocal consolidation, abscesses, and cavities can be observed (**Fig. 4**). In the setting of ABPA, mucus accumulation within an impacted bronchiectactic airway results in a mucocele. High attenuation of mucus is observed in up to 25% of patients and is the result of chelated calcium, iron, and manganese[8,14] (**Fig. 5**). Approximately 10% of adult

patients with CF are infected with atypical nontuberculous mycobacteria (NTM), frequently *Mycobacterium avium complex* and *Mycobacterium abscessus*, with classic HRCT findings, including centrilobular and tree-in-bud micronodules, which can wax and wane following episodes of treatment (**Fig. 6**).[6,15]

In advanced disease, repeat episodes of inflammation and long-standing bronchiectasis result in angiogenesis and hypertrophied bronchial arteries that may subsequently cause massive hemoptysis, which is observed in up to 4% of patients with CF.[16] Many patients present to the emergency department with hemoptysis and undergo a computed tomographic (CT) angiogram to identify the source of bleeding. CT angiography may demonstrate "filling defects" and flow artifacts, which can mimic acute or chronic emboli.[17] However, careful attention to the course of adjacent bronchial collaterals as well as performing a slightly delayed scan (by bolus triggering with a tracker placed over the descending thoracic aorta instead of the main pulmonary artery) may help elucidate the true nature of these "smoke-like filling defects" (**Fig. 7**).[17] Because bronchial artery embolization is the treatment of choice in such scenarios, it is paramount that hypertrophied bronchial arteries be reported in these patients to best provide a vascular roadmap for interventionalists. Additional HRCT findings of CF include mediastinal and hilar lymphadenopathy, secondary to reactive inflammation, and pneumothoraces (**Figs. 8 and 9**).[1,6]

Although several HRCT scoring systems have been reported, there is currently no consensus scoring system identified.[11,18–20] In particular, the Bhalla scoring system examines the severity and

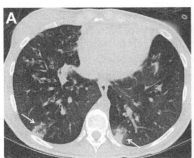
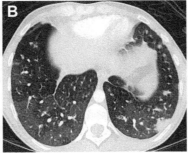
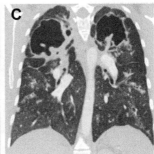

Fig. 4. A 33-year-old woman with CF, fever, and hemoptysis. (*A*) Axial lung window setting CT image demonstrates focal areas of consolidation with surrounding ground-glass and clustered nodules in both lower lobes (*arrows*) in a patient with *Pseudomonas* infection with findings superimposed on classic CF bronchiectasis. (*B, C*) Axial and coronal lung window setting CT images demonstrate a focal area of consolidation in the left lower lobe in a different CF patient with polymicrobial infection, including *Pseudomonas*, methicillin-sensitive *Staphylococcus aureus*, and *Burkholderia* with findings superimposed on classic CF findings, including severe upper lung cystic bronchiectasis, bronchial wall thickening, endobronchial mucoid impaction, clustered nodules, and air trapping.

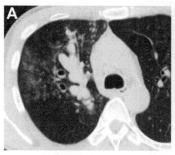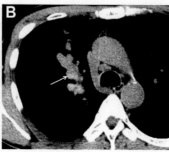

Fig. 5. A 35-year-old man with CF and shortness of breath. Axial lung window setting CT image (*A*) demonstrates completely opacified bronchiectatic airways (mucoceles) in the right upper lobe with distal centrilobular and tree-in-bud micronodules in this patient with CF with bronchoalveolar lavage demonstrating allergic bronchopulmonary aspergillosis (ABPA). Corresponding axial soft tissue window setting CT image (*B*) demonstrates high attenuation of the mucus (*arrow*) reflecting chelated minerals, a classic finding of ABPA.

extent of bronchiectasis, peribronchial thickening, extent of mucus plugging, emphysema, as well as the presence of abscesses, bubbles, and sacculations.[19] Studies have reported good correlation with the Bhalla score and pulmonary function, as determined by incentive spirometry, as well as that an increased Bhalla score had a high correlation with *Pseudomonas* infection.[21–23] However, it is ultimately the reader's responsibility in choosing a scoring system to use if using one at all.

Recently, several automated and semiautomated HRCT quantification methods have been designed to evaluate the severity of patients with CF and to monitor longitudinal progression.[24–26] However, these technologies are still in their infancy, and further studies will need to be performed to fully understand their roles in the future.

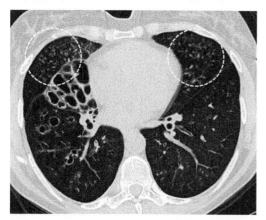

Fig. 6. A 47-year-old woman with CF and shortness of breath. Axial lung window setting CT image demonstrates classic bronchiectasis and bronchial wall thickening of CF with superimposed widespread tree-in-bud micronodules predominantly involving the right middle lobe and lingula (*dashed circles*) in this patient with CF with nontuberculous mycobacteria infection.

Emerging Imaging Techniques

Digital chest tomosynthesis

New technical developments in digital chest tomosynthesis have led to its emergence as a potential alternative imaging modality in the evaluation of CF.[27] Chest tomosynthesis images are generated from several low-dose exposures obtained during breath-hold by a moving radiograph tube over a short arc. Images are then reconstructed into a tomographic composite image consisting of up to 60 coronal images with a slice thickness of 3 mm in children and 4 mm in adults.[27] Compared with HRCT, tomosynthesis allows for higher spatial resolution with a comparatively lower radiation dose (0.1 to 0.2 msV vs 4 to 8 msV).[27,28]

Tomosynthesis findings of CF are similar to that of conventional chest radiographs and include hyperinflation, bronchiectasis, peribronchial thickening, mucus plugging, and consolidation.[27] However, unlike conventional radiographs, tomosynthesis allows for superior evaluation of the airways and vascular tree. Although central bronchiectasis is present on both radiographs and tomosynthesis, peripheral bronchiectasis can be more easily detected on tomosynthesis studies. Classification of bronchiectasis (cylindrical, varicoid, or cystic) can be easily characterized with tomosynthesis compared with chest radiographs. Areas of endobronchial mucus impaction and clustered nodules are more readily evident on tomosynthesis and may only appear as vague or blurred shadows on radiography (**Fig. 10**). Infectious complications, such as abscesses and consolidation, and noninfectious complications, such as bulla and pneumothoraces, are also more easily detectable on tomosynthesis and may be missed on conventional radiographs.

Currently, two scoring systems exist for digital chest tomographic evaluation of CF. Vult von Steyern and colleagues[29] developed a scoring

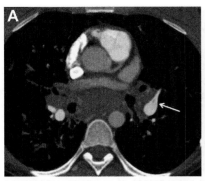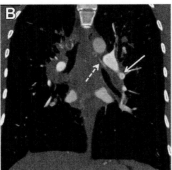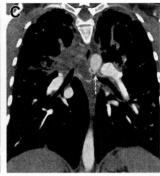

Fig. 7. A 37-year-old woman with CF and chest pain. Axial (*A*) and coronal (*B, C*) soft tissue window setting CT angiography images demonstrate an apparent filling defect in the left lower lobe pulmonary artery in keeping with a "smoke artifact" (*solid arrows*) in the presence of hypertrophied bronchial arteries (*dashed arrows*).

system incorporating increased lung volumes, bronchial wall thickening, bronchestasis, mucus plugging, and atelectasis/consolidation and reported good correlation with radiographs scored with the Brasfield scoring system. A second scoring system developed by Gunnell and colleagues[30] demonstrated superior correlation to forced expiratory volume in one second (FEV_1) when compared with Brasfield scored chest radiographs.

Several technical limitations of tomosynthesis are present when compared with HRCT and include decreased depth resolution, susceptibility to image degradation by artifact from support device hardware, longer imaging times, requirement for anesthesia in younger patients, and inability to construct multiplanar reformatted images. In particular, in severely dyspneic patients, the breath-hold of 10 seconds required for tomosynthesis may not be easily achievable. In addition, early findings of CF, such as areas of air trapping manifesting as mosacism on HRCT, may be occult on

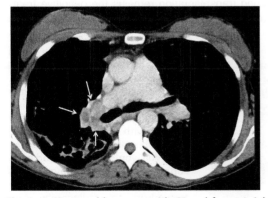

Fig. 8. A 40-year-old woman with CF and fever. Axial soft tissue window setting CT image shows enlarged right hilar lymph nodes (*arrows*); these are thought to be secondary to reactive inflammation.

tomosynthesis, leading to a delayed diagnosis. Despite these limitations, tomosynthesis offers superior evaluation for CF when compared with conventional radiography with a comparatively lower radiation dose increase between chest radiographs (0.01 mSv) and tomosynthesis (0.1–0.2 mSv) when compared with HRCT (4–8 mSv).[28,29] A potential emerging role for tomosynthesis in the evaluation of patients with CF might be as an intermediate imaging modality to further characterize abnormalities detected on surveillance chest radiographs in such scenarios whereby the detail of HRCT is not required as a means to mitigate radiation dose.

Magnetic resonance imaging

A major limitation of chest radiographs, HRCT, and digital chest tomosynthesis is its use of ionizing radiation, especially for longitudinal monitoring because several repeat studies are necessary to monitor CF disease progression and treatment over several years and decades. MR imaging avoids this limitation with several imaging techniques recently introduced to evaluate pulmonary function, including (1) hyperpolarized gas MR imaging and (2) noncontrast MR imaging techniques.[31–35]

Hyperpolarized gas MR imaging

First reported in 1999, ventilation MR imaging using hyperpolarized gases (either helium-3 [He-3] or xenon-129 [Xe-129]) has been investigated as an alternative imaging modality to HRCT in the evaluation of CF.[31,36] He-3 was the first reported hyperpolarized ventilation gas agent with MR imaging performed using a breath-hold technique following administration. By quantifying the region of lung containing low or absent signal (the ventilation defect) and comparing it to the total lung area, a ventilation defect percentage can be obtained (**Fig. 11**). Previous studies have demonstrated that the ventilation defect percentage has good

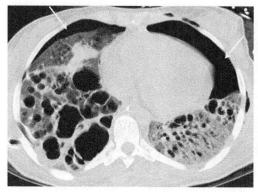

Fig. 9. A 49-year-old woman with CF and chest pain. Axial lung window setting CT image shows bilateral pneumothoraces (*arrows*); these were recurrent per the clinical history.

correlation with the degree of pulmonary dysfunction as determined by incentive spirometry and can be used to accurately assess early disease progression or treatment response.[31,37–40] Disadvantages of He-3 gas MR include the necessity for on-site production of hyperpolarized gas, scarcity of He-3, breath-hold technique in particularly dyspneic patients, and the comparatively low spatial resolution compared with HRCT.

To circumvent some of these limitations, Xe-129 has more recently been investigated as a promising alternative to He-3. In addition to evaluating and quantifying ventilation defects, newer techniques using hyperpolarized Xe-129 gas, such as diffusion-weighted imaging (DWI) and xenon alveolar capillary transfer imaging, are more sophisticated methods for real-time imaging-based quantification of pulmonary physiology and make hyperpolarized Xe-129 MR imaging an attractive and promising alternative to conventional HRCT imaging and spirometry in patients with CF.[31,32] Some disadvantages of Xe-129 MR imaging in addition to those of He-3 MR imaging include comparatively less signal compared with He-3

and anesthetic properties at higher doses with a significantly narrower safety profile.[31,41]

Noncontrast MR imaging techniques

Outside of academic or research centers, accessibility to hyperpolarized gas agents may be limited. In such scenarios, several noncontrast MR imaging techniques have been investigated in the evaluation of patients with CF, including arterial spin labeling (ASL), DWI, and normalized T1 MR imaging[41]

ASL is a novel technique that uses RF pulses to magnetically label protons within arterial blood, allowing for assessment of pulmonary perfusion in the absence of intravenous contrast. In 1 study, mean perfusion values derived from the ASL technique were found to be considerably lower in patients with CF and outcomes correlated strongly with FEV_1.[33,42]

In addition to using DWI sequences for evaluating perfusion in patients undergoing MR imaging with hyperpolarized Xe-129, areas of elevated diffusion on noncontrast MR imaging have been shown to correlate strongly with areas of mucus plugging corresponding to areas of restricted diffusion.[34] Degree of restricted diffusion also correlated strongly with FEV_1.[34]

Normalized T1 MR imaging uses a modified Look-Locker imaging sequence and images the lung parenchyma using numerous single measurements over several fixed inversion pulses. Using mathematical regression, a quantitative T1 map can be derived and subsequent lung tissue homogeneity can be estimated.[31,35] At least 1 study has reported that patients with CF demonstrate more inhomogeneous T1 maps as well as good correlation between normalized T1 values and FEV_1.[35]

PRE–LUNG TRANSPLANT EVALUATION FOR CYSTIC FIBROSIS PATIENTS

Lung transplantation remains the definitive treatment for end-stage CF. In addition to a thorough

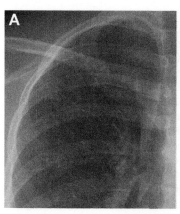
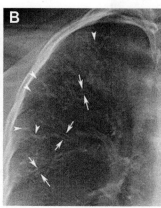

Fig. 10. A 14-year-old girl with CF. (*A*) Frontal chest radiograph demonstrates increased interstitial markings. (*B*) Corresponding digital chest tomosynthesis clearly depicts bronchiectasis and bronchial wall thickening (*arrows*) with endobronchial mucoid impaction (*arrowheads*). (*Adapted from* Vult von Steyern K, Björkman-Burtscher I, Geijer M. Tomosynthesis in pulmonary cystic fibrosis with comparison to radiography and computed tomography: a pictorial review. Insights Imaging. 2012 Feb;3(1):81-9; with permission.)

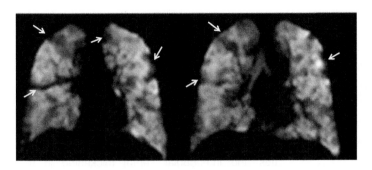

Fig. 11. Young adult patient with CF. Coronal hyperpolarized He-3 MR images demonstrate several ventilation defects (*arrows*). (*Adapted from* Altes TA, Johnson M, Fidler M, Botfield M, Tustison NJ, Leiva-Salinas C, de Lange EE, Froh D, Mugler JP 3rd. Use of hyperpolarized helium-3 MRI to assess response to ivacaftor treatment in patients with cystic fibrosis. J Cyst Fibros. 2017 Mar;16(2):267-274; with permission.)

medical history, laboratory tests, and psychosocial evaluation, HRCT is a fundamental part of the pre-transplant evaluation. Therefore, it is paramount that radiologists are aware of the key findings to report that determine eligibility for lung transplantation as well as those that can predict postoperative outcomes.

Recently, a quantitative HRCT scoring system to determine severity of CF was developed, termed the severe advanced lung disease system.[43] This system classifies areas of lung parenchyma into the following four categories: (1) infectious/inflammatory sequela (bronchiectasis, airway wall thickening, mucus, and consolidations); (2) air trapping/hypoperfusion; (3) cysts/bulla; or (4) normal/hyperperfused tissue. The fraction of total lung volume affected by each of the aforementioned categories is then determined. Belle-van Meerkerk and colleagues[44] used this system to demonstrate that dominant infectious/inflammatory disease was associated with a higher mortality following lung transplantation in patients with CF. It is, therefore, paramount that infectious/inflammatory findings be highlighted in HRCT reports when considering patients with CF for lung transplantation for appropriate risk stratification. In addition, during the pre-transplant process, any new consolidation or classic imaging findings of atypical infection detected on HRCT should prompt a workup for microorganism identification. Although colonization with methicillin-resistant *Staphylococcus aureus* or *Pseudomonas* species is not an absolute contraindication to lung transplantation, *Burkholderia* and NTM infections have been associated with poor post-transplant outcomes, and candidacy for these patients should be evaluated on a case-to-case basis.[45]

Enlarged mediastinal lymph nodes should be reported because these can limit intraoperative dissection and result in significant mediastinal bleeding.[45] Similarly, hypertrophied bronchial artery collaterals, commonly seen in advanced disease, should be conveyed given the increased risk of bleeding. Pleural thickening and adhesions have also been shown to be associated with increased intraoperative bleeding and should therefore be mentioned when present.[44,45] Reactive adenopathy can be quite prominent in patients with CF given recurrent episodes of infections and inflammation since childhood. However, because more patients are benefiting from lung transplantation and surviving to the fourth and fifth decades of life, the radiologist must be vigilant while reviewing serial scans to assess for asymmetric or single-station adenopathy or sudden increase in size of a group of lymph nodes, because the incidence of malignancies increases later in life and reactive nodal enlargement may mask early detection of malignancy.

The presence of a hiatal hernia or a patulous esophagus suggesting dysmotility should be reported because chronic gastroesophageal reflux disease has been linked to an increased development of chronic lung allograft dysfunction (CLAD) secondary to aspirated bile salts resulting in an inflammatory cascade and eventual irreversible fibrosis.[46] When a hiatal hernia or esophageal dysmotility is suspected, further evaluation with a fluoroscopic barium esophagram can be conducted and intraoperative repair and/or medication prophylaxis may be subsequently decided.

Although severe deformities of the chest wall and spine are generally considered absolute contraindications for lung transplantation, many patients with CF frequently have scoliosis, which in and of itself should not preclude these patients from transplantation.[47] Osteoporosis can be a contraindication for lung transplantation because it has been associated with poorer sternal wound healing and associated with an increased rate of post-sternotomy surgical complications.[48] In such scenarios, a Robicsek closure or plate-and-screw fixation may be considered to close the sternal defect.[48]

Additional absolute contraindications for lung transplantation include malignant disease within 2 years and multiorgan damage.[45]

POST–LUNG TRANSPLANT EVALUATION FOR CYSTIC FIBROSIS PATIENTS
Early Complications

Common noninfectious early complications of lung transplantation include primary graft dysfunction (PGD), pleural complications, and acute cellular rejection.

PGD is a noncardiogenic acute lung injury characterized by diffuse alveolar damage and is thought to be secondary to insults to lung parenchyma during the transplantation process.[49] In addition to non-CF specific risk factors (female gender, intraoperative bypass, extracorporeal membrane oxygenation), prolonged graft ischemic time and white race have both been implicated as specific risk factors for the development of PGD in the CF population.[50,51] The HRCT findings of PGD in patients with CF are identical to those of patients without CF and include mid- and lower-lung-predominant ground-glass opacities, consolidations, and bronchial wall thickening with a peak incidence at postoperative day 4 and typically with gradual resolution in the following weeks (**Fig. 12**).[52]

Pleural complications include pneumothoraces (the most common) and pleural fluid collections (effusion, hemothorax, empyema) with a reported rate of 22% to 34%.[52,53] Patients with CF have an increased risk of hemothorax development secondary to the presence of pleural adhesions, mediastinal lymphadenopathy, and hypertrophied native bronchial arteries. Therefore, careful attention for high-attenuating pleural blood products on HRCT is important in the immediate postoperative setting for these patients.

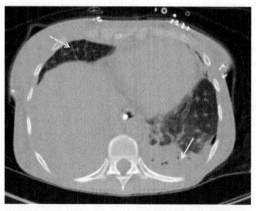

Fig. 12. A 29-year-old woman with CF and shortness of breath, 3 days after lung transplantation. Axial lung window setting CT image demonstrates left lower lobe consolidation (*solid arrow*), bilateral pleural effusions, and interlobular septal thickening (*dashed arrow*) in keeping with primary graft dysfunction.

Acute cellular rejection affects approximately 50% of lung transplant patients within the first year with a higher rate in patients with CF attributed to enhanced immune activation and younger age.[54] Although the HRCT findings may overlap with PGD and include ground-glass opacities, interlobular septal thickening, and consolidation, acute cellular rejection tends to have a delayed onset and usually manifests after postoperative day 7.[53] The combination of ground-glass opacities and interlobular septal thickening in the absence of features of fluid overload has recently been reported to have up to a 90% positive predictive value for the diagnosis of acute cellular rejection.[55] Conversely, the absence of ground-glass opacities is thought to virtually exclude the diagnosis.[52]

Infection

Infections are a leading cause of morbidity and mortality following lung transplantation and have been implicated as a risk factor for the development of CLAD. In the early postoperative period, bacterial infections are the most common and have been isolated from up to 80% of lung transplant patients.[56] Patients with CF are particularly at risk for *Pseudomonas* infection with a higher frequency compared with patients without CF, thought to be secondary to extrapulmonary reservoirs (eg, the sinuses) within the recipient as well as defective innate immunity.[56,57] According to one study, the most common bacterial pathogens isolated from CF transplant patients in order of frequency were *Pseudomonas*, *Mycobacteria*, and *Staphylococcus*.[57] Although the incidence and prognosis of patients infected with *Burkholderia* species are variable, it has been associated with a significantly higher rate of mortality in the posttransplant setting.[58] Bacterial infections will typically manifest on HRCT as consolidation, bronchial wall thickening, centrilobular micronodules, and pleural effusion (**Fig. 13**).[52,58]

Viral infections typically do not manifest until at least 2 weeks following transplantation, usually occurring between 1 and 6 months after transplantation. The most common viral pathogen is cytomegalovirus (CMV) with the seropositive donor and seronegative recipient combination having the highest risk for developing postoperative infection.[59] Patients with CF are at higher risk for developing drug-resistant CMV infections following transplantation with the underlying pathophysiology thought to be secondary to subtherapeutic antiviral drug concentrations because of disease-related pancreatic enzyme insufficiency.[60] HRCT features of viral infection include geographic areas

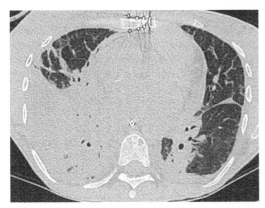

Fig. 13. A 32-year-old man with CF, 3 months after lung transplantation, with new fever. Axial lung window setting CT image demonstrates consolidations in the right greater than left lower lobes. Respiratory cultures confirmed *Pseudomonas* infection.

of ground-glass, superimposed interlobular septal thickening, bronchial wall thickening, and micronodules.[53]

Fungal infections affect up to 8.6% of patients following lung transplantation with patients at highest risk during two post-transplant timeframes: (1) in the first 3 months following transplantation, there is an increased risk for anastomotic fungal infection (eg, tracheeitis); and (2) between 6 and 12 months, there is an increased risk for angioinvasive fungal infection.[59,61] The most common fungal infections in order of frequency include *Aspergillus*, *Candida*, *Scedosporium*, and *Mucorales*.[61] Because of the presence of underlying structural abnormalities and pre-transplant colonization, patients with CF are at higher risk for developing fungal infections (most commonly angioinvasive *Aspergillus*) with one study reporting a 4-fold increased rate in angioinvasive *Aspergillus* infection following lung transplantation. The classic HRCT findings for angioinvasive fungal infections are a solid nodule or mass with a surrounding ground-glass halo (reflecting hemorrhage). Additional patterns include ground-glass opacities with surrounding consolidation, focal nodules, cavities, and micronodules.[53] Fungal mediastinitis and pleural disease are rare and may present as mediastinal fat stranding with or without fluid collections or loculated pleural effusions with or without pleural thickening and enhancement.[48,61]

Airway Complications

Large-airway complications following lung transplantation include bronchial dehiscence (mucosal ulceration and necrosis), bronchial stenosis, and tracheobronchomalacia.[62] Bronchial dehiscence

occurs within the first month of lung transplantation and is typically the result of bronchial ischemia because the anastomosed bronchial arteries are reliant on retrograde blood flow and collateral formation. HRCT findings classically demonstrate focal bronchial wall defects and perianastomotic air collections. In advanced cases, a bronchopleural fistula may form and presents as an enlarging or nonresolving pneumothorax. Bronchial stenosis and tracheobronchomalacia tend to occur months after transplant with bronchial stenosis presenting as a fixed greater than 50% in the airway luminal cross-sectional diameter, and tracheobronchomalacia, which presents as a greater than 70% reduction in anteroposterior diameter between inspiratory and expiratory phase images or bowing of the posterior membrane on expiratory imaging.

Late Complications

CLAD is defined as a drop in FEV_1 < 80% of baseline and is the leading cause of mortality in the long-term post-transplant setting.[46] Although CLAD encompasses a heterogeneous group of several disease processes, this section focuses on the two most common forms: bronchiolitis obliterans syndrome (BOS) and restrictive allograft dysfunction (RAS).[46]

BOS is the most common form of CLAD and is characterized by irreversible small airway obstruction secondary to development of intraluminal fibrosis resulting in obstructive physiology. CF has been implicated with a higher development of BOS likely as a result of an increased incidence of PGD, acute cellular rejection, and airway colonization with *Aspergillus*.[46,63] On HRCT, findings of post-transplant BOS for patients with CF are identical to those of patients without CF and include geographic areas of mosaic perfusion secondary to air trapping, bronchiectasis, and bronchial wall thickening (**Fig. 14**). Centrilobular and tree-in-bud micronodules may also be present. Although the presence of air trapping is the most sensitive imaging finding of BOS, it is imperative that obstructive physiology be present because the sensitivity of the presence of air trapping to diagnose BOS markedly decreases in its absence. Quantitative techniques using voxel-to-voxel comparison of inspiratory and expiratory phase images to assess severity of air trapping have shown promise and are still in development.[64–66]

RAS is the second-most common form of CLAD and characterized by fibroelastosis affecting the visceral pleura, alveolar interstitium, and interlobular septa resulting in a restrictive physiology. The two following clinical patterns of disease exist: (1) a stepwise decline in function; and (2) stable

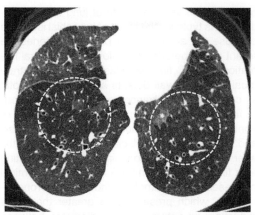

Fig. 14. A 32-year-old man with CF, 2 years following double lung transplantation, with progressive shortness of breath and obstructive physiology on spirometry. Axial lung window setting CT image demonstrates bronchiectasis and bronchial wall thickening with mosaic perfusion (*dashed circles*) in keeping with air trapping. Corresponding incentive spirometry demonstrated an obstructive physiologic pattern with the overall findings compatible with bronchiolitis obliterans syndrome.

disease followed by sudden decompensation. Classic HRCT imaging features of RAS are upper lung predominant subpleural reticulation (early phases) that progresses into dense pleuroparenchymal fibrosis (later phases) with volume loss

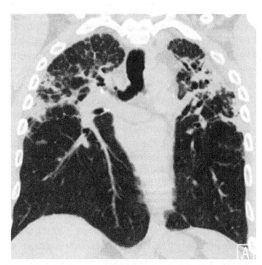

Fig. 15. A 51-year-old woman with CF, 6 years following double lung transplantation, with progressive shortness of breath and restrictive physiology on spriometry. Coronal lung window setting CT image shows upper lung predominant fibrosis, bronchiectasis, and hilar retraction. Corresponding incentive spirometry demonstrated a restrictive physiologic pattern with the overall findings in keeping with restrictive allograft syndrome.

resulting in hilar retraction with traction bronchiectasis and bronchiolectasis (**Fig. 15**).[46] During episodes of acute exacerbation, areas of ground-glass opacity and superimposed interlobular septal thickening may be observed.

SUMMARY

Pulmonary imaging continues to play a vital role in the evaluation of CF in both the pre-transplant and the post-transplant settings. With an increasing number of CF patients surviving to adulthood, it is paramount for the radiologist to not only be familiar with the diagnostic imaging features of CF, but to understand and recognize the distinct imaging features associated with poor lung transplant outcomes to best guide treatment. Emerging technologies, including machine learning and HRCT quantification as well as newer imaging techniques, such as digital chest tomosynthesis and MR imaging, have shown promise. Further studies are warranted to best define their roles in the future.

DISCLOSURE

The authors have nothing to disclose.

REFERENCES

1. Averill S, Lubner MG, Menias CO, et al. Multisystem imaging findings of cystic fibrosis in adults: recognizing typical and atypical patterns of disease. AJR Am J Roentgenol 2017;209(1):3–18.
2. Cystic fibrosis registry. Available at: https://www.cff.org/Research/Researcher-Resources/Patient-Registry/2017-Patient-Registry-Annual-Data-Report.pdf. Accessed July 21. , 2019.
3. Morrissey BM, Schock BC, Marelich GP, et al. Cystic fibrosis in adults: current and future management strategies. Clin Rev Allergy Immunol 2003;25:275–87.
4. Lugo-Olivieri CH, Soyer PA, Fishman EK. Cystic fibrosis: spectrum of thoracic and abdominal CT findings in the adult patient. Clin Imaging 1998;22:346–54.
5. Weiser G, Kerem E. Early intervention in CF: how to monitor the effect. Pediatr Pulmonol 2007;42(11):1002–7.
6. Sequeiros IM, Jarad NA. Radiological features of cystic fibrosis. In: Sriramulu D, editor. Cystic fibrosis–renewed hopes through research. IntechOpen; 2012. p. 31–50.
7. Kioumis IP, Zarogoulidis K, Huang H, et al. Pneumothorax in cystic fibrosis. J Thorac Dis 2014;6(Suppl 4):S480–7.
8. Martinez S, Heyneman LE, McAdams HP, et al. Mucoid impactions: finger-in-glove sign and other CT and radiographic features. Radiographics 2008;28(5):1369–82.

9. Terheggen-Lagro S, Truijens N, van Poppel N, et al. Correlation of six different cystic fibrosis chest radiograph scoring systems with clinical parameters. Pediatr Pulmonol 2003;35(6):441–5.

10. Zucker EJ, Barnes ZA, Lungren MP, et al. Deep learning to automate Brasfield chest radiographic scoring for cystic fibrosis. J Cyst Fibros 2019;19(1):131–8.

11. Brody AS, Klein JS, Molina PL, et al. High-resolution computed tomography in young patients with cystic fibrosis: distribution of abnormalities and correlation with pulmonary function tests. J Pediatr 2004;145(1): 32–8.

12. Brody AS, Sucharew H, Campbell JD, et al. Computed tomography correlates with pulmonary exacerbations in children with cystic fibrosis. Am J Respir Crit Care Med 2005;172(9):1128–32.

13. Judge EP, Dodd JD, Masterson JB, et al. Pulmonary abnormalities on high-resolution CT demonstrate more rapid decline than FEV1 in adults with cystic fibrosis. Chest 2006;130(5):1424–32.

14. Ward S, Heyneman L, Lee MJ, et al. Accuracy of CT in the diagnosis of allergic bronchopulmonary aspergillosis in asthmatic patients. AJR Am J Roentgenol 1999;173:937–42.

15. Roux AL, Catherinot E, Ripoll F, et al, Jean-Louis Herrmann for the OMA Group. Multicenter study of prevalence of nontuberculous mycobacteria in patients with cystic fibrosis in france. J Clin Microbiol 2009;47(12):4124–8.

16. Flume PA, Yankaskas JR, Ebeling M, et al. Massive hemoptysis in cystic fibrosis. Chest 2005;128:729–38.

17. Henry TS, Hammer MM, Little BP, et al. Smoke: how to differentiate flow-related artifacts from pathology on thoracic computed tomographic angiography. J Thorac Imaging 2019. [Epub ahead of print].

18. Sileo C, Corvol H, Boelle PY, et al. HRCT and MRI of the lung in children with cystic fibrosis: comparison of different scoring systems. J Cyst Fibros 2014; 13(2):198–204.

19. Bhalla M, Turcios N, Aponte V, et al. Cystic fibrosis: scoring system with thin-section CT. Radiology 1991;179(3):783–8.

20. de Jong PA, Tiddens HA. Cystic fibrosis specific computed tomography scoring. Proc Am Thorac Soc 2007;4(4):338–42.

21. Sasihuseyinoglu AS, Altıntaş DU, Soyupak S, et al. Evaluation of high resolution computed tomography findings of cystic fibrosis. Korean J Intern Med 2019; 34(2):335–43.

22. Davis SD, Fordham LA, Brody AS, et al. Computed tomography reflects lower airway inflammation and tracks changes in early cystic fibrosis. Am J Respir Crit Care Med 2007;175:943–50.

23. Carpio C, Albi G, Rayon-Aledo JC, et al. Changes in structural lung disease in cystic fibrosis children over 4 years as evaluated by high-resolution computed tomography. Eur Radiol 2015;25:3577–85.

24. Mumcuoglu EÜ, Prescott J, Baker BN, et al. "Image analysis for cystic fibrosis: Automatic lung airway wall and vessel measurement on CT images," in Engineering in Medicine and Biology Society, Annual International Conference of the IEEE. Minneapolis (MN), September 3-6, 2009.

25. Mumcuoglu EÜ, Long FR, Castile RG, et al. Image analysis for cystic fibrosis: computer-assisted airway wall and vessel measurements from low-dose, limited scan lung CT images. J Digit Imaging 2013;26(1):82–96.

26. Naseri Z, Sherafat S, Abrishami Moghaddam H, et al. Semi-automatic methods for airway and adjacent vessel measurement in bronchiectasis patterns in lung HRCT images of cystic fibrosis patients. J Digit Imaging 2018;31(5):727–37.

27. Vult von Steyern K, Björkman-Burtscher I, Geijer M. Tomosynthesis in pulmonary cystic fibrosis with comparison to radiography and computed tomography: a pictorial review. Insights Imaging 2012;3(1):81–9.

28. Ferrari A, Bertolaccini L, Solli P, et al. Digital chest tomosynthesis: the 2017 updated review of an emerging application. Ann Transl Med 2018;6(5):91.

29. Vult von Steyern K, Björkman-Burtscher IM, Höglund P, et al. Description and validation of a scoring system for tomosynthesis in pulmonary cystic fibrosis. Eur Radiol 2012;22:2718–28.

30. Gunnell ET, Franceschi DK, Inscoe CR, et al. Initial clinical evaluation of stationary digital chest tomosynthesis in adult patients with cystic fibrosis. Eur Radiol 2019;29(4):1665–73.

31. Kołodziej M, de Veer MJ, Cholewa M, et al. Lung function imaging methods in cystic fibrosis pulmonary disease. Respir Res 2017;18(1):96.

32. Driehuys B, Cofer GP, Pollaro J, et al. Imaging alveolar-capillary gas transfer using hyperpolarized 129Xe MRI. Proc Natl Acad Sci 2006;103:18278–83.

33. Schraml C, Schwenzer NF, Martirosian P, et al. Noninvasive pulmonary perfusion assessment in young patients with cystic fibrosis using an arterial spin labeling MR technique at 1.5 T. MAGMA 2012;25: 155–62.

34. Ciet P, Serra G, Andrinopoulou ER, et al. Diffusion weighted imaging in cystic fibrosis disease: beyond morphological imaging. Eur Radiol 2016;26:1–10.

35. Donnola SB, Dasenbrook EC, Weaver D, et al. Preliminary comparison of normalized T1 and noncontrast perfusion MRI assessments of regional lung disease in cystic fibrosis patients. J Cyst Fibros 2017;16:283–90.

36. Donnelly LF, MacFall JR, McAdams HP, et al. Cystic fibrosis: combined hyperpolarized 3He-enhanced and conventional proton MR imaging in the lung—preliminary observations. Radiology 1999;212: 885–9.

37. Altes TA, Johnson M, Fidler M, et al. Use of hyperpolarized helium-3 MRI to assess response to ivacaftor

treatment in patients with cystic fibrosis. J Cyst Fibros 2017;16(2):267–74.

38. van Beek EJ, Hill C, Woodhouse N, et al. Assessment of lung disease in children with cystic fibrosis using hyperpolarized 3-Helium MRI: comparison with Shwachman score, Chrispin-Norman score and spirometry. Eur Radiol 2007;17(4):1018–24.

39. Sun Y, O'Sullivan BP, Roche JP, et al. Using hyperpolarized 3He MRI to evaluate treatment efficacy in cystic fibrosis patients. J Magn Reson Imaging 2011;34:1206–11.

40. Paulin GA, Svenningsen S, Jobse BN, et al. Differences in hyperpolarized 3He ventilation imaging after 4 years in adults with cystic fibrosis. J Magn Reson Imaging 2015;41:1701–7.

41. Lilburn DM, Pavlovskaya GE, Meersmann T. Perspectives of hyperpolarized noble gas MRI beyond 3 He. J Magn Reson 2013;229:173–86.

42. Miller GW, Mugler JP 3rd, Sá RC, et al. Advances in functional and structural imaging of the human lung using proton MRI. NMR Biomed 2014;27(12): 1542–56.

43. Loeve M, van Hal PT, Robinson P, et al. The spectrum of structural abnormalities on CT scans from patients with CF with severe advanced lung disease. Thorax 2009;64(10):876–82.

44. Belle-van Meerkerk G, de Jong PA, de Valk HW, et al. Pretransplant HRCT characteristics are associated with worse outcome of lung transplantation for cystic fibrosis patients. PLoS One 2015;10(12): e0145597.

45. Hirche TO, Knoop C, Hebestreit H, et al. Practical guidelines: lung transplantation in patients with cystic fibrosis. Pulm Med 2014;2014:621342.

46. Hota P, Dass C, Kumaran M, et al. High-resolution CT findings of obstructive and restrictive phenotypes of chronic lung allograft dysfunction: more than just bronchiolitis obliterans syndrome. AJR Am J Roentgenol 2018;211(1):W13–21.

47. Su JW, Mason DP, Murthy SC, et al. Successful double lung transplantation in 2 patients with severe scoliosis. J Heart Lung Transplant 2008;27(11):1262–4.

48. Hota P, Dass C, Erkmen C, et al. Poststernotomy complications: a multimodal review of normal and abnormal postoperative imaging findings. AJR Am J Roentgenol 2018;211(6):1194–205.

49. Montefusco CM, Veith FJ. Lung transplantation. Surg Clin North Am 1986;66(3):503–15.

50. Felten ML, Sinaceur M, Treilhaud M, et al. Factors associated with early graft dysfunction in cystic fibrosis patients receiving primary bilateral lung transplantation. Eur J Cardiothorac Surg 2012; 41(3):686–90.

51. Martin JA, Porteous MK, Cantu E, et al. Risk factors for primary graft dysfunction in patients with cystic fibrosis receiving lung transplants. J Heart Lung Transplant 2019;38(4):S147.

52. Krishnam MS, Suh RD, Tomasian A, et al. Postoperative complications of lung transplantation: radiologic findings along a time continuum. Radiographics 2007;27(4):957–74.

53. Madan R, Chansakul T, Goldberg HJ. Imaging in lung transplants: checklist for the radiologist. Indian J Radiol Imaging 2014;24(4):318–26.

54. Calabrese F, Lunardi F, Nannini N, et al. Higher risk of acute cellular rejection in lung transplant recipients with cystic fibrosis. Ann Transplant 2015;20: 769–76.

55. Park CH, Paik HC, Haam SJ, et al. HRCT features of acute rejection in patients with bilateral lung transplantation: the usefulness of lesion distribution. Transplant Proc 2014;46:1511–6.

56. Remund KF, Best M, Egan JJ. Infections relevant to lung transplantation. Proc Am Thorac Soc 2009;6(1): 94–100.

57. Bonvillain RW, Valentine VG, Lombard G, et al. Postoperative infections in cystic fibrosis and non-cystic fibrosis patients after lung transplantation. J Heart Lung Transpl 2007;26(9):890–7.

58. Lynch JP, Sayah DM, Belperio JA, et al. Lung transplantation for cystic fibrosis: results, indications, complications, and controversies. Semin Respir Crit Care Med 2015;36(2):299–320.

59. Nosotti M, Tarsia P, Morlacchi LC. Infections after lung transplantation. J Thorac Dis 2018;10(6):3849–68.

60. Gagermeier JP, Rusinak JD, Lurain NS, et al. Subtherapeutic ganciclovir (GCV) levels and GCV-resistant cytomegalovirus in lung transplant recipients. Transpl Infect Dis 2014;16(6):941–50.

61. Kennedy CC, Razonable RR. Fungal infections after lung transplantation. Clin Chest Med 2017;38(3): 511–20.

62. Santacruz JF, Mehta AC. Airway complications and management after lung transplantation ischemia, dehiscence, and stenosis. Proc Am Thorac Soc 2009;6:79–93.

63. Varghese NP, Schecter MG, Heinle JS, et al. 486: cystic fibrosis is an independent risk factor for the development of bronchiolitis obliterans syndrome in pediatric lung transplant recipients. J Heart Lung Transplant 2009;28(2):S235.

64. Luong ML, Chaparro C, Stephenson A, et al. Pretransplant Aspergillus colonization of cystic fibrosis patients and the incidence of post-lung transplant invasive aspergillosis. Transplantation 2014;97(3): 351–7.

65. Siegel MJ, Bhalla S, Gutierrez FR, et al. Post-lung transplantation bronchiolitis obliterans syndrome: usefulness of expiratory thin-section CT for diagnosis. Radiology 2001;220:455–62.

66. de Jong PA, Dodd JD, Coxson HO, et al. Bronchiolitis obliterans following lung transplantation: early detection using computed tomographic scanning. Thorax 2006;61:799–804.

Interstitial Lung Diseases in Children, Adolescents, and Young Adults
Different from Infants and Older Adults

Teresa I-Han Liang, MD, FRCPC[a,1], Edward Y. Lee, MD, MPH[b,*]

KEYWORDS

- Interstitial lung disease (ILD) • Childhood interstitial lung disease (chILD) • Diffuse lung disease
- High-resolution computed tomography (HRCT)

KEY POINTS

- Interstitial lung disease (ILD) in children, adolescents, and young adults is a heterogeneous group of disorders with diverse clinical and imaging manifestations.
- Although childhood ILD (chILD) pathologies in infants and young children do overlap with ILD in adults, major differences in pathology and clinical presentations exist.
- ILD in this population remains a challenging and multidisciplinary diagnosis, with no standardized approach to diagnosis and management.
- It is imperative to establish the immune status of the patient when evaluating suspected ILD in this population, as it affects the pathology that can manifest and prognosis.

INTRODUCTION

Interstitial lung disease (ILD) consists of a large and heterogeneous group of rare pulmonary disorders, characterized by abnormalities involving the alveoli and airway.[1–4] However, as many of these pathologies involve beyond or do not involve the interstitium at all, ILD in children and infants (chILD) is often considered a syndrome of diffuse ILD.[5] Underlying chILD pathologies are markedly different from adult ILD. For example, the adult ILD idiopathic pulmonary fibrosis, or the corresponding pathologic diagnosis of usual interstitial pneumonia, has not been convincingly reported in children or teenagers,[3] and conversely, the chILD disorders neuroendocrine cell hyperplasia in infancy (NEHI) and pulmonary interstitial glycogenosis have not been reported in adults.[3]

The widely accepted chILD classification was initially developed and published in 2007, through the multidisciplinary collaborative efforts of the chILD Research Co-operative of North America (chILDRN), based on review of lung biopsies of 187 infants from 11 pediatric institutions with diffuse lung disease.[3,4] Although this classification was widely accepted and incorporated into official American Thoracic Society (ATS) clinical practice guidelines in 2013, it only systematized patients younger than 2 years.

Subsequently in 2015, chILDRN published an expanded classification to include older children from 2 to 18 years of age.[3] The updated classification was based on a retrospective review of lung biopsies in 191 patients between 2 and 18 years of age from 12 North American institutions with diffuse lung disease.[3] This classification divides patients into immunocompromised and immunocompetent clinical status (Table 1), and further classifies the immunocompetent patients into primary lung disease, lung disease related to

[a] Department of Radiology, University of Alberta, Stollery Children's Hospital, Edmonton, Alberta, Canada;
[b] Department of Radiology, Boston Children's Hospital, Harvard Medical School, Boston, MA, USA
[1] Present address: #203 11010 – 101 St. NW, Edmonton, Alberta T5H 4B9, Canada.
* Corresponding author. Department of Radiology, 300 Longwood Avenue, Boston, MA 02115.
E-mail address: Edward.Lee@childrens.harvard.edu

Radiol Clin N Am 58 (2020) 487–502
https://doi.org/10.1016/j.rcl.2020.01.001
0033-8389/20/© 2020 Elsevier Inc. All rights reserved.

Table 1
Adapted 2015 chILD Research Co-operative of North America Classification of childhood interstitial disease (chILD) in children to young adults

Category	Disease
Immunocompetent:	
Primary lung disease in immunocompetent host	1. Infectious/Postinfectious constrictive obliterative bronchiolitis 2. Hypersensitivity pneumonitis 3. Aspiration syndromes and exogenous lipoid pneumonia 4. Eosinophilic pneumonia 5. Idiopathic pulmonary hemosiderosis
Lung disease related to systemic disease	1. Immune-related disease; for example, vasculitis, connective tissue disease, and autoimmune pulmonary alveolar proteinosis 2. Storage diseases; for example, Gaucher disease 3. Sarcoidosis 4. Langerhans cell histiocytosis
Sequelae and ongoing disorders of infancy	1. Surfactant deficiency 2. Neuroendocrine hyperplasia of infancy
Immunocompromised:	
Immunocompromised host	1. Lymphocytic interstitial pneumonitis with human immunodeficiency virus/AIDS or combined immunodeficiency 2. Treatment-related disorders: organizing pneumonia 3. Disorders related to rejection: bronchiolitis obliterans

Adapted from Fan LL, Dishop MK, Galambos C, et al. Diffuse lung disease in biopsied children 2 to 18 years of age. Application of the chILD Classification Scheme. Ann Am Thorac Soc 2015;12(10):1498-505.

systemic disease, and patients with sequelae or diagnoses of disorders of infancy (see **Table 1**). Immunocompromised patients had the highest reported mortality rate of 52.8%,[3] whereas immunocompetent patients had markedly improved mortality rates, with reported mortality rates ranging from 7.1% to 20.0% in the subgroups.[3]

Patients with chILD most commonly present with cough, exercise intolerance, dyspnea, hypoxemia, crackles, and tachypnea, although rarely, patients can present with a normal examination.[3,6] Interestingly, Fan and colleagues[3] reported that clinical symptoms are less common in the older population, in comparison with the previously reported prevalence in infants younger than 2 years, implying that older children may have more insidious symptoms and present later in disease,[6] making the clinical diagnosis a challenge.

Given its rarity and diverse imaging manifestations, and in conjunction with an often nonspecific clinical examination, chILD in children and teenagers presents a challenge to the clinicians and radiologist. Therefore, this article discusses the utility of available imaging techniques and the associated common imaging findings, and reviews

the 2015 chILD classification scheme with clinical examples highlighting the imaging features to help the general radiologist aid in an efficient and accurate multidisciplinary diagnosis of chILD.

IMAGING TECHNIQUES
Chest Radiography

Chest radiography is an excellent initial screening imaging modality for patients with suspicion of chILD, as it uses low radiation dose, is easily reproducible, and readily accessible.[4,7] Once a chILD diagnosis has been established, it also can be used to follow the course of disease.[4,7–9] The most commonly seen radiographic abnormality is hyperinflation, although chest radiographic findings remain nonspecific, and a normal chest radiograph does not exclude a diagnosis of chILD.[4,9,10] Prior studies have reported an inferior degree of confidence and accuracy of chest radiography in the assessment of diffuse pediatric lung disease, with reported accuracies as low as 34%.[8] Therefore, further characterization to improve diagnostic accuracy and confidence with computed tomography (CT) is typically necessary.[11]

Computed Tomography

CT, usually without intravenous contrast and ideally performed as high-resolution CT (HRCT) technique, has become the standard imaging modality for evaluation of suspected chILD, as it allows confirmation of disease, superior characterization of the extent and distribution of disease, and identification of any unique imaging features.[4,8–10] In addition, as chILD can often be patchy, CT can recommend an ideal biopsy site and guide preoperative planning.[4,8–10]

In more recent years with the CT technologic advances, volumetric high-resolution scanning of the entire chest can be performed in seconds.[4,9] Thus, older patients typically do not need to be sedated, and can be imaged during quiet respiration or following breath-hold maneuvers,[4,9,10] as general anesthetic should be avoided because it is invasive, expensive, subject to procedural risks, and possibly associated with adverse neurocognitive effects.[10,12,13] Another challenge in imaging children with general anesthesia is that the pathology can be obscured, as children are particularly prone to atelectasis due to high chest wall compliance and underdeveloped collateral ventilation system (pores of Kohn and channels of Lambert).[10,12] Additional challenges in the younger child include lower lung volumes, associated with poor inspiration, small patient size, and rapid respiratory motion.[4]

CT imaging manifestations of chILD remains diverse, but typically includes nodules, ground-glass opacification, consolidation, air-trapping, cysts, interlobular and intralobular septal thickening, linear and reticular markings, and architectural distortion and traction bronchiectasis in fibrotic disease.[4,7,10] These CT imaging descriptors have specific terminology and definitions as per the Nomenclature Committee of Fleischner Society.[14]

Pulmonary nodule

Pulmonary nodules can be classified according to their distribution as either centrilobular, miliary, perilymphatic, and random. Centrilobular nodules are found centrally within the secondary pulmonary lobule, and can be seen in infectious and inflammatory entities involving the small airways, such as infectious bronchiolitis or hypersensitivity pneumonitis. In contrast, perilymphatic nodules are found along the interlobular septa, fissures, and bronchovascular bundles, and can be seen in sarcoidosis (Fig. 1). Miliary and random nodular patterns are not commonly seen in chILD.

Ground-glass opacification

Ground-glass opacification is visualized as hazy air space opacification with preservation of the bronchovascular structures, whereas consolidation represents solid air space opacification[10,14]; however, both imaging characteristics are nonspecific. Ground-glass opacification can be seen in underinflated lungs, especially in the lung bases when imaged in expiration or with shallow inspiration.[10] When ground-glass opacification is seen with superimposed interlobular and intralobular septal thickening, it is described as a "crazy-paving" pattern (Fig. 2), and can be associated with a diverse range of entities, including pulmonary alveolar proteinosis (PAP), pulmonary hemorrhage syndromes, lipoid pneumonia, diffuse alveolar disease, organizing pneumonia, and pneumocystis pneumonia.[7,10]

Air-trapping

Air-trapping appears as hypodense regions with less than normal increase in attenuation and lack of normal volume reduction with expiration (Fig. 3).[14] It is not uncommon to see a few subsegmental (lobular) hypodense foci in the lungs of healthy children, especially in the posterior juxtapleural region, and should not be confused with pathology.[10]

Cyst

Cysts appear as round hypodense, well-defined structures that usually contain air, but can contain fluid or solid material.[14] Cysts can be seen in multiple chILD entities, including pulmonary

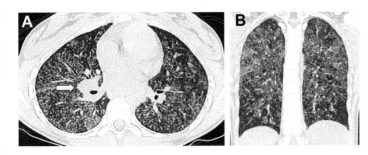

Fig. 1. A 17-year-old girl with sarcoidosis, who presented with fatigue and weight loss, and found to have an elevated ACE level. Noncontrast axial (A) and coronal (B) CT images demonstrate hilar lymphadenopathy (arrow), diffuse nodular and confluent ground-glass opacities, and peri-lymphatic nodules in the interlobular septa and bronchovascular bundles, strongly supporting the diagnosis of sarcoidosis.

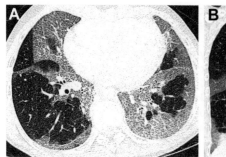
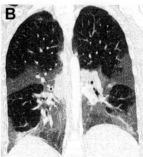

Fig. 2. A 13-year-old boy with chILD of uncertain etiology. Noncontrast axial (*A*) and coronal (*B*) CT images demonstrate bilateral multifocal geographic ground-glass opacities with superimposed interlobular and intralobular septal thickening affecting all lobes in keeping with a crazy-paving CT pattern.

Langerhans cell histiocytosis (LCH) (**Fig. 4**) and disorders of surfactant metabolism (see **Fig. 19**).[10]

Pulmonary fibrosis

Pulmonary fibrosis associated with chILD and ILD can develop, and manifest on CT as thicker-walled stacked cysts known as honeycombing, in addition to traction bronchiectasis and architectural distortion (**Fig. 5**).[10,15]

Magnetic Resonance Imaging

MR imaging is a superb imaging modality for assessment of the mediastinum and chest wall, and offers the absence of ionizing radiation. However, it remains limited in the imaging of chILD. This is mainly due to a combination of low proton content in the lungs, inevitable respiratory motion artifact as the images are obtained over a period of free breathing, and inferior spatial resolution relative to CT.[4] Sodhi and colleagues[16] previously investigated the utility of MR imaging in the evaluation of chILD in comparison with HRCT, and found that 3T MR imaging was able to detect consolidation (**Fig. 6**), parenchymal bands, and fissural thickening, but remained limited in evaluation of septal thickening, ground-glass opacity, nodules (**Fig. 7**), and cysts, which often are diagnostic and differentiating features of chILD. Therefore, at the current time, MR imaging remains limited in the clinical application of chILD, particularly for initial evaluation.

CHALLENGING ASPECTS OF INTERSTITIAL LUNG DISEASE IN ADOLESCENTS AND YOUNG ADULTS FOR GENERAL RADIOLOGISTS IN 2019

chILD remains a complex diagnosis, and the reported accuracy and diagnostic confidence of a correct diagnosis using HRCT in children is lower than in adults,[11] mostly thought to reflect the greater diversity of lung diseases in the pediatric population.[11] In addition, it is important to recognize that the ability to determine the correct diagnosis is dependent on the type of disease, the quality of the study, and the expertise of the interpreter. Even pediatric thoracic radiologists may only achieve a correct first-choice diagnosis of chILD in fewer than 50% of cases,[17] although prior diagnostic performance studies are confounded by inconsistent results and imprecise and outdated histopathologic classification schemes.[10] Therefore, it is imperative to use a multidisciplinary approach among the clinician, radiologist, and pathologist in the assessment of patients with suspected chILD to optimize diagnosis and management.

Although challenging due to the diverse pathologies and variable imaging manifestations, the essential role as a radiologist is to identify any unique features to suggest a favored or narrowed differential diagnosis. This can direct the next appropriate serologic assay, bronchoalveolar lavage (BAL), or genetic test, and potentially

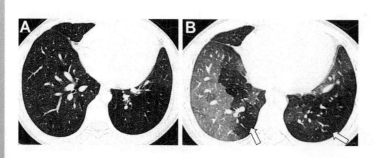

Fig. 3. A 13-year-old boy with asthma who presented with shortness of breath. Noncontrast axial inspiratory (*A*) and expiratory (*B*) CT images demonstrate patchy and geographic mosaic attenuation, which on the expiratory CT image does not increase in attenuation nor decrease in volume, most pronounced in the bilateral lobes (*arrows*), in keeping with air-trapping.

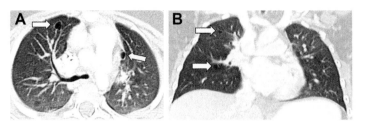

Fig. 4. A 3-year-old girl with LCH, status post chemotherapy. Noncontrast axial (A) and coronal (B) CT images demonstrate multiple bilateral thin-walled (mildly irregular) cysts in the lungs (arrows), in keeping with the known diagnosis of LCH.

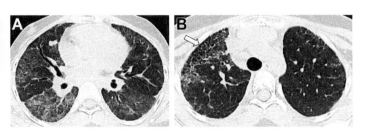

Fig. 5. A 15-year-old girl with systemic sclerosis and diffuse fibrotic pulmonary disease. Noncontrast axial (A, B) CT images demonstrate subpleural cystic changes, in keeping with honeycombing (arrow), traction bronchiectasis, patchy ground-glass opacification, interlobular septal thickening, and subpleural linear reticular markings, consistent with diffuse pulmonary fibrosis.

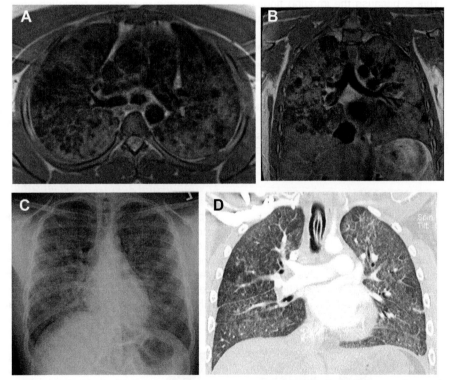

Fig. 6. An 18-year-old boy with pulmonary alveolar proteinosis (PAP) and pulmonary hemorrhage after full lung lavage. Noncontrast axial T1-weighted (A) and coronal T1-weighted (B) MR images demonstrate diffuse bilateral airspace opacification. Frontal chest radiograph (C) demonstrates dependent airspace and interstitial opacities within the left greater than right lungs, and noncontrast coronal CT image (D) demonstrates diffuse ground-glass opacification with interlobular septal thickening, in keeping with a crazy-paving pattern, compatible with the diagnosis of PAP.

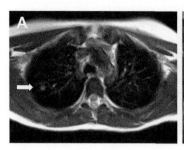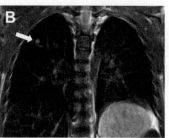

Fig. 7. A 9-year-old girl with history of acute myelocytic leukemia status post treatment. Axial (A) and coronal (B) T2-weighted Half Fourier Single Shot Turbo Spin Echo (HASTE) MR images demonstrate multiple nodules (arrows) in the right upper lobe.

obviate the need for a lung biopsy, such as in the setting of NEHI or bronchiolitis obliterans in the appropriate clinical setting.[4,10,18,19] It can be highly beneficial when extrapulmonary imaging manifestations, such as thymic enlargement and calcification in LCH, esophageal dysfunction in systemic sclerosis or aspiration, and pectus excavatum in chronic surfactant dysfunction related to ABCA3 gene mutation are present and help suggest the diagnosis.[10]

The other challenge lies in the substantial variation and absence of clear guidelines for monitoring patients with chILD with diagnostic imaging.[10] This is because the imaging findings on CT do not always correlate with pulmonary function testing (PFT), or predict response to treatment or outcome.[10] For example, patients with asymptomatic connective tissue disease with normal PFT often have ILD on imaging.[10,20,21] Conversely, it is not unusual for asymptomatic HRCT lung abnormalities to persist in LCH for many years after treatment.[22,23] In addition, there are no specific HRCT findings to predict which patients progress to clinically significant pulmonary fibrosis.[10,20,21]

SPECTRUM OF INTERSTITIAL DISEASE
Primary Lung Disease in an Immunocompetent Host

Infectious/postinfectious: constrictive obliterative bronchiolitis
Postinfectious constrictive obliterative bronchiolitis (COB) is a chronic respiratory condition characterized by severe and fixed lower respiratory airway obstruction due to inflammatory tissue and fibrosis, and associated with sequelae of prior infection from various respiratory viruses, but particularly with adenovirus.[7,24]

On chest radiographs, hyperinflation is the most common abnormality, with additional findings including atelectasis and bronchial thickening, but milder disease also can have a normal chest radiograph.[7,10,24] HRCT demonstrates characteristic mosaic attenuation, due to vascular shunting in the hypoventilated areas and reduced perfusion due to constriction of vessels from tissue hypoxia. On expiratory images, air-trapping is present, reflecting small airways disease, and mild to marked bronchiectasis, reflecting larger airways disease (Fig. 8).[10,24] Although definitive diagnosis remains by lung biopsy, a 3-part COB diagnostic scoring system with a diagnostic specificity of 100% has been proposed, potentially obviating the need for lung biopsy, with points given for a typical clinical history of postinfectious COB, history of prior adenovirus infection, and characteristic mosaic attenuation on HRCT.[10,24,25]

Environmental agents: hypersensitivity pneumonitis
Hypersensitivity pneumonitis (HP), also known as extrinsic allergic alveolitis, is a form of immune-mediated ILD that develops in response to repeated inhalation of finely dispersed organic antigens. Acute, subacute, and chronic forms have been described, with repeated exposures potentially leading to irreversible lung damage.[26] HP

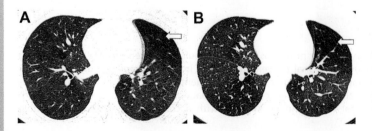

Fig. 8. An 18-year-old girl with prior history of adenovirus and diagnosis of postinfectious constrictive obliterative bronchiolitis (COB). Noncontrast axial inspiratory (A) and expiratory (B) CT images demonstrate mosaic attenuation with multiple areas of air-trapping (arrows), most prominent in the lingula in keeping with postinfectious COB.

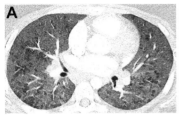 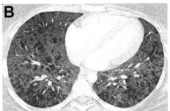

Fig. 9. A 14-year-old boy diagnosed with hypersensitivity pneumonitis (HP) to birds, who responded well to steroid treatment. Noncontrast axial (A, B) CT images demonstrate bilateral diffuse ground-glass opacities with mild septal thickening and lobular spared areas, compatible with the diagnosis of acute HP.

remains uncommon in childhood, with nonspecific symptoms often resulting in a delay in diagnosis. Affected pediatric patients with acute HP can present with symptoms mimicking a flu-like illness, including high fever, chills, dry cough, dyspnea, and malaise, whereas children with chronic HP, the more commonly reported form of HP, present with progressive and insidious nonspecific symptoms of exercise intolerance, cough, weight loss, and fever.[7,26] Although it can manifest identically on imaging to the adult form, in contrast to adult HP, which can result from a wide variety of occupational and environmental exposures to microbes, animal and plant proteins, and chemicals, HP in children most commonly results from repeated exposures to an array of birds, and is associated with an overall excellent prognosis.[26] Additional antigens in HP in children include mold spores and methotrexate.[7,26]

On chest radiographs and HRCT, acute HP classically shows ground-glass opacities (Fig. 9), which can resemble pulmonary edema or pneumonia.[7,10] In the subacute phase of HP, HRCT shows poorly defined centrilobular nodules, ground-glass opacities, and evidence of air-trapping.[7,10] There is relative sparing of the upper lung zones in both the acute and subacute phases. In chronic HP, subpleural reticular markings, architectural distortion, and honeycombing related to pulmonary fibrosis are seen.[7,10] Although clinical symptoms typically resolve within a few days of starting treatment and ceasing exposure to the inciting antigen, HRCT findings of acute and subacute HP may persist for several weeks.[10] Also, HRCT findings of pulmonary fibrosis may persist and potentially progress, even despite removal of the offending antigen.[10,26,27]

Aspiration syndromes and exogenous lipoid pneumonia

Chronic aspiration is commonly seen in children with recurrent lower respiratory tract infections, and is predicted to be present in 26% to 49% of children with chILD.[6,7,28] CT findings typically include bronchial wall thickening, centrilobular or tree-in-bud nodules, or consolidation in the dependent (posterior and basal) portions of the lung (Fig. 10).[7,29] The presence of bronchiectasis and fibrosis has been suggested to correlate with cases with greater severity and chronicity.[29] Imaging findings suggestive of esophageal dysfunction, such as a patulous or dilated esophagus, may further suggest the presence of chronic aspiration (see Fig. 10).[29]

Exogenous lipoid pneumonia in the pediatric population is most commonly associated with aspiration of mineral oil used to treat chronic constipation.[7] Affected pediatric patients may remain asymptomatic or present with nonspecific clinical symptoms, such as cough, chest pain, tachypnea, and fever.[30,31] Risk factors and comorbidities include gastroesophageal reflux, aspiration syndromes, force-feeding, choking, feeding in a recumbent position, neurologic conditions, intractable seizures, and gastrointestinal conditions, such as chronic constipation, obstruction, Hirschsprung disease, and malnutrition.[31]

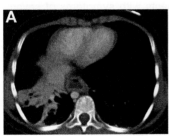 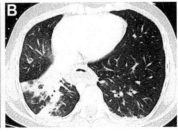

Fig. 10. An 11-year-old girl with Rubinstein-Taybi syndrome, developmental delay, failure to thrive, and chronic aspiration and respiratory symptoms. Contrast-enhanced axial CT images in soft tissue window setting (A) and lung window setting (B) demonstrate ground-glass opacities and more confluent consolidation in right greater than left lobes with bronchial wall thickening, mucous plugging, bronchiectasis, and a patulous esophagus with an air-fluid level, consistent with chronic aspiration.

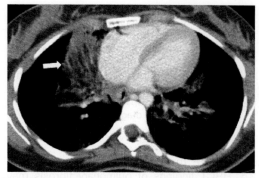

Fig. 11. A 17-year-old girl with cerebral palsy who presented with a low-grade fever and cough. Contrast-enhanced axial CT image demonstrates right middle lobe consolidation (*arrow*) with negative fat density Hounsfield units, in keeping with exogenous lipoid pneumonia. (*Courtesy of* Dr Ricardo Restrepo, Department of Radiology, Nicklaus Children's Hospital, Miami, FL.)

The most frequent imaging findings include airspace and ground-glass opacification,[30,31] and less frequently on CT, interstitial septal thickening and a crazy-paving appearance can be observed. However, lipoid pneumonia can be definitively diagnosed on CT when the consolidated lung parenchyma, typically in the bilateral lower lobes or right upper lobe, demonstrates negative Hounsfield unit values corresponding to fat density, typically between −21 and −90 HU (Fig. 11).[7,30]

Eosinophilic pneumonia

Eosinophilic pneumonia (EP) is characterized by significant eosinophil infiltration of the alveolar spaces and interstitium,[32] and can be categorized into primary EP with an unknown cause, and secondary EP related to a known cause, such as parasite infection, allergic bronchopulmonary aspergillosis, or drugs.[32] Primary idiopathic EP can occur in an acute or chronic setting (IAEP and ICEP, respectively), and are both reported to be extremely rare in the pediatric and teenage populations, with an estimated IAEP prevalence of less than 1 in a million.[32] IAEP is often associated with respiratory distress and smoke or irritant exposure, whereas in the chronic setting, it may be isolated (ICEP) or accompanied by systemic manifestations, such as in eosinophilic granulomatosis with polyangiitis (EGPA), previously known as Churg-Strauss syndrome, an uncommon necrotizing medium-vessel vasculitis, typically associated with asthma, allergic rhinitis, and peripheral eosinophilia.[7,32] Unlike adults, EGPA is rare and more severe in children with variable presentations, more frequently associated with cardiomyopathy, and can be antineutrophil cytoplasmic antibody negative in up to 40% of cases.[7,32]

Although imaging findings often are nonspecific with diffuse or local pulmonary infiltrates, the presence of classic features of multifocal peripheral pulmonary consolidation, often with perilesional halos of ground-glass (Fig. 12) and pleural effusions, can favor the diagnosis of EP. However, diagnosis still depends on the presence of peripheral blood eosinophilia (although not always present), and most importantly, alveolar eosinophilia on BAL.[32]

Idiopathic pulmonary hemosiderosis

Idiopathic pulmonary hemosiderosis (IPH), first described by Virchow in 1864, is characterized by alveolar capillary hemorrhage with deposition and accumulation of hemosiderin in the lungs.[33,34] The pathophysiology remains unclear, but multiple hypotheses, including autoimmune, environmental, allergic, and genetic theories, have been proposed.[34] Although the exact incidence is largely unknown, it has been reported to occur between 0.24 and 1.26 patients per million in select pediatric populations.[33] Recent literature suggests that patients with Down syndrome are at a higher risk for developing pulmonary hemosiderosis and are associated with more severe disease.[35] In contrast to adults, children with IPH have a more rapid and severe prognosis, with mortality rates estimated up to 50%.[33,35] Two distinct phases have been described in IPH: an acute phase and a chronic phase. The acute phase is characterized by alveolar hemorrhage, and potentially respiratory failure, whereas in the chronic phase, the patient typically presents with symptoms of severe disease, such as cyanosis or clubbing, and right heart failure due to pulmonary fibrosis.[34]

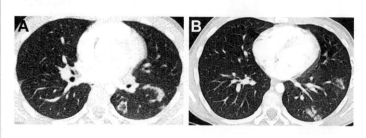

Fig. 12. An 11-year-old boy with elevated immunoglobulin E and serum eosinophils. Noncontrast axial CT images (A, B) demonstrate multiple peripheral consolidative opacities with relative central clearing and adjacent ground-glass opacities in the left lower lobe, compatible with a diagnosis of eosinophilic pneumonia.

Diagnosis of IPH in children is often delayed or misdiagnosed because of the variable and insidious presentation and lack of awareness of the condition.[33,34] Clinical symptoms include cough, hemoptysis, fever, and dyspnea, with the classic clinical triad of hemoptysis, iron deficiency anemia, and pulmonary infiltrates on chest imaging.[33] Although the presence of hemoptysis is useful for diagnosis, its absence does not exclude IPH. In fact, hemoptysis remains rare in children, likely secondary to the inability to expectorate, with reported rates of up to 62% at time of diagnosis.[33] Given the challenging diagnosis, confirmation usually requires bronchoscopy with BAL to identify hemosiderin-laden macrophages, or potentially a lung biopsy to exclude other disease processes.[34]

Imaging findings remain nonspecific and dependent on the phase involved. In the acute phase of IPH, findings include airspace opacities (**Fig. 13**) and/or consolidation reflecting alveolar hemorrhage, in a predominantly hilar, perihilar, and lower lobe distribution, with relative sparing of the lung apices and costophrenic sulci.[34] The airspace opacities and consolidation usually decrease or clear within 3 days of presentation, at which time reticular opacities may become evident.[34] Interstitial deposition of the hemosiderin-laden macrophages can result in interlobular and intralobular septal thickening, which can manifest as the crazy-paving pattern when superimposed on a background of ground-glass opacification.[34] In patients with repeated pulmonary hemorrhage in the chronic phase, findings of pulmonary fibrosis can be seen.[34] Pleural involvement is uncommon in IPH, but can manifest as a hemothorax, potentially with a fluid-fluid level of layering blood products, and nonresolving or recurrent hemothoraces may result in formation of a fibrothorax, which appears as pleural thickening and calcification and can result in a persistently collapsed "trapped" lung.[34]

Lung Disease Related to Systemic Disease

Immune-related disease
Disorders related to systemic immune-mediated disease, as per the ATS proposed classification, includes pulmonary vasculitis syndromes and connective tissue disorders, nonspecific interstitial pneumonia (NSIP), pulmonary hemorrhage, autoimmune PAP, and other diagnoses.[3]

Pulmonary vasculitis syndromes: systemic lupus erythematosus Vasculitis disorders of childhood include a spectrum of disorders, including granulomatous polyangiitis (GPA, formerly known as Wegner granulomatosis) and systemic lupus erythematosus (SLE).[10] Unlike adult-onset SLE, interstitial disease is uncommon in childhood-onset SLE, with only 8% of patients reported to have abnormal imaging findings, suggesting that asymptomatic children with SLE do not require HRCT screening.[10,36] When pulmonary disease is present in childhood-onset SLE, it is frequently in the form of vasculitis with pulmonary hemorrhage.[10] Acute pulmonary hemorrhage can be identified with the presence of ill-defined fluffy ground-glass opacities, sparing the lung periphery (**Fig. 14**). With repeated hemorrhage, mild interstitial fibrosis and interlobular septal thickening can be seen.[7,37]

Connective tissue disorders: systemic sclerosis The connective tissue disorders of childhood are frequently associated with pulmonary disease. For example, pulmonary disease has been reported in up to 90% of pediatric patients with juvenile systemic sclerosis (scleroderma).[38] Systemic sclerosis is a rare autoimmune connective tissue disorder with proliferative small vessel vasculopathy and obliterative microvascular disease. Juvenile systemic sclerosis is a rare subgroup, with disease onset in patients younger than 16 years old.[38] The main prognostic factor in systemic sclerosis in both the juvenile and adult populations is the involvement of the cardiopulmonary system, with the development of ILD being most common, as well as pulmonary arterial hypertension and heart failure.[38] On HRCT, these patients often present with an NSIP pattern, described as fine reticular markings and ground-glass opacities in the lower lobes with subpleural sparing and in an apicobasal gradient distribution.[38] CT also may

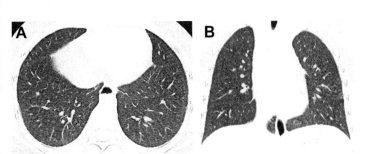

Fig. 13. A 9-year-old girl with recurrent pulmonary hemorrhage, but no active hemorrhage. Noncontrast axial (*A*) and coronal (*B*) CT images demonstrate diffuse subtle nodular ground-glass opacities and innumerable cysts, compatible with idiopathic pulmonary hemosiderosis.

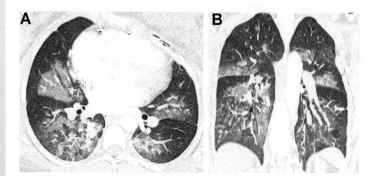

Fig. 14. A 22-year-old woman with systemic lupus erythematosus who presented with intermittent chest pain and hemoptysis. Noncontrast axial (*A*) and coronal (*B*) CT images demonstrate bilateral ground-glass and reticular opacities, sparing the periphery of the lung in the upper and lower lobes, in keeping with alveolar hemorrhage.

reveal mediastinal lymphadenopathy, esophageal dilatation, and pleural effusions,[38] although the incidence of these findings is lower in the pediatric population, possibly due to shorter disease duration.[38] If the patient develops progressive pulmonary fibrosis, subpleural cysts, traction bronchiectasis, and honeycombing may be observed (see **Fig. 5**).

Autoimmune pulmonary alveolar proteinosis

PAP comprises of a broad group of rare diseases characterized by the accumulation of pulmonary surfactants in the alveolar space.[39] This can be caused by altered surfactant production, removal, or both. Although much rarer in children, autoimmune PAP is typically secondary to disruption of the granulocyte-macrophage colony-stimulating factor receptor (GM-CSF) signaling via neutralization of the GM-CSF autoantibodies.[39] Serology testing has excellent sensitivity and specificity, and can be used to help diagnose patients with autoimmune PAP.[39] On HRCT, the crazy-paving pattern is characteristic, but not specific for PAP (see **Fig. 6**); therefore, BAL and sometimes lung biopsies are required for definitive diagnosis and exclusion of alternative diagnoses.[39]

Storage disease

Lysosomal storage disorders composes a large group of inherited metabolic diseases characterized by lipid-laden "foamy" macrophage accumulation in various tissues resulting from enzyme deficiencies, with Gaucher and Niemen-Pick diseases representing the most well-known entities.[7,10] Gaucher disease is the most common lysosomal storage disease, and estimated to affect 1 in 100,000 live births (although markedly more common in those of Ashkenazi Jewish descent).[7] Gaucher disease is due to the deficient activity of the enzyme β-glucocerebrosidase, resulting in glucocerebroside within the macrophages (Gaucher cells) in the spleen, liver, bone marrow, brain, osteoclasts, and less commonly

the lungs, skin, kidneys, conjunctivae, and heart.[40–42] Pulmonary involvement, although infrequent, is correlated with severe forms of disease, and is secondary to the deposition of the Gaucher cells within the alveolar, interstitial, subpleural, and peribronchovascular spaces.[42,43] In addition, arteriovenous shunting, most commonly as a complication of chronic liver disease (hepatopulmonary syndrome), can be observed.[42]

Chest radiographs may demonstrate reticulonodular opacities, and on HRCT, interstitial thickening (both interlobular and intralobular), ground-glass opacities, consolidation, and bronchial wall thickening can be seen[41,42] (**Fig. 15**A). Hilar and mediastinal lymphadenopathy, thymic, hepatic, and splenic enlargement (**Fig. 15**B, C) can further support the diagnosis of Gaucher disease.[41] Although children receiving enzyme replacement therapy for Gaucher disease may see gradual improvement of pulmonary abnormalities on imaging, it is important to be aware that imaging findings may not completely resolve.[43]

Sarcoidosis

Sarcoidosis is characterized by the presence of noncaseating granulomas,[44] and is well recognized and characterized in the adult population. In contrast, pediatric (juvenile) sarcoidosis remains markedly rare, estimated to affect children 10 times less frequently, and with an equal gender distribution.[44–47] Pediatric sarcoidosis is most commonly diagnosed in adolescents, but has been reported in infants and young children.[44] In younger children, pediatric sarcoidosis typically manifests as the clinical triad of rash, arthritis, and uveitis,[45] whereas in older children, sarcoidosis manifests similar to the adult form as a multisystem disorder, with lungs being the most commonly involved, in up to 92%.[44,45,47] The predominant symptom in the older patients is a mild, dry, chronic cough.[45] Similar to the adult patients, serum angiotensin-converting enzyme (ACE) levels are often

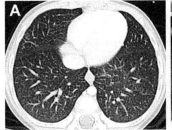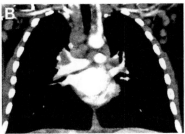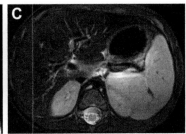

Fig. 15. A 3-year-old boy with type 1 Gaucher disease on enzyme replacement therapy, who presented for workup of an incidental hepatic mass (not shown). Contrast-enhanced axial CT image in lung window setting (A) demonstrates diffuse ground-glass opacities and mild interlobular and intralobular septal thickening. Axial CT image in soft tissue window setting (B) demonstrates bilateral mediastinal, hilar, and axillary lymphadenopathy. Axial T2-weighted MR image with fat suppression (C) demonstrates splenomegaly, supporting the diagnosis of Gaucher disease.

elevated, and should be measured when a diagnosis of sarcoidosis is considered; however, it is nonspecific and can be elevated in multiple conditions.[44–47]

When pulmonary involvement is present, the most common imaging pattern is hilar lymphadenopathy, usually bilateral (see Fig. 1).[44,45] Parenchymal disease occurs in approximately 65% of children, but isolated parenchymal disease remains rare, and typically involves the interstitium.[44] Typical sarcoidosis parenchymal imaging findings include peribronchovascular and interstitial thickening and peribronchovascular nodules[44,46] (see Fig. 1). Although imaging findings can be indicative, pediatric sarcoidosis remains a diagnosis of exclusion, suggested by clinical and imaging manifestations, but usually requiring confirmation with histopathology.[46]

Langerhans cell histiocytosis
LCH is characterized by accumulation of dendritic cells (Langerhans cells) in various organs, which can result in fibrosis, scarring, and cyst formation.[48] In contrast to the adult form of LCH, which is typically related to smoking and involves the lungs, LCH in children is often a multisystem disease potentially involving all organs, including the bones, skin, liver, spleen, and central nervous system.[23,48] Pulmonary involvement, especially isolated, is seen in only a minority of cases, with reported estimates of approximately 20% to 50%.[48] Clinical presentation can vary, and up to a quarter of patients remain asymptomatic; common presentations include dyspnea, nonproductive cough, and constitutional symptoms.[49]

Pulmonary LCH imaging findings in children are similar to adults, with the presence of nodular or diffuse reticulonodular opacities and cysts, often irregular in shape (see Fig. 4). The lung bases near the costophrenic angles are almost always

involved in children, but are spared in adults.[49,50] The peripheral cysts can rupture, resulting in spontaneous pneumothoraxes, a well-recognized complication in approximately 10% to 20%.[49] Rarely, pneumomediastinum from air leakage from the pulmonary interstitium may occur.[49] As parenchymal destruction and fibrosis progresses, pulmonary arterial hypertension and cor pulmonale may result, eventually leading to end-stage disease and death.[49] The presence of a thymic mass or calcification may help favor the diagnosis of LCH.[23] HRCT imaging allows a confident prospective diagnosis, and imaging findings are thought to correlate well with severity of functional impairment and pathologic findings, although not predictive of prognosis, and is recommended in all patients newly diagnosed with LCH.[49]

Immunocompromised Host

Lymphocytic interstitial pneumonitis
Lymphocytic interstitial pneumonia (LIP) is a rare disorder confined to the lungs, characterized by dense alveolar septal and interstitial reactive lymphocyte and plasma cell infiltrates.[51] LIP has been strongly associated with infection, and in children, LIP is particularly common, but not exclusive to children with human immunodeficiency virus (HIV), estimated to occur in approximately 30% to 40%.[51,52] Patients older than 2 years typically have an insidious clinical presentation, with a nonproductive cough, mild hypoxemia, generalized lymphadenopathy, and finger clubbing.[52–54]

The US Centers for Disease Control and Prevention (CDC) has previously established characteristic clinical and radiological features to obviate the need for a lung biopsy.[52] The radiological criteria were defined by the persistence of diffuse, symmetric, reticulo-nodular or nodular pulmonary opacification (Fig. 16), with or without mediastinal adenopathy for at least 2 months, without an

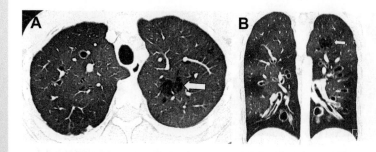

Fig. 16. A 15-year-old girl with lymphocytic interstitial pneumonia (LIP) and history of human immunodeficiency virus on retroviral therapy. Noncontrast axial (A) and coronal (B) CT images demonstrate multiple ground-glass opacities, diffuse bronchiectasis, and multiple cysts (arrows) in the left upper lobe, in keeping with diagnosis of LIP.

identifiable pathogen or response to antibiotic therapy.[52,54] Additional findings include characteristic cysts; subpleural, interlobular, and peribronchovascular micronodules; bronchiectasis, and less frequently ground-glass opacities (see Fig. 16) and pleural effusions.[51–53] There has been conflicting literature regarding the clinical implications of resolved radiographic LIP findings in the HIV-infected pediatric patient, with no definitive correlation identified.[54]

Treatment-related disorders: organizing pneumonia

Organizing pneumonia occurs as a pulmonary response to injury, incited by secondary causes such as infection, asthma, drug reaction, aspiration pneumonia, autoimmune disease, chemotherapy, transplantation, or other disorders, with resultant intraluminal inflammatory granulation tissue and fibrosis in the bronchi, alveolar ducts, and airspaces.[55,56] When no identifiable cause is identified, this is described as cryptogenic organizing pneumonia.[56]

Organizing pneumonia has variable imaging manifestations. However, the most frequent pattern is bilateral asymmetric patchy airspace opacities, often in a subpleural, peribronchial, or bandlike distribution.[55,56] These lesions may be migratory on follow-up studies.[56] Additional imaging findings may include ground-glass opacities, consolidation with air bronchograms, small nodular or linear ill-defined opacities, bronchial wall thickening and dilatation, or larger nodules or masses.[56] The reversed halo "atoll" sign, defined as a focal rounded ground-glass

opacification surrounded by a ring of consolidation, is seen infrequently (Fig. 17), approximately 20%, but felt to be relatively specific, although it can be seen in other entities, such as invasive fungal infections, GPA, pulmonary infarct, and lymphoproliferative disorders.[14,55–57] Mediastinal lymphadenopathy and pleural effusions also can be infrequently seen.[55,56]

Disorders related to rejection: bronchiolitis obliterans

Bronchiolitis obliterans (BO) is a serious late irreversible and progressive complication, thought to represent chronic rejection after allogeneic bone marrow/stem cell or lung transplantation, clinically defined by chronic airflow obstruction and pathologically characterized by fibrosis and obliteration of bronchioles.[58,59] The clinical correlate (without histopathology diagnosis) of airflow obstruction, based on spirometry criteria (forced expiratory volume in 1 second [FEV_1]/forced vital capacity of less than 0.7 or FEV_1 less than 75% of predicted value) or imaging findings, and with the exclusion of respiratory tract infection, is BO syndrome (BOS).[58–60] Affected pediatric patients with BO/BOS present with nonspecific and insidious symptoms of dyspnea, cough, exercise intolerance, and wheezing.[59] Multiple risk factors are associated with BO; however, the most important is the presence of chronic graft versus host disease (GVHD).[60,61]

On imaging, findings of bronchiolitis, with mosaic attenuation and air-trapping, bronchiectasis, and peribronchial thickening, are seen[58–60] (Fig. 18). Siegel and colleagues[62] have previously

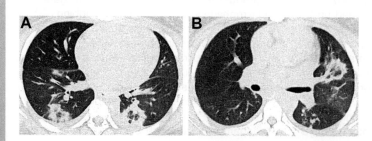

Fig. 17. An 18-year-old girl previously healthy, with biopsy-proven organizing pneumonia. Noncontrast axial (A, B) CT images demonstrate bilateral reverse halo "atoll" lesions in the left upper and bilateral lower lobes, in keeping with the diagnosis of organizing pneumonia.

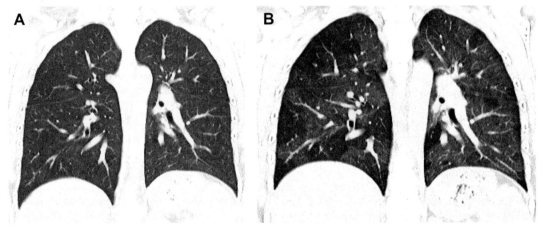

Fig. 18. An 11-year-old girl with history of acute myeloid leukemia status post bone marrow treatment 2 years ago, complicated by chronic graft versus host disease (GVHD). Noncontrast coronal inspiratory (A) and expiratory (B) CT images demonstrate diffuse bilateral lobular air-trapping in keeping with bronchiolitis obliterans (BO).

demonstrated the superior sensitivity of expiratory thin-section CT, in comparison with inspiratory thin-section CT scans in older children and teenagers, and more recently, Togni Filho and colleagues[61] have recommended the exclusion of inspiratory phase in the HRCT protocol, and to only use the expiratory phase for the diagnosis of BO to minimize radiation exposure in children.

Sequelae and Ongoing Disorders of Infancy

Surfactant deficiency disorders
Surfactant dysfunction disorders can be attributed to mutations in multiple genes, including genes for surfactant protein B (SFTPB), surfactant protein C (SFTPC), and adenosine triphosphate-binding cassette transporter protein A3 (ABCA3).[4] Although these diseases typically present early in the neonatal periods, SFTPC and ABCA3 mutations can have variable clinical presentations, and may remain asymptomatic until later in childhood or adulthood.[4,63] Although genetic testing may identify many known mutations in surfactant disorders, histopathological confirmation is typically sought to confirm diagnosis.[4]

On imaging, there may be diffuse ground-glass opacification, interlobular septal thickening, and a crazy-paving pattern on HRCT.[4] In older patients, the ground-glass opacities may appear diffuse or patchy, the septal thickening can appear fine or coarse with architectural distortion, and pulmonary cysts may develop and progress over time (Fig. 19).[10] Associated pectus excavatum has been reported, and hypothesized to represent sequelae of chronic restrictive lung disease in the developing chest wall.[4,64]

Neuroendocrine cell hyperplasia of infancy
NEHI, characterized by abnormally increased bombesin-immunopositive airway neuroendocrine cells in the absence of additional abnormalities, is typically diagnosed in full-term infants before the age of 2 years.[4,65] Affected patients usually present with a prolonged course of tachypnea, hypoxia, and retractions that do not improve with corticosteroids.[4,66] Due to the nonspecific presentation, diagnosis up to the age of 4 years has been reported.[67] However, most of these patients present early, and typically improve within 1 to 2 years.[65,66] Interestingly, Lukkarinen and colleagues[67] recently followed patients with NEHI

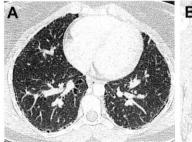

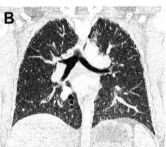

Fig. 19. A 21-year-old woman who presented with a 6-year history of dyspnea on exertion and found to have a surfactant protein C mutation. Noncontrast axial (A) and coronal (B) CT images demonstrate innumerable subpleural and paraseptal cysts and septal thickening, compatible with surfactant dysfunction interstitial lung disease.

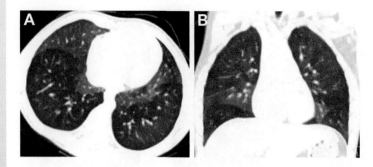

Fig. 20. A 4-year-old boy with chronic increased work of breathing without an infectious etiology and not improving on steroids. Noncontrast axial (*A*) and coronal (*B*) CT images demonstrate diffuse ground-glass opacification within the right middle lobe and lingula, compatible with a diagnosis of neuroendocrine cell hyperplasia of infancy (NEHI).

up to the age of 10 years, and found 6 of the 9 patients developed nonatopic asthma, suggesting its relationship to bronchial obstruction, which is not definitively seen on histopathology.

NEHI characteristically presents with ground-glass opacities within the right middle lobe and lingula and diffuse air-trapping, without airway or additional parenchymal abnormalities (**Fig. 20**).[4,65] HRCT has been reported to have up to 100% specificity, potentially obviating the need for lung biopsies in patients with classic symptoms and imaging findings, although HRCT remains unable to exclude NEHI as a potential diagnosis.[4,18] Recently, an increased apical anterior-posterior lung diameter has also been recommended to support a diagnosis of NEHI.[68]

SUMMARY

chILD in the older child and teenagers can pose a diagnostic challenge given the rarity and variable and often nonspecific clinical and imaging manifestations. On review of the available imaging techniques with emphasis on HRCT and of the recommended chILD classification in this population with imaging examples to highlight unique features, the general radiologist should feel more confident, in conjunction with the multidisciplinary team, to expedite an appropriate and accurate diagnosis.

DISCLOSURE

The authors have nothing to disclose.

REFERENCES

1. Clement A, Nathan N, Epaud R, et al. Interstitial lung diseases in children. Orphanet J Rare Dis 2010;5:22.
2. Das S, Langston C, Fan LL. Interstitial lung disease in children. Curr Opin Pediatr 2011;23:325–31.
3. Fan LL, Dishop MK, Galambos C, et al. Diffuse lung disease in biopsied children 2 to 18 years of age.

Application of the chILD classification scheme. Ann Am Thorac Soc 2015;12(10):1498–505.
4. Liang T, Vargas SO, Lee EY. Childhood interstitial (diffuse) lung disease: pattern recognition approach to diagnosis in infants. AJR Am J Roentgenol 2019; 212:1–10.
5. Deterding R. Evaluating infants and children with interstitial lung disease. Semin Respir Crit Care Med 2007;28:333–41.
6. Deutsch GH, Young LR, Deterding RR, et al, Pathology Cooperative Group, ChILD Research Co-operative. Diffuse lung disease in young children: application of a novel classification scheme. Am J Respir Crit Care Med 2007;176:1120–8.
7. Semple TR, Ashworth MT, Owens CM. Interstitial lung disease in children made easier...well, almost. Radiographics 2017;37:1679–703.
8. Copley SJ, Coren M, Nicholson AG, et al. Diagnostic accuracy of thin section CT and chest radiography of pediatric interstitial lung disease. AJR Am J Roentgenol 2000;174:549–54.
9. Lee EY. Interstitial lung disease in infants: new classification system, imaging technique, clinical presentation and imaging findings. Pediatr Radiol 2013;43:3–13.
10. Guillerman RP. Imaging of childhood interstitial lung disease. Pediatr Allergy Immunol Pulmonol 2010;23: 43–68.
11. Lynch DA, Hay T, Newell JD Jr, et al. Pediatric diffuse lung disease: diagnosis and classification using high resolution CT. AJR Am J Roentgenol 1999;173:713–8.
12. Long FR. High-resolution CT of the lungs in infants and young children. J Thorac Imaging 2001;16:251–8.
13. Schneuer FJ, Bentley JP, Davidson AJ, et al. The impact of general anesthesia on child development and school performance: a population-based study. Paediatr Anaesth 2018;28(6):528–36.
14. Hansell DM, Bankier AA, MacMahon H, et al. Fleischner Society: glossary of terms for thoracic imaging. Radiology 2008;246:697–722.
15. Deterding RR. Children's interstitial and diffuse lung disease - progress and future horizons. Ann Am Thorac Soc 2015;12(10):1451–7.

16. Sodhi KS, Sharma M, Lee EY, et al. Diagnostic utility of 3T lung MRI in children with interstitial lung disease: a prospective pilot study. Acad Radiol 2018; 25:380–6.

17. Schneebaum N, Blau H, Soferman R, et al. Use and yield of chest computed tomography in the diagnostic evaluation of pediatric lung disease. Pediatrics 2009;124:472–9.

18. Brody AS, Guillerman RP, Hay TC, et al. Neuroendocrine cell hyperplasia of infancy: diagnosis with high-resolution CT. AJR Am J Roentgenol 2010; 194:238–44.

19. Moonnumakal SP, Fan LL. Bronchiolitis obliterans in children. Curr Opin Pediatr 2008;20:272–8.

20. Panigada S, Ravelli A, Silvestri M, et al. HRCT and pulmonary function tests in monitoring of lung involvement in juvenile systemic sclerosis. Pediatr Pulmonol 2009;44:1226–34.

21. Wells AU. High-resolution computed tomography in the diagnosis of diffuse lung disease: a clinical perspective. Semin Respir Crit Care Med 2003;24: 347–56.

22. Ha SY, Helms P, Fletcher M, et al. Lung involvement in Langerhans' cell histiocytosis: prevalence, clinical features, and outcome. Pediatrics 1992;89: 466–9.

23. Odame I, Li P, Lau L, et al. Pulmonary Langerhans cell histiocytosis: a variable disease in childhood. Pediatr Blood Cancer 2006;47:889–93.

24. Colom AJ, Teper AM. Post-infectious bronchiolitis obliterans. Pediatr Pulmonol 2019;54(2):212–9.

25. Yalçin E, Dogru D, Haliloglu M, et al. Postinfectious bronchiolitis obliterans in children: clinical and radiological profile and prognostic factors. Respiration 2003;70:371–5.

26. Fan LL. Hypersensitivity pneumonitis in children. Curr Opin Pediatr 2002;14(3):323–6.

27. Hartman TE. The HRCT features of extrinsic allergic alveolitis. Semin Respir Crit Care Med 2003;24: 419–26.

28. Fan LL, Mullen AL, Brugman SM, et al. Clinical spectrum of chronic interstitial lung disease in children. J Pediatr 1992;121(6):867–72.

29. Cardasis JJ, MacMahon H, Husain AN. The spectrum of lung disease due to chronic occult aspiration. Ann Am Thorac Soc 2014;11(6):865–73.

30. Zanetti G, Marchiori E, Gasparetto TD, et al. Lipoid pneumonia in children following aspiration of mineral oil used in the treatment of constipation: high-resolution CT findings in 17 patients. Pediatr Radiol 2007;37(11):1135–9.

31. Marangu D, Gray D, Vanker A, et al. Exogenous lipoid pneumonia in children: a systematic review. Paediatr Respir Rev 2019. https://doi.org/10.1016/j.prrv.2019.01.001.

32. Giovanni-Chami L, Blanc S, Hadchouel A, et al. Eosinophilic pneumonitis in children: a review of the epidemiology, diagnosis, and treatment. Pediatr Pulmonol 2016;51(2):203–16.

33. Zhang Y, Luo F, Wang N, et al. Clinical characteristics and prognosis of idiopathic pulmonary hemosiderosis in pediatric patients. J Int Med Res 2019; 47(1):293–302.

34. Khorashadi L, Wu CC, Betancourt SL, et al. Idiopathic pulmonary haemosiderosis: spectrum of thoracic imaging findings in the adult patient. Clin Radiol 2015;70(5):459–65.

35. Alimi A, Taytard J, Taam RA, et al. Pulmonary hemosiderosis in children with Down syndrome: a national experience. Orphanet J Rare Dis 2018; 13(1):60.

36. Lilleby C, Aalokeen TM, Johansen B, et al. Pulmonary involvement in patients with childhood-onset systemic lupus erythematosus. Clin Exp Rheumatol 2006;24:203–8.

37. Guillerman RP, Brody AS. Contemporary perspectives on pediatric diffuse lung disease. Radiol Clin North Am 2011;49(5):847–68.

38. Valeur NS, Stevens AM, Ferguson MR, et al. Multimodality thoracic imaging of juvenile systemic sclerosis: emphasis on clinical correlation and high-resolution CT of pulmonary fibrosis. AJR Am J Roentgenol 2015;204(2):408–22.

39. Griese M. Pulmonary alveolar proteinosis: a comprehensive clinical perspective. Pediatrics 2017;140(2) [pii:e20170610].

40. Copley SJ, Padley SP. High-resolution CT of paediatric lung disease. Eur Radiol 2001;11:2564–75.

41. McHugh K, Olsen EØE, Vellodi A. Gaucher disease in children: radiology of non-central nervous system manifestations. Clin Radiol 2004;59:117–23.

42. Gulhan B, Ozcelik U, Gurakan F, et al. Different features of lung involvement in Niemann-Pick disease and Gaucher disease. Respir Med 2012;106(9): 1278–85.

43. Goitein O, Elstein D, Abrahamov A, et al. Lung involvement and enzyme replacement therapy in Gaucher's disease. QJM 2001;94:407–15.

44. Keesling CA, Frush DP, O'Hara SM, et al. Clinical and imaging manifestations of pediatric sarcoidosis. Acad Radiol 1998;5:122–32.

45. Fretzayas A, Moutsaki M, Vougiouka O. The puzzling clinical spectrum and course of juvenile sarcoidosis. World J Pediatr 2011;7(2):103–10.

46. Nathan N, Sileo C, Calender A, et al. Paediatric sarcoidosis. Paediatr Respir Rev 2019;29:53–9.

47. Hoffmann AL, Milman N, Byg KE. Childhood sarcoidosis in Denmark 1979-1994: incidence, clinical features and laboratory results at presentation in 48 children. Acta Paediatr 2004;93(1):30–6.

48. Smets A, Mortele K, de Praeter G, et al. Pulmonary and mediastinal lesions in children with Langerhans cell histiocytosis. Pediatr Radiol 1997; 27(11):873–6.

49. Bano S, Chaudhary V, Narula MK, et al. Pulmonary Langerhans cell histiocytosis in children: a spectrum of radiologic findings. Eur J Radiol 2014;83(1):47–56.

50. Seely JM, Salahudeen S Sr, Cadaval-Goncalves AT, et al. Pulmonary Langerhans cell histiocytosis: a comparative study of computed tomography in children and adults. J Thorac Imaging 2012;27(1):65–70.

51. Panchabhai TS, Farver C, Highland KB. Lymphocytic interstitial pneumonia. Clin Chest Med 2016;37:463–74.

52. Pitcher RD, Beningfield SJ, Zar HJ. Chest radiographic features of lymphocytic interstitial pneumonitis in HIV-infected children. Clin Radiol 2010;65:150–4.

53. Becciolini V, Gudinchet F, Cheseaux JJ, et al. Lymphocytic interstitial pneumonia in children with AIDS: high-resolution CT findings. Eur Radiol 2001;11:1015–20.

54. Lynch JL, Blickman JG, terMeulen DC, et al. Radiographic resolution of lymphocytic interstitial pneumonitis (LIP) in children with human immunodeficiency virus (HIV): not a sign of clinical deterioration. Pediatr Radiol 2001;31:299–303.

55. Mehrjardi MZ, Kahkouee S, Pourabdollah M. Radio-pathological correlation of organizing pneumonia (OP): a pictorial review. Br J Radiol 2017;90:20160723.

56. Long NM, Plodkowski AJ, Schor-Bardach R, et al. Computed tomographic appearance of organizing pneumonia in an oncologic patient population. J Comput Assist Tomogr 2017;41:437–41.

57. Kim SJ, Lee KS, Ryu YH, et al. Reversed halo sign on high-resolution CT of cryptogenic organizing pneumonia: diagnostic implications. AJR Am J Roentgenol 2003;180:1251–4.

58. Uhlving HH, Anderson CB, Christensen IJ, et al. Biopsy-verified bronchiolitis obliterans and other noninfectious lung pathologies after allogenic hematopoetic stem cell transplantation. Biol Blood Marrow Transplant 2015;21(3):531–8.

59. Kurland G, Michelson P. Bronchiolitis obliterans in children. Pediatr Pulmonol 2005;39:193–208.

60. Bergeron A, Cheng GS. Bronchiolitis obliterans syndrome and other late pulmonary complications after allogeneic hematopoietic stem cell transplantation. Clin Chest Med 2017;38(4):607–21.

61. Togni Filho PH, Casagrande JLM, Lederman HM. Utility of the inspiratory phase in high-resolution computed tomography evaluations of pediatric patients with bronchiolitis obliterans after allogenic bone marrow transplant: reducing patient radiation exposure. Radiol Bras 2017;50(2):90–6.

62. Siegel MJ, Bhalla S, Gutierrez FR, et al. Post-lung transplantation bronchiolitis obliterans syndrome: usefulness of expiratory thin-section CT for diagnosis. Radiology 2001;220(2):455–62.

63. Gower WA, Nogee LM. Surfactant dysfunction. Paediatr Respir Rev 2011;12:223–9.

64. Doan ML, Guillerman RP, Dishop MK, et al. Clinical, radiological and pathological features of ABCA3 mutations in children. Thorax 2008;63(4):355–73.

65. Brody AS, Crotty EJ. Neuroendocrine cell hyperplasia of infancy (NEHI). Pediatr Radiol 2006;36:1328.

66. Soares JJ, Deutsch GH, Moore PE, et al. Childhood interstitial lung diseases: an 18-year retrospective analysis. Pediatrics 2013;132(4):684–91.

67. Lukkarinen H, Pelkonen A, Lohi J, et al. Neuroendocrine cell hyperplasia of infancy: a prospective follow-up of nine children. Arch Dis Child 2013;98:141–4.

68. Mastej EJ, DeBoer EM, Humphries SM, et al. Lung and airway shape in neuroendocrine cell hyperplasia of infancy. Pediatr Radiol 2018;48:1745–54.

Repaired Congenital Heart Disease in Older Children and Adults

Up-to-Date Practical Assessment and Characteristic Imaging Findings

Varuna K. Gadiyaram, MD[a], Caterina B. Monti, MD[b], Anurag Sahu, MD[c], Peter D. Filev, MD[a], Giuseppe Muscogiuri, MD[d], Francesco Secchi, MD, PhD[b,e], Francesco Sardanelli, MD[b,e], Arthur E. Stillman, MD, PhD[a], Carlo N. De Cecco, MD, PhD[a,*]

KEYWORDS

- Aortic coarctation • Heart defects • Congenital • Magnetic resonance imaging
- Multidetector computed tomography • Tetralogy of Fallot • Transposition of great vessels

KEY POINTS

- Continuous advancements in diagnostic and therapeutic techniques have led to an increased long-term survival of patients with congenital heart disease.
- Imaging of repaired congenital heart disease is becoming a common routine in radiology practice.
- General radiologists need to be familiar with the most common congenital heart disease, surgical techniques, and complications.

INTRODUCTION

Congenital heart disease (CHD) has a prevalence of 4 to 10 per 1000 live births. The median age of patients with CHD in the United States has increased from 11 to 17 years between 1985 and 2000, and continues to increase today.[1] Since the first successful repair of CHD with cardiopulmonary bypass more than 70 years ago, survival of children with CHD has greatly improved: from an estimate of 20% of patients reaching adulthood, survival rose to 80% to 85%.[2] Today, in the United States, there are more adults living with CHD than there are children.[3] Adult patients

with CHD present a challenge to the general radiologist because of the unique anatomy and physiology, which is often associated with their disease processes.[4]

The overarching goal of this review article was to provide general radiologists with an insight into the main issues of imaging patients with repaired CHD, and the most common findings and complications of each individual pathology and its repair, focusing on tetralogy of Fallot (ToF), transposition of the great vessels, functional univentricular heart, aortic coarctation, anomalous pulmonary venous return, and atrial septal defects (ASDs).

a Division of Cardiothoracic Imaging, Department of Radiology and Imaging Sciences, Emory University Hospital, 1364 Clifton Road, Atlanta, GA 30307, USA; b Department of Biomedical Sciences for Health, Università degli Studi di Milano, Via Mangiagalli 31, Milano 20133, Italy; c Cardiac Intensive Care Unit, Emory University Hospital, 1364 Clifton Road, Atlanta, GA 30307, USA; d Centro Cardiologico Monzino, IRCCS, Via Carlo Parea 4, Milano 20138, Italy; e Department of Radiology, IRCCS Policlinico San Donato, Via Morandi 30, San Donato Milanese, Milan 20097, Italy
* Corresponding author. Division of Nuclear Medicine and Molecular Imaging, Emory University Hospital, 1364 Clifton Road Northeast, Atlanta, GA 30307.
E-mail address: carlo.dececco@emory.edu

Radiol Clin N Am 58 (2020) 503–516
https://doi.org/10.1016/j.rcl.2019.12.004

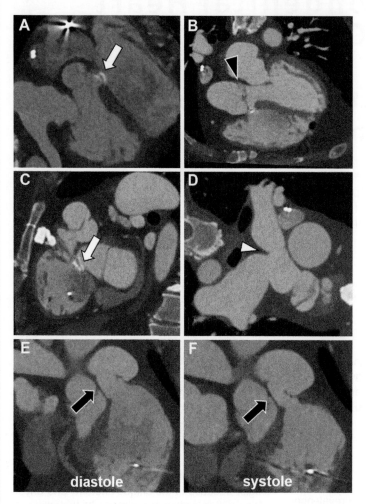

diastole   systole

Fig. 1. CCT of an 18-year-old male patient with repaired ToF, highlights repaired VSD (*A, C, white arrow*), RV hypertrophy with overriding aorta (*B, black arrowhead*), pulmonary artery stenosis (*D, white arrowhead*), narrowing of the RVOT with incomplete opening of the pulmonary leaflet throughout the cardiac cycle (*E*: diastole, *F*: systole, *black arrows*).

IMAGING TECHNIQUES

Although serial electrocardiograms (ECG) and echocardiograms continue to be important first-line modalities to evaluate patients with CHD, and catheterization represents the invasive reference standard, cardiac computed tomography (CCT) and magnetic resonance (CMR) are indispensable noninvasive second-level tests for a comprehensive evaluation of such individuals.[5] Specifically, CCT and CMR are superior to echocardiography when analyzing the right ventricle (RV), great vessels, pulmonary circulation, coronary arteries, and cardiac valves.[6]

Computed Tomography

In more recent years, use of CCT has become increasingly prevalent for the evaluation of patients with CHD, because of advancements that allow for faster scans, with very low radiation doses.[7] CCT is most useful in those particular cases when CMR is not feasible: for instance in the presence of CMR-unsafe devices, or in the case or claustrophobic, obese, critically ill, or unstable patients, as well as when coronary arteries, prosthetic valve integrity, or calcifications are under consideration.[8]

It is common for CCT protocols in patients with CHD to include an ECG-synchronized unenhanced scan in case of suspected acute aortic pathology, in the evaluation of calcifications or postsurgical or degenerative modifications. Furthermore, in certain cases, the administration of contrast agent may be contraindicated.[9] However, contrast-enhanced scans are the mainstay of CCT protocols in CHD. Iodinated contrast volumes range from 1 to 2 mL/kg in children to approximately 120 mL in adults. They should be acquired at the appropriate time after injection with regard to the structure that is the main objective of the examination.[10]

Contrast-enhanced CCT can provide valuable morpho-functional information, including measurements of ventricular volumes and ejection

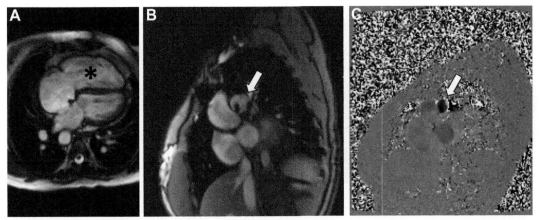

Fig. 2. CMR of a 26-year-old male patient with repaired ToF, with cine sequences shows dilated RV (*black asterisk, A*) as a consequence of pulmonary regurgitation (PR) and bioprosthetic pulmonary valve (*white arrow, B*), and phase-contrast sequence highlighting PR (*white arrow, C*).

fraction with a reliability comparable to that of CMR. It is the current reference standard for an in vivo evaluation of cardiac and vascular anatomy, because of its high spatial and temporal resolution.[11] Another potential advantage of CCT is that, because examinations take less time, sedation may be needed less often than in CMR, where it is recommended for every patient younger than 8 years.[12] This may be a significant advantage in patients with CHD, as most of them need second-level imaging studies during childhood, and they may be more prone to comorbidities or side effects secondary to sedation.

One of the major concerns associated with CCT in patients with CHD is radiation exposure, as these patients are frequently subjected to repeated examinations over the course of their lifetimes.[13] In this view, a proper choice for image acquisition synchronization is a main issue, as prospective gating is useful for the evaluation of great vessels, whereas retrospectively ECG-gated scans may provide more detailed information, especially regarding coronary arteries, albeit with a trade-off in terms of higher radiation exposure.[14] In this regard, scanners commonly found in clinical settings, from 64-row multidetector CCT to more recent scanners using cutting-edge technology, are able to provide reasonably low radiation doses.[12]

Magnetic Resonance Imaging

Along with CCT, CMR is an important second-line diagnostic test used in patients with CHD: the 2018 American Heart Association guidelines for the management of adult CHD report a class I recommendation for serial CMR examinations in patients who are at risk of developing RV dysfunction.[15]

CMR examinations in patients with CHD typically include nonenhanced stacks of cine sequences of the heart on long-axis and short-axis, phase-contrast sequences for the evaluation of flows in specific planes, unenhanced CMR angiography, and contrast-enhanced sequences for the evaluation of fibrotic scars, the so-called late gadolinium enhancement (LGE), and myocardial perfusion studies.[16] Cine sequences allow for the evaluation of morpho-functional parameters, such as ventricular volumes and ejection fraction, with a precision superior to that of echocardiography, especially with regard to the RV, and comparable to that of CCT.[17] The main exclusive advantage of CMR, however, is the possibility to quantify flows: phase-contrast sequences are designed for the assessment of flow volumes and velocities through imaging planes, thus providing insight on valve function and possible stenosis or regurgitation.[18] CMR angiography provides an accurate anatomic outline of the heart and vessels, whereas LGE and myocardial perfusion offer information concerning myocardial viability.[19]

More recently, novel CMR sequences have been introduced to better assess the 3-dimensional morphology and the functionality of the heart and its vessels. Among those, free-breathing whole heart magnetic resonance angiography, which allows for excellent visualization of finer structures, such as coronary arteries,[20] and 4-dimensional flow, which may add additional information regarding blood flow compared with phase-contrast sequences.[21]

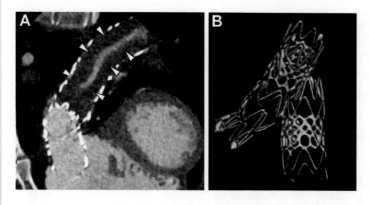

Fig. 3. CCT of a 21-year-old female patient shows left pulmonary artery (PA) stent thrombosed (*white arrowheads, A*), and 3-dimensional reconstruction (*B*) of bilateral PA stents.

Nearly all of the recent implantable devices are CMR-safe or at least CMR-conditional; however, they often produce significant imaging artifacts.[22] The typical contrast-enhanced CMR examination requires the intravenous administration of a gadolinium-based contrast agent; doses ranging from 0.1 to 0.2 mmol/kg are reported in the literature; however, considering the risk of potential accumulations of gadolinium in the brain, due to the frequency of repeated examinations in these patients, doses not exceeding 0.1 mmol/kg should be used.[23]

SPECTRUM OF REPAIRED CONGENITAL HEART DISEASE
Tetralogy of Fallot

ToF is the most common cyanotic CHD in children, occurring in approximately 5 in 10,000 live births, and representing 5% to 7% of all CHD.[24] ToF is caused by anterosuperior deviation of the conal septum, and this malalignment results in overriding of the interventricular septum by the aortic roof,

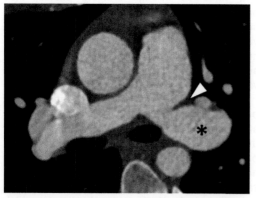

Fig. 4. CCT of a 22-year-old female patient with repaired ToF shows narrowing of the proximal left pulmonary artery (*white arrowhead*), with distal dilation (*black asterisk*).

obstruction of the pulmonary outflow tract, interventricular defect, and RV hypertrophy.[25] Right-sided aortic arch, atrial septal defect (ASD), a secondary ventricular septal defect (VSD), or atrioventricular canal defects also can be associated with ToF. With regard to coronary anomalies, the most significant is the left anterior descending artery arising anteriorly off the right coronary artery. When present, it travels anterior to the right ventricular outflow tract (RVOT) and is at risk of injury during sternal entry, it is seen in 3% of ToF cases. As such, any 3-dimensional imaging performed in this patient population should mention the coronary anatomy. Progressive aortic root dilation also may occur.[26]

The nature and timing of surgical repair has changed over the past few decades. In the current era, patients undergo primary repair typically by the first year of life or when they develop symptoms.[27] A palliative approach may be considered when surgical repair is not immediately possible, with its aim being the establishment of a reliable source of pulmonary blood flow, thereby reducing the cyanosis.[28] Palliative treatment consists of creation of shunts between systemic and pulmonary circulation, the most common of which are the Blalock-Taussig shunt, connecting the subclavian artery directly to a pulmonary artery, and especially in more recent years, the modified Blalock-Taussig shunt, which uses a Gore-Tex interposition graft.[29] Pulmonary artery distortion is often seen in patients with prior palliative shunts and thus architecture of the branch pulmonary artery should be evaluated.

Surgical repair in patients with ToF involves closure of the VSD and relief of the RVOT obstruction (**Fig. 1**).[30] In prior decades, repair was done through a large RV incision and placement of a transannular patch. This routinely resulted in RV dysfunction and free pulmonic insufficiency. In the modern era, large transannular patches are

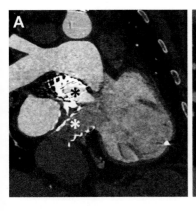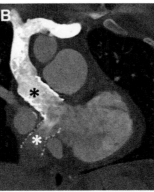

Fig. 5. CCT of a 36-year-old male patient (*A*) and a 24-year-old male patient (*B*) with D-TGA s/p Mustard/Senning repair, show superior and inferior vena cava baffles with stents (*black* and *white asterisks*).

avoided and a full degree of competency of the pulmonary valve is the aim.[31]

General radiologists should be aware of the possible anatomic findings they might face while imaging a patient with ToF at any repair stage, namely before palliation, between palliation and surgery, or after surgery, and of the possible complications of every stage. When imaging a patient who underwent ToF palliation without complete repair, it is important to assess the status of the shunts and their patency, as the preservation of a constant source of blood to the pulmonary circulation is of utmost importance. In current era of adults with repaired ToF, the most common complication related to surgical ToF repair is severe pulmonary regurgitation. The primary purpose of advanced imaging focuses on this point, as timing of pulmonary valve replacement, as well as the nature of the surgical or percutaneous intervention, is dependent on 3-dimensional imaging.[32]

CMR represents the most common technique for the morpho-functional assessment of the RV in patients with repaired ToF through cine sequences.[33] It is important to report RV volumes, ejection fraction, and degree of pulmonary regurgitation. Regurgitant fraction of greater than 48% is considered severe. MR angiography is also considered standard in the evaluation of repaired ToF. In asymptomatic patients, indications for pulmonary valve replacement (PVR) in the presence of moderate to severe pulmonary regurgitation often include RV end diastolic volume index of greater than 160 mL/m^2 or evidence of RV dysfunction (**Fig. 2**).[34] Contrast-enhanced CMR also allows the assessment of myocardial scar and diffuse fibrosis, where myocardial scar has been shown to relate to systolic dysfunction, and both scar and diffuse fibrosis are related to the insurgence of arrhythmias.[35]

CCT also can provide accurate estimates of cardiac volumes and function. In patients with repaired ToF, it is well suited to evaluate for coronary artery anomalies or coronary disease. It is also commonly used in postoperative assessment of patients with ToF (**Fig. 3**).[36] Structurally, CCT

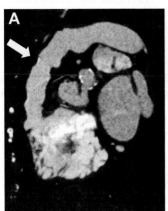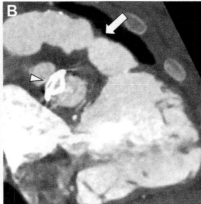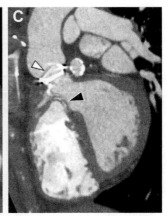

Fig. 6. CCT of a 27-year old male patient (*A*) and of a 25-year-old female patient (*B, C*) after Rastelli procedure with conduit placement (*white arrow*), mechanical aortic valve (*white arrowhead*), and VSD closure (*black arrowhead*).

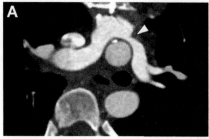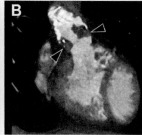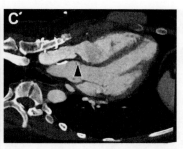

Fig. 7. CCT of a 25-year-old male patient with repaired TGA, depicts proximal left pulmonary artery narrowing (*white arrowhead, A*), large vegetation on pulmonary valve (*black arrowheads, B and C*) with decreased leaflets mobility (*C*).

well defines the anatomy of the RVOT, pulmonary valve annulus, and the branch pulmonary arteries (**Fig. 4**). The severity and distribution of pulmonary artery calcifications and relationship between the RVOT and coronary arteries are well seen.[33]

Transposition of the Great Arteries

Transposition of the great arteries (TGA) is a CHD in which the aorta arises from the RV and the pulmonary artery arises from the left ventricle (5% of all patients with CHD).[37] Commonly associated defects include VSDs, left ventricular outflow tract obstruction, and coarctation of the aorta. In addition, the anatomy of the coronary arteries is variable.

The most common form of TGA is dextro-TGA (D-TGA), in which atrial-ventricular concordance is preserved, but the resultant ventriculo-arterial discordance results in cyanosis. In essence, there are 2 parallel circulations of blood flow with deoxygenated blood remaining in the systemic circuit, and oxygenated blood remaining in the pulmonary circuit.

Initial surgical palliations of D-TGA involved the creation of an atrial-level baffle in which blood from the systemic veins (inferior vena cava and superior vena cava) is rerouted to the posterior

left ventricle and blood from the pulmonary veins is rerouted to the anterior RV. The RV remains the systemic ventricle and the left ventricle remains the subpulmonic ventricle. Two types of repairs are described, in the Mustard procedure, the atrial septum is excised, and pericardial tissue is used to create the atrial-level baffle. The Senning procedure is considered more complicated, but results in the same final solution. From an advanced imaging standpoint, they look nearly identical, and without operative history are difficult to distinguish.

Current era surgical repair for D-TGA is arterial switch, in which the aorta and the main pulmonary artery are cut above their sinuses and transposed with the pulmonary artery placed anterior to the aorta (**Fig. 5**).[38] The coronary arteries are detached from the native aorta with some surrounding tissue and then sutured into place on the posterior neoaortic root. The Rastelli procedure is a surgical intervention that palliates TGA along with VSD and left ventricular outflow tract obstruction when such concomitant issues are present (**Fig. 6**).[39]

Complications of TGA repair are directly related to the type of surgical repair. In those with Mustard/Senning repairs, narrowing of the atrial baffles or baffle leaks may occur, although the

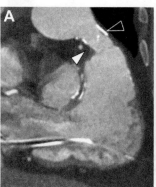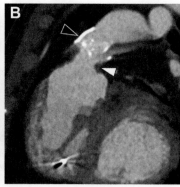

Fig. 8. CCT of a 33-year-old female patient with repaired TGA shows a narrowed RV to pulmonary artery conduit, with thickening (*white arrowheads, A and B*) and calcifications (*black arrowheads, A and B*).

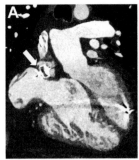
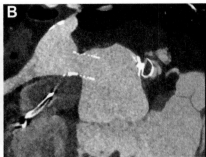

Fig. 9. CCT of a 19-year-old female patient with repaired TGA, shows Amplatzer (*white arrow*, A) and stented pulmonary vein baffle to the left ventricle (*B*).

most sinister finding is the development of systemic RV dysfunction. In patients with an arterial switch, coronary ostial stenosis related to the arterial anastomosis or supravalvular obstruction at the site of the aortic/pulmonic transection may occur. Systemic valvular disease, tricuspid valve regurgitation, is also common. Branch pulmonary stenosis also can be seen (**Fig. 7**).[37]

In patients with repaired TGA, CCT can provide accurate information with regard to cardiovascular anatomy and function, and it can help identify narrowing in baffles or baffle leaks, and calcifications (**Fig. 8**).[36,40] Moreover, CCT can be used to assess coronary arteries and pulmonary arteries in view of a potential compression or stenosis due to surgical intervention (**Fig. 9**).[41] CCT is especially indicated in those patients who have implanted cardiac devices, as they may cause image artifacts, which account for up to 15% of individuals with repaired TGA, and in those in whom noncardiac thoracic pathology is likely to be a major issue.[42]

CMR provides reliable functional information regarding the cardiac ventricles, valves, and great arteries in patients with repaired TGA, and it is recommended to include it in the follow-up of such patients whenever possible.[42] The key feature of CMR is its ability to detect baffle leaks or residual shunting, by quantification of the pulmonary flow divided by the systemic flow (Qp/Qs ratio) from phase-contrast sequences.[43] Assessment of LGE may show myocardial scars, and stress-CMR may highlight perfusion defects as a result of

coronary artery pathologies arising from TGA correction.[44]

Functional Univentricular Heart

Functional univentricular heart (FUV) encompasses different anatomic abnormalities that share the inability of either ventricle to sustain its typically defined anatomic circulation[45]: double inlet ventricles, hearts with absent atrioventricular connections, or hearts with single ventriculoarterial connections (**Fig. 10**).[46] FUV can be palliated through surgery with the Fontan procedure, thus establishing a total cavo-pulmonary connection and leaving the FUV to serve as the systemic ventricle.[47] Long-term complications of this repair are numerous and include Fontan baffle stenosis, thrombosis of the Fontan, branch pulmonary artery stenosis, ventricular dysfunction, development of veno-veno collaterals, and valvular heart disease, to name a few (**Fig. 11**).[15]

When imaging a patient with repaired FUV, it is important to understand the surgical palliation the patient has undergone. Given the variation in single-ventricle palliations and the heterogeneity of complications, evaluation of the anatomic and physiologic complications is challenged without review of the operative record or other record of surgical/catheterization history.

CCT can be useful in the assessment of volumes and function, of patency of the anastomoses, narrowing or obstruction of the venous return, and in

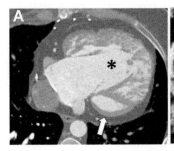
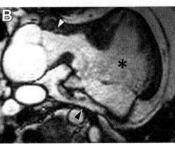

Fig. 10. (*A*) CCT of a single-ventricle 26-year-old female patient with double-outlet RV (*black asterisk*), and hypoplastic left heart (*white arrow*). (*B*) CMR of a 23-year-old male patient with double-outlet RV (*black asterisk*), with pulmonary veins (*black arrowhead*) and aorta (*white arrowhead*).

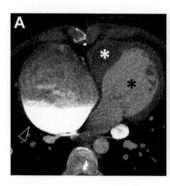 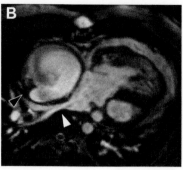

Fig. 11. CCT of a 38-year-old male patient (*A*) with Fontan circulation after atrio-pulmonary Fontan, shows markedly dilated right atrium (*black arrowhead*), hypertrophic left ventricle (*black asterisk*), and hypoplastic RV (*white asterisk*). CMR of a 38-year-old male patient (*B*) with Fontan circulation after atrio-pulmonary Fontan, shows compression of the pulmonary veins (*white arrowhead*) secondary to markedly dilated right atrium (*black arrowhead*).

the detection of abnormal communications, due to its excellent anatomic resolution.[48] However, due to the peculiarities of the venous return in Fontan physiology, it might be hard to obtain the desired contrast enhancement at CCT.[49] Thus, CCT is considered as mainly an alternative imaging modality in repaired FUV, when CMR is contraindicated, or when the presence of devices might severely hinder the quality of CMR.[50]

CMR is a pillar for the follow-up of patients with repaired FUV.[51] CMR allows for an accurate depiction of cardiovascular anatomy in repaired FUV through cine sequences, along with reliable noninvasive quantification of morphology and functionality of the ventricle. Phase-contrast sequences allow for quantification of flows throughout the Fontan circulation, thus screening for possible overloads or valvular pathologies, which would lead to potential ventricular dysfunction.[52] MR angiography is also a standard part of the anatomic evaluation. After injection of gadolinium-based contrast agents, many patients with repaired FUV show myocardial scars, whose amount has been linked to adverse clinical outcomes.[36]

Aortic Coarctation

Aortic coarctation (CoA) is a CHD characterized by segmental constriction of the aorta, with

thickening of the media and infolding of both medial and intimal tissue.[53] CoA is most often found immediately distal to the left subclavian artery, near the ductal remnant.[54] CoA is fairly common, accounting for 5% to 8% of all CHD, and it may either present as isolated, or be accompanied by other cardiac anomalies, such as a bicuspid aortic valve.[55] Repair of CoA can be performed through surgery, removing or grafting a stent over the narrowed segment, balloon angioplasty, or stent placement.[56] After repair, the likelihood of residual recoarctation may be as high as 60%, and more than 50% of patients may develop subsequent hypertension.[57] Thus, even when CoA has already been repaired, follow-up imaging at 5-year intervals using CCT or CMR bears a class I-B recommendation, to monitor possible recoarctation, aneurysm formation, dissection, stent rupture or displacement, or cardiac morpho-functional abnormalities (**Fig. 12**).[15] Morpho-functional evaluation of the cardiac chambers is paramount, as left ventricular hypertrophy might present secondary to hypertension, and the aortic arch may present with additional anomalies in patients with CoA.[58]

In patients with repaired CoA, CCT has been found to be especially useful in evaluating stent-related postoperative complications due to its high spatial resolution, as it can precisely identify

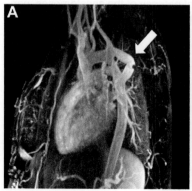 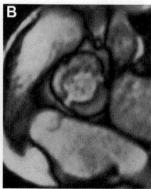

Fig. 12. T1-weighted, contrast-enhanced CMR angiography of a 24-year-old man shows severe aortic coarctation treated with a jump graft to descending aorta (*A*, *arrow*), and bicuspid aortic valve associated with aortic coarctation (*B*).

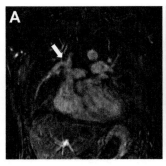
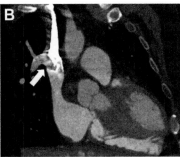

Fig. 13. Two cases of partial APVR. CMR (*A*) and CCT (*B*) show the connection of the right pulmonary vein to the superior vena cava (*arrows*).

the extent of stent damage, its position, and its relation to the aortic wall.[59] Moreover, 3-dimensional reconstructions have further enhanced the role of CCT in the follow-up of CoA, allowing for more precise anatomic representations.[60]

CMR, likewise, has an important role in the follow-up of patients with repaired CoA, typically including phase-contrast sequences, for the assessment of nature of flow and pressure gradients and relapse of CoA.[61] Contrast-enhanced CMR angiography may provide additional information, for instance with regard to collateral branches, allowing for more accurate appraisal of the vascular lumens.[62] Stents may produce artifacts in patients with CoA undergoing CMR.[63]

Anomalous Pulmonary Venous Return

Anomalous pulmonary venous return (APVR) is a rare CHD, accounting for 1% to 3% of all CHDs diagnosed after birth, and it is characterized by either partial or total connection of the pulmonary venous system to the systemic venous system, depending on whether only some or all pulmonary veins drain into the systemic venous system (Fig. 13).[64] APVR is often associated to interatrial

defects, or other cardiac anomalies, such as right atrial isomerism.[65] APVR repair consists of creating an anastomosis of the misplaced pulmonary veins and the left atrium.[66] After APVR repair, some patients may experience pulmonary venous stenosis, obstruction, and pulmonary hypertension, and require reintervention, particularly those with higher intraoperative pressure gradients.[67]

In patients with repaired APVR, morphofunctional evaluation through CCT may show RV dilation and progressive dysfunction, whereas CCT angiography may provide the highest-resolution anatomic depiction of the pulmonary vessels, thus potentially highlighting postintervention pulmonary stenoses or obstructions.[68] Furthermore, as CCT allows the best noninvasive evaluation of lung disease, it could help identify previous APVR as a possible origin of pulmonary hypertension, as opposed to other causes.[69]

In patients with repaired APVR, as per functional evaluation via CCT, CMR cine sequences may help highlight possible RV dilation, and lead to a detection of postoperative complications earlier than that allowed by echocardiography.[70] Moreover, phase-contrast sequences could allow calculation of the Qp/Qs ratio, by estimating

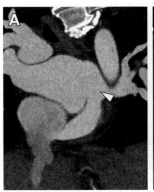
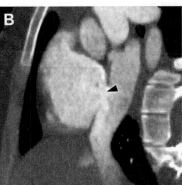
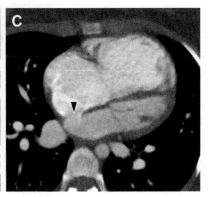

Fig. 14. CCT of a 37-year-old male patient shows coronary sinus atrial septal defect (*white arrowhead* in A). CCT of a 38-year-old male patient demonstrates sinus venosus atrial septal defect shown from lateral view and long axis (*black arrowheads* in B and C).

Table 1
List of the 6 common congenital heart diseases, along with their main repair techniques, postrepair imaging findings, and possible complications that can be detected at computed tomography or magnetic resonance imaging

Congenital Heart Disease	Main Repair Techniques	Postrepair Imaging Findings	Complications Detected at Imaging
Tetralogy of Fallot	Surgical, infundibulectomy, valvulectomy, patch and defect closure	After palliation, shunt between systemic and pulmonary circulation, with residual ventricular septal defect and obstruction of the right ventricular outflow tract. After surgery, closure of the ventricular septal defect, disobstructed right ventricular outflow tract.	After palliation, shunt obstruction. After surgery, pulmonary regurgitation and consequent right ventricular dilation and failure.
Transposition of the great arteries	Surgical, atrial switch or arterial switch	Great arteries originating from the contralateral ventricle.	Narrowing of baffles, baffle leaks, valvular dysfunction, aortic root dilation, coronary artery disease.
Single-ventricle palliation	Surgical, Norwood procedure with shunting, or Glenn shunt and Fontan	Fontan circulation, with the systemic veins connected to the pulmonary arteries, and presence of only 1 functional ventricle.	Narrowing of anastomoses of the pulmonary arteries with consequent dilation of the right ventricle, narrowing of the shunts, valvular dysfunction.
Aortic coarctation	Surgical repair through anastomosis, graft, or patch, percutaneous treatment with angioplasty or stent	Loss of continuity in the aortic profile, or aortic grafts.	Recoarctation, left ventricular hypertrophy.
Anomalous pulmonary venous return	Surgical, anastomosis between pulmonary veins and left atrium	Residual connections between the pulmonary and systemic veins in case of partial residual anomalous pulmonary venous return, ectopic connection between the pulmonary veins and left atrium.	Pulmonary hypertension with possible consequent right ventricular dilation.
Atrial septal defects	Surgical or percutaneous defect closure	Closure of the defect.	Device thrombosis, erosion through the atrial wall.

pulmonary blood flow from the pulmonary artery and systemic blood flow from the aorta, thus detecting potential obstructions.[71]

Atrial Septal Defects

ASDs represent the CHD most frequently diagnosed in adulthood.[72] There are 4 main types of ASD, namely *ostium primum*, *ostium secundum*, *unroofed coronary sinus,* and *sinus venosus defects* (**Fig. 14**). ASD may lead to dangerous complications, such as embolism due to passage of blood clots, or pulmonary hypertension.[73] The treatment for ASD consists of the closure of the defect and is performed in case of hemodynamically significant shunt.[6] ASD closure can be surgical or transcatheter, depending on the type. Coronary sinus and sinus venosus must be repaired surgically, whereas secundum ASDs may possibly be approached percutaneously depending on certain anatomic considerations.[73] It is important to note that 10% to 15% of secundum defects have an associated anomalous pulmonary vein, which would then exclude such patients from percutaneous repair.[74] Among long-term complications of percutaneous ASD closure are device thrombosis or erosion through the atrial wall or aortic root,[75] although these are remarkably uncommon when patients are selected appropriately.

When CCT is performed in a patient with previously corrected ASD, it may highlight the status of the device used for closure, and whether it is causing issues with cardiac or vascular walls.[76] All devices used for ASD closure are either CMR-compatible or conditional, and, although to a lesser extent compared with CCT because of lower anatomic resolution, CMR may show problems connected to devices.[22]

SUMMARY

Both CCT and CMR are important in diagnosing and potentially preventing complications in the follow-up of patients with repaired CHD, as summarized in **Table 1**. On the whole, although CCT and CMR can be used interchangeably for the evaluation of cardiovascular anatomy, morphology, and function, CCT can bring such information to a higher level of spatial resolution, whereas CMR has the advantage of providing information with regard to blood flow characteristics. The clinical value of these two imaging techniques also has been amplified by the considerable increase in survival rates of such patients. This result of cardiac surgery opened new issues related to the aging process in these patients, also involving body systems other than the cardiovascular system, for instance a possibly faster brain aging, a topic now under investigation, which is beyond the scope of this article.

It is expected that general radiologists will encounter more and more adult patients with CHD in their clinical practice, either referred for specific follow-up cardiac evaluation or for body evaluation including the heart for suspected or already ascertained comorbidities. To guide the execution of a high-quality CCT and/or CMR examination in these patients, and to provide a first assessment of the modified cardiovascular anatomy and function, as well as to know when to ask for further investigations are important professional duties to be accomplished.

DISCLOSURE

C.N. De Cecco receives institutional research support and/or honorarium as speaker from Siemens and Bayer. F. Sardanelli received institutional research support and honorarium as speaker from Bracco, Bayer, and General Electric. The other authors have no conflicts of interest to disclose.

REFERENCES

1. Marelli AJ, Mackie AS, Ionescu-Ittu R, et al. Congenital heart disease in the general population: changing prevalence and age distribution. Circulation 2007;115(2):163–72.

2. Triedman JK, Newburger JW. Trends in congenital heart disease: the next decade. Circulation 2016; 133(25):2716–33.

3. Marelli AJ, Ionescu-Ittu R, Mackie AS, et al. Lifetime prevalence of congenital heart disease in the general population from 2000 to 2010. Circulation 2014;130(9):749–56.

4. Gaydos SS, Varga-Szemes A, Judd RN, et al. Imaging in adult congenital heart disease. J Thorac Imaging 2017;32(4):205–16.

5. Puchalski MD, Williams RV, Askovich B, et al. Assessment of right ventricular size and function: echo versus magnetic resonance imaging. Congenit Heart Dis 2007;2(1):27–31.

6. Warnes CA, Williams RG, Bashore TM, et al. ACC/AHA 2008 guidelines for the management of adults with congenital heart disease: a report of the American College of Cardiology/American Heart Association Task Force on Practice Guidelines (Writing Committee to Develop Guidelines on the Management of Adults With Congenital Heart Disease). Developed in collaboration with the American Society of Echocardiography, Heart Rhythm Society, International Society for Adult Congenital Heart Disease, Society for Cardiovascular Angiography and

Interventions, and Society of Thoracic Surgeons. J Am Coll Cardiol 2008;52(23):e143–263.

7. Han BK, Lesser AM, Vezmar M, et al. Cardiovascular imaging trends in congenital heart disease: a single center experience. J Cardiovasc Comput Tomogr 2013;7(6):361–6.

8. Han BK, Rigsby CK, Hlavacek A, et al. Computed tomography imaging in patients with congenital heart disease part I: rationale and utility. An expert consensus document of the Society of Cardiovascular Computed Tomography (SCCT): endorsed by the Society of Pediatric Radiology (SPR) and the North American Society of Cardiac Imaging (NASCI). J Cardiovasc Comput Tomogr 2015;9(6): 475–92.

9. Suranyi P, Varga-Szemes A, Hlavacek AM. An overview of cardiac computed tomography in adults with congenital heart disease. J Thorac Imaging 2017; 32(4):258–73.

10. Rajiah P, Saboo SS, Abbara S. Role of CT in congenital heart disease. Curr Treat Options Cardiovasc Med 2017;19(1):6.

11. Han BK, Rigsby CK, Leipsic J, et al. Computed tomography imaging in patients with congenital heart disease, part 2: technical recommendations. An expert consensus document of the Society of Cardiovascular Computed Tomography (SCCT): endorsed by the Society of Pediatric Radiology (SPR) and the North American Society of Cardiac Imaging (NASCI). J Cardiovasc Comput Tomogr 2015;9(6):493–513.

12. Cannao PM, Secchi F, Ali M, et al. High-quality low-dose cardiovascular computed tomography (CCT) in pediatric patients using a 64-slice scanner. Acta Radiol 2018;59(10):1247–53.

13. Bonnichsen C, Ammash N. Choosing between MRI and CT imaging in the adult with congenital heart disease. Curr Cardiol Rep 2016;18(5):45.

14. Halliburton SS, Abbara S, Chen MY, et al. SCCT guidelines on radiation dose and dose-optimization strategies in cardiovascular CT. J Cardiovasc Comput Tomogr 2011;5(4):198–224.

15. Stout KK, Daniels CJ, Aboulhosn JA, et al. 2018 AHA/ACC guideline for the management of adults with congenital heart disease: a report of the American College of Cardiology/American Heart Association Task Force on Clinical Practice Guidelines. Circulation 2019;139(14):e698–800.

16. Kilner PJ, Geva T, Kaemmerer H, et al. Recommendations for cardiovascular magnetic resonance in adults with congenital heart disease from the respective working groups of the European Society of Cardiology. Eur Heart J 2010;31(7):794–805.

17. Wheeler M, Leipsic J, Trinh P, et al. Right ventricular assessment in adult congenital heart disease patients with right ventricle-to-pulmonary artery conduits. J Am Soc Echocardiogr 2015;28(5):522–32.

18. Sahu A, Slesnick TC. Imaging adults with congenital heart disease part II: advanced CMR techniques. J Thorac Imaging 2017;32(4):245–57.

19. Harris MA, Johnson TR, Weinberg PM, et al. Delayed-enhancement cardiovascular magnetic resonance identifies fibrous tissue in children after surgery for congenital heart disease. J Thorac Cardiovasc Surg 2007;133(3):676–81.

20. Albrecht MH, Varga-Szemes A, Schoepf UJ, et al. Coronary artery assessment using self-navigated free-breathing radial whole-heart magnetic resonance angiography in patients with congenital heart disease. Eur Radiol 2018;28(3):1267–75.

21. De Cecco CN, Muscogiuri G, Varga-Szemes A, et al. Cutting edge clinical applications in cardiovascular magnetic resonance. World J Radiol 2017;9(1):1–4.

22. Shellock FG. Reference manual for magnetic resonance safety, implants, and devices: edition 2019. Los Angeles (CA): Biomedical Research Publishing Group; 2019.

23. Kanda T, Nakai Y, Oba H, et al. Gadolinium deposition in the brain. Magn Reson Imaging 2016;34(10): 1346–50.

24. Liu Y, Chen S, Zuhlke L, et al. Global birth prevalence of congenital heart defects 1970-2017: updated systematic review and meta-analysis of 260 studies. Int J Epidemiol 2019;48(2):455–63.

25. Delius RE, Kumar RV, Elliott MJ, et al. Atrioventricular septal defect and tetralogy of Fallot: a 15-year experience. Eur J Cardiothorac Surg 1997;12(2):171–6.

26. Bailliard F, Anderson RH. Tetralogy of Fallot. Orphanet J Rare Dis 2009;4:2.

27. Al Habib HF, Jacobs JP, Mavroudis C, et al. Contemporary patterns of management of tetralogy of Fallot: data from the Society of Thoracic Surgeons Database. Ann Thorac Surg 2010;90(3):813–9 [discussion: 819–20].

28. Yamada Y, Ishizu T, Tsuneoka H, et al. A long-term survivor with tetralogy of Fallot treated only with the classical Blalock-Taussig shunt. Case Rep Cardiol 2018;2018:5262745.

29. Singh SP, Chauhan S, Choudhury M, et al. Modified Blalock Taussig shunt: comparison between neonates, infants and older children. Ann Card Anaesth 2014;17(3):191–7.

30. Alassal M, Ibrahim BM, Elrakhawy HM, et al. Total correction of tetralogy of Fallot at early age: a study of 183 cases. Heart Lung Circ 2018;27(2):248–53.

31. Sen DG, Najjar M, Yimaz B, et al. Aiming to preserve pulmonary valve function in tetralogy of Fallot repair: comparing a new approach to traditional management. Pediatr Cardiol 2016;37(5):818–25.

32. Secchi F, Resta EC, Cannao PM, et al. Biventricular heart remodeling after percutaneous or surgical pulmonary valve implantation: evaluation by cardiac magnetic resonance. J Thorac Imaging 2017;32(6): 358–64.

33. Valente AM, Cook S, Festa P, et al. Multimodality imaging guidelines for patients with repaired tetralogy of Fallot: a report from the American Society of Echocardiography: developed in collaboration with the Society for Cardiovascular Magnetic Resonance and the Society for Pediatric Radiology. J Am Soc Echocardiogr 2014;27(2):111–41.

34. Lee C, Kim YM, Lee CH, et al. Outcomes of pulmonary valve replacement in 170 patients with chronic pulmonary regurgitation after relief of right ventricular outflow tract obstruction: implications for optimal timing of pulmonary valve replacement. J Am Coll Cardiol 2012;60(11):1005–14.

35. Cochet H, Iriart X, Allain-Nicolai A, et al. Focal scar and diffuse myocardial fibrosis are independent imaging markers in repaired tetralogy of Fallot. Eur Heart J Cardiovasc Imaging 2019;20(9):990–1003.

36. De Cecco CN, Muscogiuri G, Madrid Perez JM, et al. Pictorial review of surgical anatomy in adult congenital heart disease. J Thorac Imaging 2017;32(4):217–32.

37. Warnes CA. Transposition of the great arteries. Circulation 2006;114(24):2699–709.

38. Haeffele C, Lui GK. Dextro-transposition of the great arteries: long-term sequelae of atrial and arterial switch. Cardiol Clin 2015;33(4):543–58, viii.

39. Brawn WJ, Barron DJ. Technical aspects of the Rastelli and atrial switch procedure for congenitally corrected transposition of the great arteries with ventricular septal defect and pulmonary stenosis or atresia: results of therapy. Semin Thorac Cardiovasc Surg Pediatr Card Surg Annu 2003;6:4–8.

40. Lu JC, Dorfman AL, Attili AK, et al. Evaluation with cardiovascular MR imaging of baffles and conduits used in palliation or repair of congenital heart disease. Radiographics 2012;32(3):E107–27.

41. Han BK, Lesser JR. CT imaging in congenital heart disease: an approach to imaging and interpreting complex lesions after surgical intervention for tetralogy of Fallot, transposition of the great arteries, and single ventricle heart disease. J Cardiovasc Comput Tomogr 2013;7(6):338–53.

42. Cohen MS, Eidem BW, Cetta F, et al. Multimodality imaging guidelines of patients with transposition of the great arteries: a report from the American Society of Echocardiography developed in collaboration with the Society for Cardiovascular Magnetic Resonance and the Society of Cardiovascular Computed Tomography. J Am Soc Echocardiogr 2016;29(7):571–621.

43. Geva CWS, Ioannis G, Matthew TW, et al. Cardiovascular magnetic resonance findings late after the arterial switch operation. Circ Cardiovasc Imaging 2016;9(9) [pii:e004618].

44. Ntsinjana HN, Hughes ML, Taylor AM. The role of cardiovascular magnetic resonance in pediatric congenital heart disease. J Cardiovasc Magn Reson 2011;13:51.

45. Anderson RH, Cook AC. Morphology of the functionally univentricular heart. Cardiol Young 2004;14(Suppl 1):3–12.

46. Frescura C, Thiene G. The new concept of univentricular heart. Front Pediatr 2014;2:62.

47. Yoo SJ, Prsa M, Schantz D, et al. MR assessment of abdominal circulation in Fontan physiology. Int J Cardiovasc Imaging 2014;30(6):1065–72.

48. Ghadimi Mahani M, Agarwal PP, Rigsby CK, et al. CT for assessment of thrombosis and pulmonary embolism in multiple stages of single-ventricle palliation: challenges and suggested protocols. Radiographics 2016;36(5):1273–84.

49. Prabhu SP, Mahmood S, Sena L, et al. MDCT evaluation of pulmonary embolism in children and young adults following a lateral tunnel Fontan procedure: optimizing contrast-enhancement techniques. Pediatr Radiol 2009;39(9):938–44.

50. Han BK, Huntley M, Overman D, et al. Cardiovascular CT for evaluation of single-ventricle heart disease: risks and accuracy compared with interventional findings. Cardiol Young 2018;28(1):9–20.

51. Lewis G, Thorne S, Clift P, et al. Cross-sectional imaging of the Fontan circuit in adult congenital heart disease. Clin Radiol 2015;70(6):667–75.

52. Ginde S, Goot BH, Frommelt PC. Imaging adult patients with Fontan circulation. Curr Opin Cardiol 2017;32(5):521–8.

53. Nigro G, Russo V, Rago A, et al. Heterogeneity of ventricular repolarization in newborns with severe aortic coarctation. Pediatr Cardiol 2012;33(2):302–6.

54. Warnes CA. Bicuspid aortic valve and coarctation: two villains part of a diffuse problem. Heart 2003;89(9):965–6.

55. Dijkema EJ, Leiner T, Grotenhuis HB. Diagnosis, imaging and clinical management of aortic coarctation. Heart 2017;103(15):1148–55.

56. Schafer M, Morgan GJ, Mitchell MB, et al. Impact of different coarctation therapies on aortic stiffness: phase-contrast MRI study. Int J Cardiovasc Imaging 2018;34(9):1459–69.

57. Lee MGY, Babu-Narayan SV, Kempny A, et al. Long-term mortality and cardiovascular burden for adult survivors of coarctation of the aorta. Heart 2019;105(15):1190–6.

58. Muscogiuri G, Secinaro A, Ciliberti P, et al. Utility of cardiac magnetic resonance imaging in the management of adult congenital heart disease. J Thorac Imaging 2017;32(4):233–44.

59. Chakrabarti S, Kenny D, Morgan G, et al. Balloon expandable stent implantation for native and recurrent coarctation of the aorta—prospective computed tomography assessment of stent integrity, aneurysm

formation and stenosis relief. Heart 2010;96(15): 1212–6.

60. Thakkar AN, Chinnadurai P, Lin CH. Imaging adult patients with coarctation of the aorta. Curr Opin Cardiol 2017;32(5):503–12.

61. Karaosmanoglu AD, Khawaja RD, Onur MR, et al. CT and MRI of aortic coarctation: pre- and postsurgical findings. AJR Am J Roentgenol 2015;204(3): W224–33.

62. Bogaert J, Kuzo R, Dymarkowski S, et al. Follow-up of patients with previous treatment for coarctation of the thoracic aorta: comparison between contrast-enhanced MR angiography and fast spin-echo MR imaging. Eur Radiol 2000;10(12):1847–54.

63. Babu-Narayan SV, Giannakoulas G, Valente AM, et al. Imaging of congenital heart disease in adults. Eur Heart J 2016;37(15):1182–95.

64. Paladini D, Pistorio A, Wu LH, et al. Prenatal diagnosis of total and partial anomalous pulmonary venous connection: multicenter cohort study and meta-analysis. Ultrasound Obstet Gynecol 2018; 52(1):24–34.

65. Musewe NN, Smallhorn JF, Freedom RM. Anomalies of pulmonary venous connections including cor triatriatum and stenosis of individual pulmonary veins. In: Freedom RM, Benson LN, Smallhorn JF, editors. Neonatal heart disease. London: Springer; 1992. p. 309–31.

66. Lemaire A, DiFilippo S, Parienti JJ, et al. Total anomalous pulmonary venous connection: a 40 years' experience analysis. Thorac Cardiovasc Surg 2017;65(1):9–17.

67. Shi G, Zhu Z, Chen J, et al. Total anomalous pulmonary venous connection: the current management strategies in a pediatric cohort of 768 patients. Circulation 2017;135(1):48–58.

68. Files MD, Morray B. Total anomalous pulmonary venous connection: preoperative anatomy, physiology, imaging, and interventional management of postoperative pulmonary venous obstruction. Semin Cardiothorac Vasc Anesth 2017;21(2): 123–31.

69. Lang AG, Claudia G, Irene M. Distinguishing chronic thromboembolic pulmonary hypertension from other causes of pulmonary hypertension using CT. AJR Am J Roentgenol 2017;209(6):1228–38.

70. Akam-Venkata J, Turner DR, Joshi A, et al. Diagnosis and management of the unligated vertical vein in repaired total anomalous pulmonary venous connection. World J Pediatr Congenit Heart Surg 2019 [Epub ahead of print].

71. Muscogiuri G, Suranyi P, Eid M, et al. Pediatric cardiac MR imaging: practical preoperative assessment. Magn Reson Imaging Clin N Am 2019;27(2): 243–62.

72. Steele PM, Fuster V, Cohen M, et al. Isolated atrial septal defect with pulmonary vascular obstructive disease—long-term follow-up and prediction of outcome after surgical correction. Circulation 1987; 76(5):1037–42.

73. Geva T, Martins JD, Wald RM. Atrial septal defects. Lancet 2014;383(9932):1921–32.

74. Brickner ME, Hillis LD, Lange RA. Congenital heart disease in adults. First of two parts. N Engl J Med 2000;342(4):256–63.

75. Divekar A, Gaamangwe T, Shaikh N, et al. Cardiac perforation after device closure of atrial septal defects with the Amplatzer septal occluder. J Am Coll Cardiol 2005;45(8):1213–8.

76. Amin Z, Hijazi ZM, Bass JL, et al. Erosion of Amplatzer septal occluder device after closure of secundum atrial septal defects: review of registry of complications and recommendations to minimize future risk. Catheter Cardiovasc Interv 2004;63(4): 496–502.

Beyond Crohn Disease
Current Role of Radiologists in Diagnostic Imaging Assessment of Inflammatory Bowel Disease Transitioning from Pediatric to Adult Patients

Michael S. Furman, MD[a,b,*], Edward Y. Lee, MD, MPH[c]

KEYWORDS

- Inflammatory bowel disease • Gastrointestinal • Pediatric • Magnetic resonance enterography

KEY POINTS

- Inflammatory bowel disease (IBD) prevalence continues to rise in children and now there is an increased number of adults living with IBD diagnosed in their childhood.
- IBD presents differently in children compared with adults, with more aggressive, multisegmental disease. Small bowel obstruction is less common than in adults.
- As pediatric patients transition to the adult population, they begin to experience similar complications and phenotype of those who present in adulthood.
- Magnetic resonance enterography (MRE) remains the reference standard for evaluating patients with IBD, although there is a role for other imaging modalities, which should always be considered, depending on clinical presentation.
- Differentiating fibrotic from inflammatory disease is a shortcoming in current IBD imaging and an area of research.

INTRODUCTION

Inflammatory bowel disease (IBD) has become more prevalent in recent years. Although the disease is classically divided into Crohn disease (CD) and ulcerative colitis (UC), patients may also be diagnosed with unclassified IBD[1] in the pediatric population. In the United States, the prevalence of UC in adults reaches 238 per 100,000 and 201 cases of CD per 100,000.[2] Among adults, younger patients (ages 20–29) have a higher prevalence of CD.[3] Some of the increasing prevalence of IBD in recent years is on account of improving life expectancy. An added contributor, however, is the diagnosis of childhood IBD; up to 20% of patients with CD and 12% of patients with UC are diagnosed younger than 20 years old.[4] Therefore, there is now an increased number of adults living with IBD diagnosed in their childhood.

This review article discusses the role of imaging in evaluation of IBD transitioning from pediatric to adult patients. Imaging modalities and techniques currently used for evaluating IBD are reviewed. In addition, the spectrum of characteristic acute and chronic imaging findings of IBD is discussed with emphasis on what general radiologists need to clearly understand.

[a] Diagnostic Imaging, Alpert Medical School of Brown University, Providence, RI, USA; [b] Department of Diagnostic Imaging, Rhode Island Hospital, 593 Eddy Street, Providence, RI 02903, USA; [c] Department of Radiology, Boston Children's Hospital, Harvard Medical School, 300 Longwood Avenue, Boston, MA 02115, USA
* Corresponding author. 593 Eddy St. Providence, RI 02903.
E-mail address: furman.m@gmail.com

Radiol Clin N Am 58 (2020) 517–527
https://doi.org/10.1016/j.rcl.2020.01.007

ROLE OF IMAGING IN EVALUATION OF INFLAMMATORY BOWEL DISEASE: TRANSITIONING FROM PEDIATRIC TO ADULT PATIENTS

Adolescents diagnosed with IBD tend to present differently from adult patients, and this should be considered when performing imaging studies. CD is more likely to be ileocolonic, rather than confined to small bowel. Gastric involvement, although less common, is typically a feature of pediatric rather than adult disease. UC is more likely to diffusely involve the colon rather than segments of it.[5] Stricture and obstruction are more common in adults, but as IBD progresses, the risk for these complications increases in children. Children and adults exhibit extraintestinal manifestations at similar rates, and one should always be mindful to look for these complications on imaging studies.[6]

IMAGING TECHNIQUES

Until recently, there had been a lack of consensus as to the imaging modality of choice for evaluation and surveillance of IBD (Table 1). However, as technique for magnetic resonance enterography (MRE) has advanced, it has emerged as the preferred method of serial imaging pediatric patients with IBD.[7,8] Still, a meta-analysis of more than 14,000 patients revealed that all modalities have comparable detection rates of IBD in children[9]; for this reason, ultrasound remains an alternative to MRE for imaging of IBD.[10]

Radiography

When evaluating IBD, radiography serves as an entry point for clinical investigation, rather than a sole method for achieving diagnosis. Children

Table 1
Four major imaging modalities with essential techniques, advantages, and disadvantages for evaluating inflammatory bowel disease

Modality	Advantages	Disadvantages	Essential Techniques
Radiography	Easily accessible Can identify surgical emergency (ie, perforation)	Neither sensitive nor specific	Supine and upright anteroposterior abdominal radiography
Ultrasound	Low cost No radiation No sedation No gadolinium Good spatial resolution Good if MRE not available	Operator dependent Limited evaluation of sigmoid colon and rectum Limited evaluation of extraintestinal disease	Longitudinal and transverse representative images in all four quadrants with and without color Doppler High-frequency linear transducer
Computed tomography	Widely available No sedation Good spatial resolution	Ionizing radiation	Intravenous and enteric contrast Axial and coronal multiplanar reformats Neutral enteric contrast to opacify the small bowel is preferred
Magnetic resonance imaging	No ionizing radiation Excellent contrast resolution Good anatomic detail on SSFP images	Vulnerable to respiratory and susceptibility artifact Gadolinium required Spasmolytics required Sedation may be needed	SSFSE axial SSFSE coronal with cine loop Axial and coronal T2-weighted fat-suppressed Coronal T1-weighted fat-suppressed postgadolinium in 3 dynamic phases, including early mesenteric phase Diffusion weighted imaging preferred Dedicated small field of view if perineal fistula a concern

Abbreviations: MRE, magnetic resonance enterography; SSFP, steady-state free precession; SSFSE, single-shot fast spin echo.

with new-onset IBD may present with ongoing abdominal pain, for which an abdominal radiograph is often requested. Typically, images are obtained with patients in the upright and supine position.

Ultrasound

Individual protocols for evaluation of the gastrointestinal tract may vary by institution. However, to optimize the excellent spatial resolution of ultrasound, it is important to evaluate the small and large bowel with a linear high-frequency transducer. Such high-frequency transducer can demonstrate intestinal segments in longitudinal and transverse axes. Color Doppler imaging can further evaluate abnormal findings, such as hyperemia in the setting of active inflammation.[11] Unfortunately, because of the limited acoustic window, adequate sonographic interrogation of the sigmoid colon and rectum is often more difficult.

Computed Tomography

Abdominal computed tomography (CT) provides excellent spatial resolution, and rapid imaging capability obviates breath-holding.[12] Spasmolytic agents, an essential component of MRE, are not necessary with CT. An obvious disadvantage is the use of ionizing radiation. Patients with IBD require multiple studies over time, further rendering this modality suboptimal in a younger population. When evaluating IBD, it is best to opacify the small bowel with a neutral oral contrast agent. Intravenous contrast should be administered to increase the conspicuity of inflammation.

Magnetic Resonance Imaging

Magnetic resonance (MR), specifically MRE, with excellent contrast resolution, has become the cornerstone of imaging children and adolescents with IBD (**Table 2**). The field of view extends from

Table 2
Indication, protocol, and additional elements of MRE and MR imaging pelvis for evaluating inflammatory bowel disease

Exam	Indication	Full Protocol	Additional Elements
MRE	Assessment of small intestine involvement (primary) Assessment of colon (secondary) Assessment of extraintestinal manifestations (secondary) Assessment of intra-abdominal fistula	Body matrix coil Axial SSFSE Coronal T2-weighted fat-suppressed Axial T2-weighted fat-suppressed Coronal SSFSE with cine loop for peristalsis Axial diffusion weighted imaging Multiphase dynamic coronal VIBE postgadolinium Axial VIBE postgadolinium	Gadolinium (0.1 mL/kg) Glucagon Polyethylene glycol Examination time: 45 min
MR imaging pelvis	Assessment for perirectal abscess (primary) Assessment of perianal fistula (primary) Assessment of small intestine involvement (secondary, if low-lying terminal ileum) Assessment of extraintestinal manifestations (secondary, sacroiliac joints)	Body matrix coil Sagittal FSEIR Oblique axial SSFSE Oblique axial T2-weighted fat-suppressed Oblique coronal FSEIR Oblique coronal T1-weighted Oblique axial T1-weighted fat-suppressed postgadolinium Oblique coronal T1-weighted fat-suppressed postgadolinium Sagittal T1-weighted fat-suppressed postgadolinium)	Small field of view Gadolinium (0.1 mL/kg) Examination time: 78 min

Abbreviations: FSEIR, fast spin echo inversion recovery; SSFSE, single-shot fast spin echo; VIBE, volumetric interpolated breath-hold examination.

the lung bases through the perineum, with additional smaller field-of-view imaging of the perineum if there is concern for perianal fistula. Flexible phased-array body coils, and the built-in spine coil, are used.[13] Imaging may be performed on either a 1.5- or 3.0-T strength magnet. The 3.0-T magnet allows for superior spatial resolution, signal, and contrast-to-noise ratio. There is, however, greater susceptibility artifact secondary to intra-abdominal gas and surgical material.[14] Fat suppression is difficult on 3.0-T magnets, necessitating acquisition of images in two stacks (upper and lower) with separate shim boxes to reduce inhomogeneity.[15]

Fluid-sensitive sequences are rapidly acquired in the axial and coronal planes. Single-shot fast spin echo and balanced steady-state free-precession sequences optimize anatomic evaluation. Fat-suppressed MR images increase the conspicuity of inflammation. Diffusion weighted imaging, although bereft of spatial resolution, has excellent sensitivity for detection of inflammation and lymphadenopathy. Single-shot fast spin echo in the coronal plane is used to acquire cine MR imaging sequences to evaluate peristalsis.[13] Postcontrast MR imaging is performed dynamically, first in the mesenteric phase (45–55 seconds postinjection), followed by two successive acquisitions to evaluate bowel wall enhancement over time. To decrease respiratory motion artifact, breath-hold imaging is performed.[16]

Intrinsically T1 hypointense oral contrast is given to distend the small bowel, which improves the ability to detect mucosal and bowel wall disease. The media must be hyperosmolar to optimize terminal ileal distention. To reduce motion artifact caused by bowel peristalsis, paralytic agents, such as glucagon, are administered before contrast injection.[15,16] Pediatric patients may have difficulty with breath-holding instructions, and respiratory triggered or radial noncartesian acquisitions may be performed.[17]

SPECTRUM OF IMAGING FINDINGS
Acute Findings of Inflammatory Bowel Disease

In the acute setting, IBD typically manifests with bowel wall inflammation. Radiography may reveal layering fluid within segments of bowel. If there is colonic disease, edema within the bowel wall causes the thickened haustra to project into the aerated lumen (thumbprinting sign) (**Fig. 1**). In most instances, however, cross-sectional imaging is requested for further evaluation, irrespective of the radiograph findings. In more advanced cases, additional findings include peri-intestinal fat induration, and engorgement of the adjacent vasa recta (**Fig. 2**). MRE can aid clinicians in distinguishing disease amenable to medical therapy from that requiring surgical intervention. Bowel wall thickening greater than 3 mm, intramural T2 prolongation, and restricted diffusivity are sensitive for active disease requiring a pharmacologic regimen (**Fig. 3**).[18,19] Segmental arterial phase hyperenhancing bowel may also indicate active IBD (**Fig. 4**).[15]

In acute ileitis, the surrounding mesenteric fat may enhance heterogeneously. Pockets of nonenhancement may signify early abscess formation (**Fig. 5**). Fluid with a thickened, hyperenhancing, T2 hyperintense periphery with restricted diffusivity suggests a discrete fluid collection. Identifying this complication is particularly crucial, because it implies a bowel perforation, which may necessitate interventional management. Furthermore, active infection may be a contraindication to immunologic drug therapy.[13]

If the patient is in extremis, CT may be preferable to evaluate for perforation, because this may occur in the setting of acute presentations. In such an instance, intravenous contrast alone is necessary; enteric contrast as an adjunct is preferable to help differentiate abscess formation from abnormal-appearing segments of bowel, but may not be practical, depending on the level of acuity.

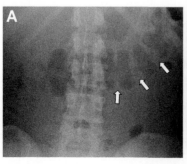
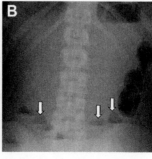

Fig. 1. A 17-year-old girl with long-standing Crohn disease who presented emergently for abdominal pain. The patient was found to have colitis on optical colonoscopy, which was confirmed on biopsy. (*A*) Frontal supine abdominal radiograph shows haustral thickening (*arrows*) in the transverse colon. (*B*) Upright abdominal radiograph shows scattered air-fluid levels (*arrows*) in the small bowel of similar size, consistent with an enteritis.

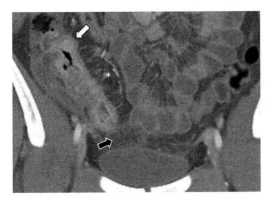

Fig. 2. A 17-year-old girl who presented with abdominal pain and weight loss. Coronal oral and enteric contrast-enhanced soft tissue setting CT enterography image shows a segment of thickened terminal ileum (*white arrow*) with hyperattenuating mucosa and thickened, edematous submucosa. Notably, the adjacent mesenteric fat is indurated and inflamed (*black arrow*). There is also engorgement of the mesenteric vasculature (vasa recta) and adjacent reactive mesenteric lymph nodes (*asterisk*).

Toxic megacolon, although uncommon, is a potentially lethal IBD complication, and should be raised as a diagnostic consideration if an acute clinical presentation is commensurate with imaging. Damaged colonic ganglia results in aperistaltic large bowel. The colon may be dilated greater than 6 cm, and as little as 4 cm in children younger than 11 years of age.[20] Radiography may suggest the finding, but cross-sectional imaging is necessary to confirm irregular wall thickening.[20,21] CT may be preferred over MRE, because this is an emergent entity. Moreover, perforation and intramural pneumatosis, both supportive findings of toxic megacolon, are more easily detected on CT (Fig. 6).

Large bowel IBD is usually evaluated by optical colonoscopy. MRE is limited in evaluating the colon, because enteric contrast does not reach the distal bowel, and intraluminal air and stool create artifact. Underdistended colon may appear falsely thickened. In the acute setting, imaging may be helpful, because severe inflammation could delay or modify a planned invasive procedure. In this instance, CT with intravenous contrast is performed, or MRE, despite the previously mentioned limitations. Uniformly enhancing, featureless segments of colon, and thickened haustra may be identified.

Chronic Findings of Inflammatory Bowel Disease

As IBD becomes a chronic condition particularly in adult patients with childhood onset of IBD, the imaging features evolve. Structural quality of the bowel wall degrades, as intramural fibrous deposition results in hypointense T2 signal.[22] Fibrous bowel wall demonstrates delayed phase enhancement, rather than the brisk arterial hyperenhancement seen in active inflammatory disease. Ultimately, fibrosis results in fixed intraluminal narrowing, behaving as a partial small bowel obstruction, with dilated adjacent proximal segments of bowel.

Identifying chronic fibrosis on MRE is challenging. Although active inflammatory and chronic fibrotic disease have separate imaging features, there is frequently overlap between these categories. Intramural T2 prolongation, therefore, obfuscates the expected findings in chronic disease. As a secondary finding, prestenotic dilatation spanning greater than 3 cm in length has been associated with transmural fibrosis (Fig. 7).[23]

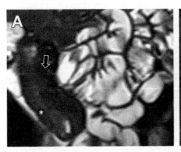
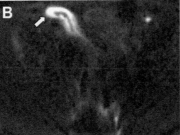
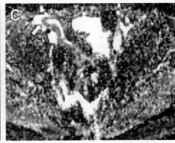

Fig. 3. A 16-year-old boy with history of crampy abdominal pain and weight loss. The imaging findings led to colonoscopy and active ileocolonic Crohn disease was visualized and confirmed on biopsy. The patient then began medical therapy. (*A*) Coronal unenhanced T2-weighted fat-suppressed MR image shows a segment of terminal ileum (*asterisk*), with intramural T2 prolongation compared with adjacent, normal-appearing segments of small bowel. The bowel wall is also thickened, measuring 1.1 cm. The vasa recta is engorged (*arrow*). (*B*) High b-value diffusion weighted MR image demonstrates that this segment of ileum is intrinsically hyperintense (*arrow*). (*C*) High b-value ADC MR image shows that the segment of ileum correspondingly loses signal (*arrow*).

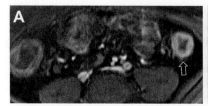
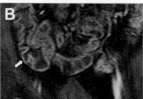

Fig. 4. A 10-year-old boy with history of ulcerative colitis who presented with abdominal pain. This patient was diagnosed with active pancolitis. (A) Axial early phase contrast-enhanced T1-weighted fat-suppressed MRE image shows a thickened and hyperintense descending colon (*arrow*). (B) Coronal early phase contrast-enhanced T1-weighted fat-suppressed MRE imaging shows a thickened, hyperintense proximal ascending colon (*arrow*).

In patients with IBD, "creeping fat" is often identified. This is essentially fibrofatty proliferation, circumferentially investing affected segments of bowel, and is seen on any cross-sectional modality, featuring the expected imaging characteristics of fat (Fig. 8). Creeping fat is a predictor of poor outcomes in patients; it implies ongoing inflammation and chronicity, and is found in patients who go on to surgical intervention.[24]

Fistulous tracts may develop in various anatomic positions, and one may identify aberrant enterovesicular, enterocutaneous, enterovaginal, or enteroenteral communications. These are best evaluated on MRE; a peripherally enhancing channel with T2 prolongation within the tract itself emanates from bowel. CT and ultrasound are less favored, but alternative modalities, particularly if a patient has difficulty holding still and there is a

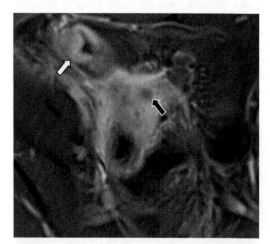

Fig. 5. An 18-year-old boy with Crohn disease who presented with abdominal pain, fever, and leukocytosis. The presence of phlegmon and early abscess formation necessitated antibiotic therapy, before further treatment. Axial contrast-enhanced T1-weighted fat-suppressed MRE image shows abnormally enhancing terminal ileum (*white arrow*). Adjacent to it is densely enhancing mesenteric fat, with a pocket of nonenhancing material (*black arrow*) contained within representing early abscess.

wish to avoid sedation. With ultrasound, power Doppler imaging shows increased vascularity about thickened echogenic material that communicates between two otherwise unrelated anatomic structures. Within the perineum, perianal fistula is a common complication. This requires MR imaging with a dedicated smaller field of view to identify a fistulous tract extending from bowel to the ischiorectal fossa or skin. This is further characterized based on how the anal sphincter is affected (Fig. 9).[25,26]

Historically, patients with IBD have been followed with clinical activity index metrics to guide management. As imaging techniques have advanced, however, incongruity between the clinical metrics and imaging findings has emerged. Clinically quiescent disease may, in fact, be active on a histologic level. Radiologic response is therefore now a management target, because it predicts decreased need for surgery, hospitalization, and corticosteroids.[27] In one single-institution retrospective study from South Korea evaluating 243 patients with known IBD who underwent MRE, of 61 patients with clinically silent disease, 72.1% had active disease on imaging.[28] Although this study focused on young adults, the same conclusions are drawn in pediatric imaging. Imaging findings can also guide treatment decisions, allowing tapering of toxic or expensive medications when feasible, and alteration of drug regimens when necessary. Mucosal healing on MRE is a finding of disease remission; this is reflected by the absence of engorged vasa recta and hyperenhancing bowel wall in pediatric patients with IBD.[29]

Over time, patients with IBD are susceptible to developing colorectal adenocarcinoma. This is monitored with surveillance by optical colonoscopy. Pediatric patients need this level of clinical care once they have entered adulthood. Although the radiologist should certainly be vigilant for evaluation of a mass-like colonic lesion, these are not evaluated or excluded by any imaging modalities, including CT colonography, at this time.

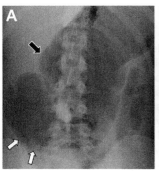
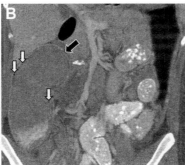

Fig. 6. A 16-year-old girl with history of ulcerative colitis who presented with worsening abdominal pain and concerning abdominal examination. The patient underwent urgent colectomy for toxic megacolon. (*A*) Supine frontal abdominal radiograph shows a markedly dilated segment of colon (*black arrow*), with areas of abnormal mucosal thickening (*white arrows*). (*B*) Coronal enteric and intravenous contrast-enhanced soft tissue setting CT image demonstrates a markedly abnormal segment of ascending colon with wall thickening (*black arrow*) and intramural pneumatosis (*white arrows*).

Extraintestinal Manifestations of Inflammatory Bowel Disease

Pediatric patients are susceptible to an array of extraintestinal manifestations of IBD, many of which are seen on MRE. A review of all extraintestinal complications is beyond the scope of this article. However, common complications that are seen in adolescent and young adult populations are described next.

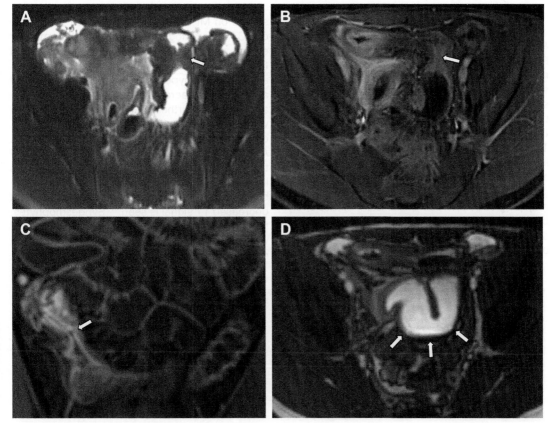

Fig. 7. An 18-year-old boy with history of unspecified inflammatory bowel disease who presented with worsening abdominal pain and elevated inflammatory markers. By MRE, it was difficult to ascertain which areas of narrowing were fibrotic and which were inflammatory, given the signal properties. The patient was found to have tandem fibrotic strictures requiring surgical resection, confirmed on histology. (*A*) Axial non-contrast-enhanced T2-weighted fat-suppressed MR image shows focal intraluminal narrowing (*arrow*) in the terminal ileum with intramural intermediate T2 signal. (*B*) Axial contrast-enhanced T1-weighted fat-suppressed MR image shows that the segment delineated in *A* is hypointense (*arrow*) relative to adjacent loops of ileum. (*C*) Coronal contrast-enhanced T1-weighted fat-suppressed MR image shows additional area of robust hyperenhancement in the terminal ileum (*arrow*). (*D*) Axial noncontrast fast imaging with steady-state precession MR image shows a long segment of prestenotic small bowel dilatation (*arrows*).

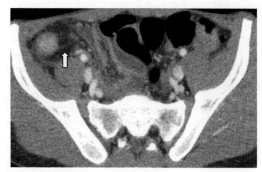

Fig. 8. A 13-year-old girl with no past medical history who presented with right lower quadrant pain. Imaging and subsequent optical colonoscopy demonstrated ileocolonic Crohn disease. Axial contrast-enhanced soft tissue setting CT image of the pelvis shows abnormal thickening and enhancement of the terminal ileum and ascending colon. There is fibrofatty proliferation, "creeping fat" (*arrow*), around the abnormal segment of bowel, implying at least some degree of chronicity.

Primary sclerosing cholangitis

Primary sclerosing cholangitis has been associated more with UC than CD. However, this complication seems related to the extent of colonic involvement and because iliocolonic CD is common in pediatric patients, one must thoroughly evaluate for this entity, regardless of the IBD subtype. Fluid-sensitive, T2-weighted sequences in MRE are most likely to illustrate primary sclerosing cholangitis; namely, alternating strictures and dilatations of the intrahepatic and extrahepatic ducts.[30] If chronic, patients may progress to portal hypertension, cirrhosis, or cholangiocarcinoma. If seen on MRE, consideration should be given to dedicated imaging of the liver and biliary tree (**Fig. 10**).

Cholelithiasis

Patients with IBD, particularly those with CD, often develop cholelithiasis. The pathogenesis is thought to be related to ileal disease, which affects bile salt absorption and enterohepatic circulation. As a result, pediatric patients with active ileal disease or who have had the ileum resected are vulnerable to gallstone formation.[31] This should be kept in mind if these patients present with upper abdominal pain; ultrasound may then be the study of choice, which can characteristically demonstrate mobile, hyperechoic calculi with posterior acoustic shadowing.

Musculoskeletal manifestations

Musculoskeletal manifestations of IBD are not uncommon in children; 4% of pediatric patients with IBD have some form of axial spondyloarthropathy. The findings of sacroiliitis are demonstrable on MRE long before they are detectable on CT or radiography. Subchondral marrow edema is best illustrated on fat-suppressed fluid-sensitive sequences; with postcontrast imaging, there is hyperenhancement of the synovial aspect of the sacroiliac joint.[32] Although detectable on MRE, further imaging may be necessary with dedicated imaging of the sacroiliac joints, depending on the clinical scenario (**Fig. 11**). Ankylosing spondylitis involves the spine and the sacroiliac joints. Patients manifest Romanus lesions, or marrow edema adjacent to the vertebral body end plates; increased T2 and decreased T1 signal is seen.[33] Syndesmophytes, thin osseous linear outgrowth along the anterior vertebral body edge, are best seen on radiography.[32]

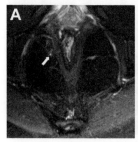
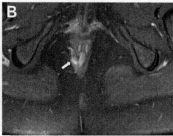
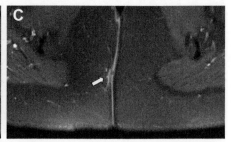

Fig. 9. A 14-year-old girl with history of Crohn disease complicated by large perirectal abscess necessitating and drainage and antibiotic therapy who presented for follow-up imaging 6 months later. No residual fluid collection is seen; however, there is a residual grade III trans-sphincteric fistula. (*A*) Axial-oblique noncontrast T2-weighted fat-suppressed MR image shows a fistulous tract (*arrow*) in its short axis in the right anterior ischiorectal fossa. (*B*) Axial contrast-enhanced T1-weighted fat-suppressed MR image shows a fistulous tract (*arrow*) with thick, hyperintense peripheral walls extending from the ischiorectal fossa through both layers of the anal sphincter. (*C*) Axial contrast-enhanced T1-weighted fat-suppressed MR image shows that the peripherally enhancing tract (*arrow*) extends to the skin surface at the posterior gluteal cleft.

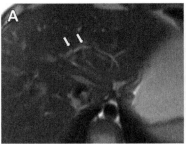
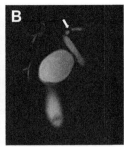
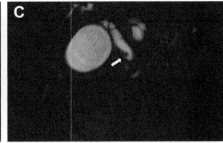

Fig. 10. An 18-year-old girl with ulcerative colitis, complicated by development of primary sclerosing cholangitis. (*A*) Axial noncontrast T2-weighted non-fat-suppressed MR image shows irregularity (*arrows*) of the left intrahepatic duct (*arrows*). (*B*) Coronal noncontrast T2-weighted three-dimensional fast spin echo non-fat-suppressed MR image then shows the irregular left intrahepatic duct (*arrow*) to have tandem areas of dilation and stricturing. (*C*) Coronal noncontrast T2-weighted three-dimensional fast spin echo non-fat-suppressed MR image also also show stricturing (*arrow*) within the extrahepatic duct.

FUTURE DIRECTIONS

Although imaging of IBD has advanced significantly in recent years, there are opportunities to continue optimizing care for pediatric patients, especially adolescents, because many require several imaging studies well into adulthood. Discerning inflammatory from fibrotic stricture is a challenge that is appropriate to address. A recent prospective study evaluated the magnetization transfer ratio in the small bowel, which depicts collagen in the intestinal wall.[34] This performed superior to diffusion weighted imaging and dynamic postcontrast imaging, when comparing with histopathologic results, and therefore, may be a useful tool for distinguishing medical and surgical patients.[34] This has not yet been studied in children. Evaluation of contrast-enhanced ultrasound and shear wave elastography to detect fibrotic bowel segments have had more mixed results.[35]

SUMMARY

There is rising prevalence of IBD among pediatric patients and now there is an increasing number of adults living with IBD diagnosed in their childhood. This is a disease that manifests differently in children and adolescents compared with adults at presentation, although, as these patients age, acute and chronic complications become similar to those seen in patients who present as adults. Although practitioners should make use of CT in children with caution given to potentially harmful ionizing radiation, there is an appropriate role for it, particularly in acutely ill patients. Still, increasing attention has been given to advancing MRE in recent years, and this is the current reference

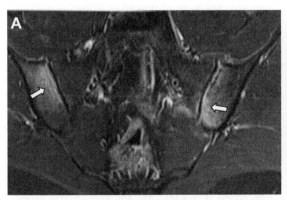
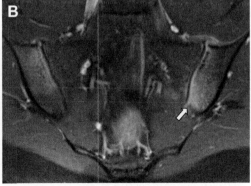

Fig. 11. A 16-year-old boy with ulcerative colitis who presented with worsening morning stiffness. He was ultimately diagnosed with ankylosing spondyloarthropathy, after active sacroiliitis was identified on MR imaging. (*A*) Coronal oblique noncontrast T2-weighted inversion recovery fat-suppressed MR image shows marrow edema in the bilateral iliac bones, adjacent to the sacroiliac joints (*arrows*). (*B*) Coronal oblique contrast-enhanced T1-weighted fat-suppressed MR image shows abnormal gadolinium enhancement of the inferior one-third of the left sacroiliac joint (*arrow*), which is lined by synovium.

standard for imaging of IBD. As techniques improve, radiologists should be vigilant to evaluate for any extraintestinal manifestations of IBD in these young patients.

DISCLOSURE

The authors have nothing to disclose.

REFERENCES

1. Levine A, Koletzko S, Turner D, et al. ESPGHAN revised porto criteria for the diagnosis of inflammatory bowel disease in children and adolescents. J Pediatr Gastroenterol Nutr 2014;58(6):795–806.
2. Kappelman MD, Rifas-Shiman SL, Kleinman K, et al. The prevalence and geographic distribution of Crohn's disease and ulcerative colitis in the United States. Clin Gastroenterol Hepatol 2007;5(12):1424–9.
3. Shivashankar R, Tremaine WJ, Harmsen WS, et al. Incidence and prevalence of Crohn's disease and ulcerative colitis in Olmsted county, Minnesota from 1970 through 2010. Clin Gastroenterol Hepatol 2017;15(6):857–63.
4. Kappelman MD, Moore KR, Allen JK, et al. Recent trends in the prevalence of Crohn's disease and ulcerative colitis in a commercially insured US population. Dig Dis Sci 2013;58(2):519–25.
5. Abraham BP, Kahn SA. Transition of care in inflammatory bowel disease. Gastroenterol Hepatol 2014;10(10):633–40.
6. Sauer CG, Kugathasan S. Pediatric inflammatory bowel disease: highlighting pediatric differences in IBD. Med Clin North Am 2010;94(1):35–52.
7. Paolantonio P, Ferrari R, Vecchietti F, et al. Current status of MR imaging in the evaluation of IBD in a pediatric population of patients. Eur J Radiol 2009;69(3):418–24.
8. Yoon HM, Suh CH, Kim JR, et al. Diagnostic performance of magnetic resonance enterography for detection of active inflammation in children and adolescents with inflammatory bowel disease: a systematic review and diagnostic meta-analysis. JAMA Pediatr 2017;171(12):1208–16.
9. Horsthuis K, Bipat S, Bennink RJ, et al. Inflammatory bowel disease diagnosed with US, MR, scintigraphy, and CT: meta-analysis of prospective studies. Radiology 2008;247(1):64–79.
10. Ahmad TM, Greer M-L, Walters TD, et al. Bowel sonography and MR enterography in children. AJR Am J Roentgenol 2016;206(1):173–81.
11. Barber JL, Zambrano-Perez A, Olsen ØE, et al. Detecting inflammation in inflammatory bowel disease: how does ultrasound compare to magnetic resonance enterography using standardised scoring systems? Pediatr Radiol 2018;48(6):843–51.
12. Callahan MJ, MacDougall RD, Bixby SD, et al. Ionizing radiation from computed tomography versus anesthesia for magnetic resonance imaging in infants and children: patient safety considerations. Pediatr Radiol 2018;48(1):21–30.
13. Schooler GR, Hull NC, Mavis A, et al. MR imaging evaluation of inflammatory bowel disease in children: where are we now in 2019. Magn Reson Imaging Clin N Am 2019. https://doi.org/10.1016/j.mric.2019.01.007.
14. Soher BJ, Dale BM, Merkle EM. A review of MR physics: 3T versus 1.5 T. Magn Reson Imaging Clin N Am 2007;15(3):277–90.
15. Mollard BJ, Smith EA, Dillman JR. Pediatric MR enterography: technique and approach to interpretation: how we do it. Radiology 2014;274(1):29–43.
16. Grand DJ, Guglielmo FF, Al-Hawary MM. MR enterography in Crohn's disease: current consensus on optimal imaging technique and future advances from the SAR Crohn's disease-focused panel. Abdom Imaging 2015;40(5):953–64.
17. Courtier J, Rao AG, Anupindi SA. Advanced imaging techniques in pediatric body MRI. Pediatr Radiol 2017;47(5):522–33.
18. Morani AC, Smith EA, Ganeshan D, et al. Diffusion-weighted MRI in pediatric inflammatory bowel disease. AJR Am J Roentgenol 2015;204(6):1269–77.
19. Greer MC. Paediatric magnetic resonance enterography in inflammatory bowel disease. Eur J Radiol 2018;102:129–37.
20. Maddu KK, Mittal P, Shuaib W, et al. Colorectal emergencies and related complications: a comprehensive imaging review–imaging of colitis and complications. AJR Am J Roentgenol 2014;203(6):1205–16.
21. Siow VS, Bhatt R, Mollen KP. Management of acute severe ulcerative colitis in children. Semin Pediatr Surg 2017;26(6):367–72.
22. Gee MS, Nimkin K, Hsu M, et al. Prospective evaluation of MR enterography as the primary imaging modality for pediatric Crohn disease assessment. AJR Am J Roentgenol 2011;197(1):224–31.
23. Barkmeier DT, Dillman JR, Al-Hawary M, et al. MR enterography–histology comparison in resected pediatric small bowel Crohn disease strictures: can imaging predict fibrosis? Pediatr Radiol 2016;46(4):498–507.
24. Althoff P, Schmiegel W, Lang G, et al. Creeping fat assessed by small bowel MRI is linked to bowel damage and abdominal surgery in Crohn's disease. Dig Dis Sci 2019;64(1):204–12.
25. Morris J, Spencer JA, Ambrose NS. MR imaging classification of perianal fistulas and its implications for patient management. Radiographics 2000;20(3):623–35 [discussion: 635–7].
26. Zwintscher NP, Shah PM, Argawal A, et al. The impact of perianal disease in young patients with

inflammatory bowel disease. Int J Colorectal Dis 2015;30(9):1275–9.

27. Deepak P, Fletcher JG, Fidler JL, et al. Radiological response is associated with better long-term outcomes and is a potential treatment target in patients with small bowel Crohn's disease. Am J Gastroenterol 2016;111(7):997–1006.

28. Lee JH, Park YE, Seo N, et al. Magnetic resonance enterography predicts the prognosis of Crohn's disease. Intest Res 2018;16(3):445.

29. Mojtahed A, Gee MS. Magnetic resonance enterography evaluation of Crohn disease activity and mucosal healing in young patients. Pediatr Radiol 2018;48(9):1273–9.

30. Chavhan GB, Roberts E, Moineddin R, et al. Primary sclerosing cholangitis in children: utility of magnetic resonance cholangiopancreatography. Pediatr Radiol 2008;38(8):868–73.

31. Navaneethan U, Shen B. Hepatopancreatobiliary manifestations and complications associated with inflammatory bowel disease. Inflamm Bowel Dis 2010;16(9):1598–619.

32. Olpin JD, Sjoberg BP, Stilwill SE, et al. Beyond the bowel: extraintestinal manifestations of inflammatory bowel disease. Radiographics 2017;37(4):1135–60.

33. Hermann K-GA, Althoff CE, Schneider U, et al. Spinal changes in patients with spondyloarthritis: comparison of MR imaging and radiographic appearances. Radiographics 2005;25(3):559–69 [discussion: 569–70].

34. Li X-H, Mao R, Huang S-Y, et al. Characterization of degree of intestinal fibrosis in patients with Crohn disease by using magnetization transfer MR imaging. Radiology 2018;287(2):494–503.

35. de Sousa HT, Brito J, Magro F. New cross-sectional imaging in IBD. Curr Opin Gastroenterol 2018;34(4):194.

Top Ten Adult Manifestations of Childhood Hip Disorders

An Up-To-Date Review for General Radiologists

Jedidiah Schlung, MD*, Scott Schiffman, MD, Apeksha Chaturvedi, MD

KEYWORDS

- Pediatric • Hip • Dysplasia • Legg-Calve-Perthes • Slipped capital femoral epiphysis
- Impingement • Osteoarthritis

KEY POINTS

- Pediatric hip pathologic conditions arise from various etiopathogeneses but frequently display common morphologic and functional outcomes.
- Specific radiographic views and quantitative imaging metrics are useful for assessing mechanics and congruity of the hip joint.
- Altered joint mechanics in the adult arising secondary to pediatric hip pathologic conditions can result in labral and chondral injury with premature osteoarthritis.

INTRODUCTION

To accurately assess the hip, the practicing radiologist should have familiarity with its anatomic components and the standard imaging techniques used to visualize them.[1–5] The hip is a ball-in-socket joint with the femoral head articulating within the acetabulum. The femoral head and acetabulum are lined with hyaline cartilage to absorb shock and decrease friction during articulation. The fibrocartilaginous labrum attached to the bony acetabular rim both stabilizes the hip and seals in joint fluid to promote even load-bearing. Any incongruence in femoral head-acetabular articulation can promote uneven cartilage wear and weight-bearing and premature cartilage breakdown. Both femoral head dysplasia and acetabular dysplasia can result in pathologic weight-bearing, early breakdown of articular cartilage, labral loading and injury, proliferative bone formation leading to CAM (an abbreviation for "camshaft," an automotive analogy describing the shape, which the femoral head and neck resembles) and pincer impingement, and premature osteoarthritis. These pathologic outcomes are common endpoints for a wide variety of different pediatric hip pathologic conditions.

This review discusses the top 10 etiopathogeneses of pediatric hip conditions and presents associated dysmorphisms in the adult on an illustrative, multimodality, case-based template. Quantitative imaging metrics and the role of advanced imaging techniques are reviewed.

Department of Imaging Sciences, Strong Memorial Hospital, Box 648, 601 Elmwood Avenue, Rochester, NY 14642, USA
* Corresponding author.
E-mail address: Jedidiah_Schlung@urmc.rochester.edu

Radiol Clin N Am 58 (2020) 529–548
https://doi.org/10.1016/j.rcl.2020.01.002

Imaging discussion is supplemented with case presentations, key radiology pearls, and discussion of treatment modalities. The ultimate goal is enhanced understanding of the expected evolution of childhood hip pathologic conditions and their associated complications for general radiologists.

IMAGING TECHNIQUES AND NORMAL ANATOMY

Five basic radiographic views are generally sufficient to accurately evaluate the adult hip: the anterioposterior (AP), lateral, frog-leg-lateral, Dunn, and false profile views[6] (Fig. 1). Radiographic technique for each of these views is summarized in Table 1. Frequently referenced anatomic hip landmarks are summarized in Fig. 2. Specific imaging metrics frequently used for quantitative analysis of plain radiographs of the hip are summarized in Table 2. Excellent pictorial summaries of these metrics have been previously published.[6–9] A summary of several of the more advanced imaging modalities commonly used to evaluate the adult hip is summarized in Table 3.[10]

Two scenarios are generally encountered when evaluating adult hip disease arising secondary to

childhood hip pathologic conditions in daily clinical practice:

The disease process and pathophysiology are known, in which case the radiologist is following hip morphology for interval change.
The disease process is unknown, and the radiologist is evaluating hip morphology to assist in diagnosis of the underlying pathologic condition.

It is most helpful, therefore, to organize commonly encountered hip pathologic conditions by both morphology (see Table 2) and etiopathogenesis (Tables 4 and 5).

SPECTRUM OF HIP DISORDERS: TOP TEN DIAGNOSIS
Developmental Hip Dysplasia

A range of femoral and acetabular dysmorphologies characterizes developmental dysplasia of the hip (DDH); these differ in configuration and severity among affected patients. Crowe[11] and Hartofilakidis[12] devised a method to characterize these dysmorphologies. A detailed discussion, however, is beyond the scope of this article. Imaging deformities range from slight lateral uncovering to subluxation to chronic dislocation of the

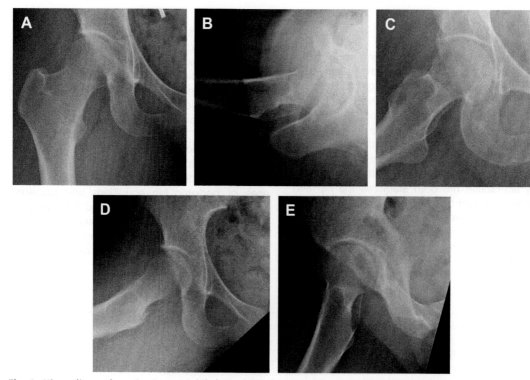

Fig. 1. Hip radiograph projections: AP (*A*), lateral (*B*), frog-leg (*C*), Dunn (*D*), and false profile (*E*).

Table 1
Radiograph technique

Projection	Patient Position	Tube Position	Clinical Utility	Quantitative Radiographic Metrics
AP	Supine Hips 15° internal rotation	Beam perpendicular to table at 120 cm Crosshairs centered between PS and ASIS	Acetabular morphology	Acetabular depth Acetabular version Acetabular index (sharp index) Tonnis angle LCEA (angle of Wiberg) Femoral head sphericity Femoral head lateralization Congruency
False profile	Standing Symptomatic hip against cassette Symptomatic foot parallel to cassette Pelvis 65° to cassette, facing beam	Beam perpendicular to patient at 102 cm Crosshairs centered on femoral head	Acetabular morphology	ACEA (angle of Lequesne) Congruency
Lateral	Supine Contralateral hip and knee flexed 80° Symptomatic hip 15° internal rotation	Beam parallel to table 45° to symptomatic limb Crosshairs centered on femoral head	Proximal femur	Femoral head sphericity Femoral head neck offset congruency
Frog-leg lateral	Supine Ipsilateral knee flexed 30°–40° Symptomatic hip abducted 45° Heel against contralateral knee	Beam perpendicular to table at 102 cm Crosshairs centered between PS and ASIS	Proximal femur	Femoral head sphericity Femoral head neck offset Alpha angle[a] Congruency
Dunn	Supine Symptomatic hip and knee flexed 90° Symptomatic hip abducted 20°	Beam perpendicular to table at 102 cm Crosshairs centered between PS and ASIS	Proximal femur	Femoral head sphericity Femoral head neck offset Congruency

Criteria for technical adequacy: coccyx in line with pubic symphysis; iliac wings, obturator foramen, and teardrops symmetric; upper border of pubic symphysis to tip of coccyx 1 to 3 cm.

Abbreviations: ACEA, anterior center edge angle; ASIS, anterior superior iliac spine; OA, osteoarthritis; PS, pubic symphysis.

[a] Approximate; true angle traditionally measured on cross-sectional oblique CT or MR imaging.

femoral head, occasionally with excessive femoral anteversion and coxa valga[13,14] (Fig. 3). Because of a lack of femoral head molding, the native acetabulum is small, with deficiencies in bony architecture around the acetabulum seen laterally, anteriorly, or posteriorly. If not corrected, these changes lead to pathologic loading of the superior-lateral acetabular rim and labrum, early degenerative osteoarthritis, and labral injury[13] (Fig. 4). Treatments of DDH focus on restoration of normal femoral coverage/articulation using techniques such as periacetabular osteotomy (Fig. 5) with hip replacement reserved for end-stage osteoarthritis.[14]

PEARLS

1. Osteoarthritis is expected to occur by the seventh decade of life in *all* hips with untreated moderate hip dysplasia (lateral center edge angle [LCEA] ≤15°).

2. DDH predisposes the affected hip to *subchondral insufficiency fractures.*

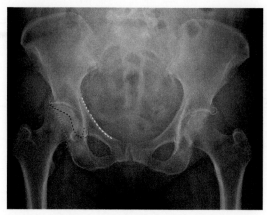

Fig. 2. Hip anatomic landmarks on an AP pelvic radiograph: posterior acetabular rim (violet); anterior acetabular rim (purple); teardrop (red); iliopectineal line (yellow); ilioischial line (green); acetabular sourcil (edges marked by light blue and yellow circles).

Table 2
Hip imaging metrics (hip pathologic condition by morphology)

	Imaging Modality	Normal	Clinical Significance (Abnormal)	Common Pertinent Hip Pathologic Conditions
CAM deformity				
Alpha angle	Axial MR imaging or CT	<55°	CAM deformity	LCPD SCFE Intraarticular osteoid osteoma of hip AIIS avulsion
Femoral head neck offset	Any lateral radiograph	>0.17	CAM deformity	LCPD SCFE Intraarticular osteoid osteoma of hip AIIS avulsion
Pincer deformity, acetabular dysplasia				
LCEA	AP radiograph	25°–40°	Decreased: structural instability Increased: pincer impingement	DDH PFFD Charcot hip Inflammatory/ infectious arthritis LCPD
ACEA	AP radiograph	20°–45°	Decreased: structural instability Increased: pincer impingement	DDH PFFD Charcot hip Inflammatory/ infectious arthritis LCPD
Acetabular depth	AP radiograph	Floor of acetabulum does not abut/cross ilioischial line on AP radiograph	Pincer impingement	Infectious/ inflammatory arthritis

(continued on next page)

Table 2
(continued)

	Imaging Modality	Normal	Clinical Significance (Abnormal)	Common Pertinent Hip Pathologic Conditions
Femoral head lateralization	AP radiograph	>10 mm	Structural instability	DDH Charcot hip
Acetabular index (Sharp index)	AP radiograph	<45°	Structural instability	DDH PFFD Charcot hip LCPD
Tonnis angle	AP radiograph	0°–10°	Increased: structural instability Decreased: pincer impingement	DDH PFFD Charcot hip LCPD
Joint alignment				
Acetabular version	AP radiograph	13°–20° anteversion	Pincer impingement	SCFE
Femoral version	Axial MR imaging or CT	8°–14° anteversion	Excessive retroversion risk factor for poor outcomes after corrective FAI surgery	DDH FAI SCFE
Joint congruity				
Femoral head sphericity	AP and lateral radiograph	Any portion of femoral head >2 mm beyond standard Mose template	Joint wear and early OA	DDH PFFD Charcot hip LCPD Infectious/inflammatory arthritis IHC

Abbreviations: ACEA, anterior center edge angle; FHC, femoral head center.

Table 3
Summary of basic and advanced hip imaging modalities

Imaging Modality	Views/Sequences	Clinical Utility
Plain radiograph	AP Lateral Frog-leg lateral Dunn False profile	Evaluate acetabular and femoral morphology and congruence Preoperative and postoperative assessment Routine surveillance imaging
CT	Axial, coronal, and sagittal views 3D modeling	Assess complex fractures and hip dysmorphologies Preoperative planning with automated hip measurements Assessment of hip version
MR imaging	Conventional 3 T imaging: dedicated hip coils, parallel imaging, isotropic MR MR arthrography, ± traction Biochemical MR imaging: dGEMRIC, T2 and T2*, T1 rho, Na+ mapping 3D modeling Virtual ROM analysis Open MR imaging (functional imaging) 3D printing Advanced metal suppression MR fingerprinting	Assessment of cartilage and labral injuries Biochemical cartilage mapping (dGEMRIC, T2/T2*, T1 rho, Na+ mapping) Automated analysis of joint parameters, for example, alpha angle via 3D modeling Subject-tailored preoperative virtual planning Dynamic ROM simulation Real time in vivo functional imaging

Abbreviations: AP, anterior posterior; dGEMRIC, delayed gadolinium-enhanced MR imaging of cartilage; Na+, sodium; ROM, range of motion.

Table 4
Hip pathologic conditions by etiopathogenesis: developmental/congenital

Etiopathogenesis	Pathophysiology/ Mechanism	Imaging Features	Abnormal Imaging Metrics	Possible Operative Findings
Developmental/congenital				
DDH	Lateralized femoral head Acetabular undercoverage	Coxa valga Femoral lateralization Hip subluxation AD Premature OA/ cartilage damage	LCEA/ACEA Acetabular index Tonnis angle	Periacetabular osteotomy Femoral varus osteotomy Hip resurfacing arthroplasty Total hip arthroplasty
PFFD	Abnormal mesenchymal development • Dysmorphic femoral head • Shortened femur Loss of developmental acetabular molding	Coxa vara Femoral head deformity Proximal femoral deficiency AD	LCEA/ACEA Acetabular index Tonnis angle	Various femoral lengthening procedures
Charcot hip[a]	Sensory/ autonomic neuropathy Insensate bone imperceptible trauma Hyperemia bone breakdown	Femoral head deformity Femoral lateralization Pseudoarticulation AD Premature OA/ cartilage damage	Acetabular index Acetabular depth Tonnis angle	Total hip arthroplasty

General assessment of the above includes AP and lateral radiographs, MR imaging (cartilage/labral assessment), and CT (3D bone morphology, operative planning, and so forth).
Abbreviations: ACEA, anterior center edge angle; AD, acetabular dysplasia; OA, osteoarthritis.
[a] Congenital neuropathic hip most frequently related to spina bifida, Chiari malformations, and syringomyelia.

Proximal Focal Femoral Deficiency

Proximal focal femoral deficiency (PFFD) is characterized by abnormal mesenchymal development of the femur (in utero insult vs idiopathic) leading to underdevelopment of the femoral head, acetabular dysplasia owing to loss of the normal femoral head molding effect, and characteristic shortening of the femoral shaft[15] (**Fig. 6**). Aitken[16] classifies PFFD into types A through D based on the presence or absence of the femoral head and acetabulum and the osseous integrity of the remainder of the femoral shaft. The least severe class, type A, is characterized by a short femur, preserved femoral head and acetabulum, and frequently a pseudoarthrosis at the femoral neck.[17,18] Class D, the most severe type of PFFD, is characterized by a shortened femur with absent femoral head and acetabulum.[17,18] Classes B and C have intermediate

morphologies. MR imaging also plays a supplemental role in evaluating physeal and cartilaginous/labral abnormalities in PFFD.[18] Distal lower-extremity defects, including hypoplasia/deficiency of the tibia, fibula, cruciate ligaments, lateral rays, and talocalcaneal coalition, are also common in patients with PFFD.[15] Treatment of PFFD focuses on hip stability and correction of leg length discrepancy, through lengthening procedures, prosthesis, and operations such as the Van Nes rotationoplasty.[15]

PEARL

1. PFFD can be associated with *missing, reduced, and/or retained primitive blood vessels.*

Table 5
Hip pathologic conditions by etiopathogenesis: acquired

Etiopathogenesis	Pathophysiology/Mechanism	Imaging Sequela	Abnormal Imaging Metrics	Possible Operative Findings
Acquired				
LCPD	Loss of blood flow to femoral head AVN Relative CAM deformity	Femoral head deformity CAM deformity AD Premature OA/cartilage damage	LCEA Acetabular index Femoral head neck offset ratio Alpha angle	Femoral varus osteotomy Periacetabular osteotomy Femoral neck lengthening Innominate osteotomy Shelf procedure
SCFE	Anterior/lateral slippage of femoral neck • Pathologic stress[a] • Pathologic physeal weakness[b] Relative CAM deformity	Femoral head deformity CAM deformity Premature OA/cartilage damage	Acetabular version Femoral head neck offset ratio Alpha angle	Femoral head pinning Proximal femoral osteotomy Femoral head/neck osteochondroplasty
Infectious/inflammatory arthritis	Inflammatory change/hyperemia • Premature triradiate/physeal closure • Femoral head erosion/AVN • Acetabular deformity Possibly idiopathic (eg, JIA)	Femoral head deformity Femoral lateralization Coxa vara/valga Leg length discrepancy AD Joint ankylosis/heterotopic bone Premature OA/cartilage damage	Femoral head sphericity Tonnis angle Acetabular index Femoral head extrusion index	Pelvic acetabuloplasty Femoral varus/valgus osteotomy Epiphysiodesis with contralateral leg lengthening Trochanteric arthroplasty Total hip arthroplasty
IHC	Idiopathic rapid destruction of hip cartilage	Symmetric joint space narrowing Periarticular osteopenia Acetabular protrusion Joint ankylosis/heterotopic bone Premature OA/cartilage damage	Acetabular depth Acetabular index Tonnis angle	Total hip arthroplasty

(continued on next page)

Table 5
(continued)

Etiopathogenesis	Pathophysiology/ Mechanism	Imaging Sequela	Abnormal Imaging Metrics	Possible Operative Findings
Osteoid osteoma of the hip	Benign bone tumor • Reactive hyperemia • Bone proliferation	Lucent nidus with surrounding sclerosis (minority of intraarticular cases) Coxa valga Widening of femoral neck (CAM deformity) Premature OA/cartilage damage	Alpha angle Femoral head neck offset ratio	Osteochondroplasty
Traumatic avulsion	Repetitive stress (athletics) Direct trauma	AIIS hypertrophy, malunion, or nonunion Heterotopic bone formation CAM deformity	Alpha angle (concurrent CAM deformity) Femoral head neck offset ratio	AIIS osteochondroplasty Femoral head/neck osteochondroplasty

General assessment of the above includes AP and lateral radiographs, MR imaging (cartilage/labral assessment), and CT (3D bone morphology, operative planning, and so forth).
Abbreviations: AVN, avascular necrosis; ROM, range of motion.
[a] Most commonly obesity.
[b] Often metabolic causes such as hypothyroidism.

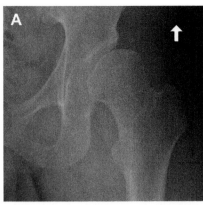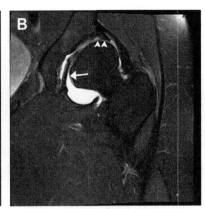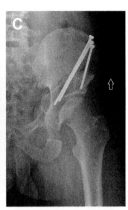

Fig. 3. DDH in a 23-year-old man who presented with left groin pain (*A*). AP radiograph of the left hip shows a flattened lateralized femoral head and acetabular dysplasia (shallow with increased inclination) (*B*). Axial SWISS T1-weighted MR arthrogram of the left hip shows an anterior superior labral tear (*arrowheads*) due to pathologic loading with associated hypertrophy of the ligamentum teres (*arrows*) (*C*). AP radiograph of the left hip shows a periacetabular osteotomy with improved femoral head coverage and acetabular orientation.

Hip Dysmorphisms Associated with Childhood Central Nervous System and Neuromuscular Diseases

Several well-known entities affecting the central nervous and neuromuscular systems in children may predispose to hip dysmorphisms. Children with neural tube defects (spina bifida) can develop several congenital and acquired deformities of the hip, including joint contractures, subluxations, and teratologic dislocations. Hip dislocations are seen in up to 30% to 50% of patients with myelomenigoceles.[19] Congenital arthrogryposis, a condition characterized by multifocal joint contractures, may also present with hip dislocation followed by progressive dysplasia.[20] Progressive hip dysplasia affects one-third of children with cerebral palsy with a higher prevalence in nonambulatory children.[21] Its pathophysiology is dominated by an underlying dynamic muscle imbalance with hip flexors and adductors overpowering hip extensors and abductors.[22] Excessive femoral anteversion and coxa valga are often present.[23] Acetabular deficiency and an increased acetabular index may be present and lead to pathologic labral loading,

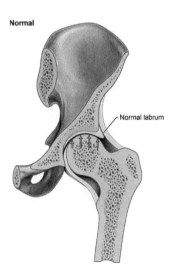

Normal

Normal labrum

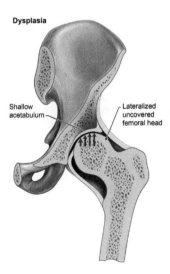

Dysplasia

Shallow acetabulum

Lateralized uncovered femoral head

Fig. 4. Schematic representation of a normal hip with physiologic loading of the acetabulum (*left*) compared to a dysplastic hip with pathologic loading of the acetabular rim and labrum (*right*). (*Courtesy of* Nadezhda Kiriyak, University of Rochester Medical Center, Rochester, NY; with permission.)

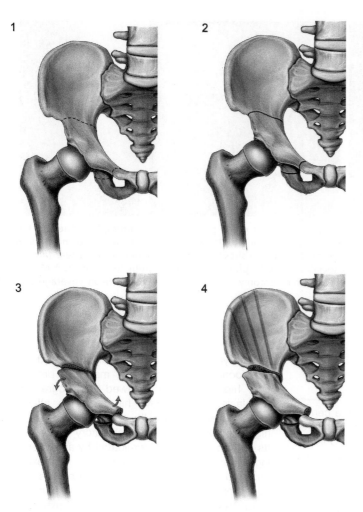

Fig. 5. Schematic demonstration of a periacetabular osteotomy (1-2) followed by mobilization of the acetabular fragment (3) and fixation (4) resulting in improved femoral head coverage and congruity. (*Courtesy of* Nadezhda Kiriyak, University of Rochester Medical Center, Rochester, NY; with permission.)

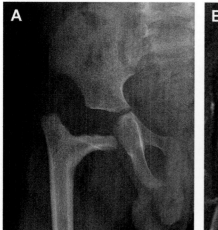
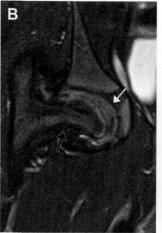
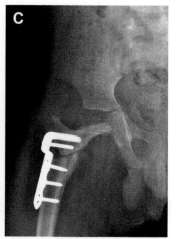

Fig. 6. PFFD in a 3-year-old boy with a history of prematurity and triplet birth (*A*). Anterior posterior radiograph of the right hip shows a dysmorphic flattened femoral head and coxa vara (*B*). Coronal nonenhanced T2-weighted MR imaging of the left hip shows a dysmorphic femoral head (*black arrow*) and articular cartilage (*white arrow*) (*C*). AP radiograph of the right hip after corrective valgus osteotomy.

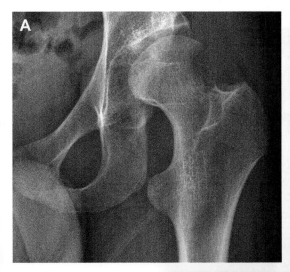
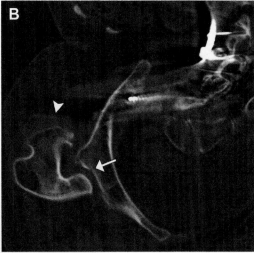
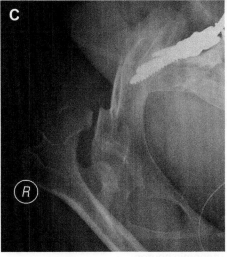

Fig. 7. Cerebral palsy with hip dysplasia, multiple cases. (*A*) AP radiograph of the left hip in a 21-year-old man with cerebral palsy shows coxa valga, a flattened lateralized femoral head, acetabular dysplasia, and a chronic acetabular rim fracture from pathologic loading. (*B*) Axial nonenhanced bone window setting CT of the right hip in a 28-year-old with cerebral palsy and scoliosis shows a subluxed dysplastic femoral head (*arrowhead*) and a shallow dysplastic acetabulum with pseudoarticulation of the lesser trochanter (*arrow*). (*C*) AP radiograph of the right hip of the 28-year-old presented in panel (*B*).

labral injury, and acetabular rim fractures[21] (Fig. 7). Although there are generally no soft tissue obstacles to reduction, recurrent deformities and subluxations frequently occur as the patient grows because of persistent muscle imbalance even after corrective surgery.[22] Management options include preventive, reconstructive, or salvage procedures.[21]

Neurofibromatosis 1 can also be associated with numerous hip manifestations, including intraarticular neurofibromas, protrusio acetabuli, coxa valga, and increased femoral offset (Fig. 8). There have been reports of hip dislocations following minor trauma in affected patients.[24–26]

PEARLS

1. The ambulatory status of patients with hip dislocations that arise secondary to neural tube defects is more closely associated with neurologic level of involvement rather than status of hip reduction.

2. Spastic hip dislocations in cerebral palsy are associated with progressive quality-of-life impairment over time; screening programs combining physical examination and radiologic assessment lead to early diagnosis and improve long-term outcomes.

3. Hip dislocations in neurofibromatosis 1 may be multifactorial, underscoring the importance of a multidisciplinary approach to diagnosis and management.

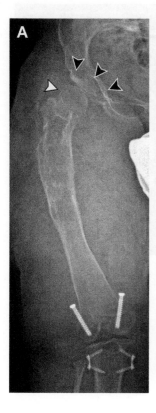 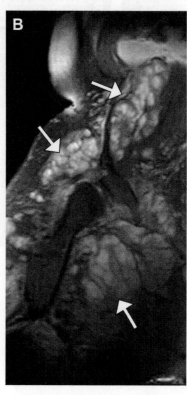

Fig. 8. Neurofibromatosis type 1 in a 17-year-old male adolescent with femoral overgrowth and plexiform neurofibromas throughout the right leg (*A*). AP radiograph of the right femur shows coxa magna and plana, a subluxed femoral head (*white arrowhead*), acetabular dysplasia (*black arrowheads*), and diffuse osseous and soft tissue hypertrophy (*B*). Coronal enhanced fat-saturated MR imaging of the right hip shows femoral and acetabular dysplasia and extensive plexiform neurofibromas surrounding the hip and throughout the leg (*arrows*).

Neuropathic (Charcot) Hip Secondary to Congenital Abnormalities of the Neuroaxis

The neuropathic arthropathies are a broad group of disorders in which denervation of the joint leads to unperceived trauma. Autonomic neuropathy may also contribute by leading to abnormal blood flow to the involved joint causing an imbalance of bone formation and reabsorption.[27] Neuropathic arthropathy of the hip (Charcot hip) may accompany congenital diseases, such as spina bifida, Chiari malformation, syringomyelia, and congenital pain insensitivity, as well as other acquired disorders, such as diabetes, tertiary neurosyphilis, and alcoholism.[27,28] Imaging features range from femoral head necrosis/deformity, acetabular dysplasia, and early degenerative arthropathy to gross bone destruction with periarticular heterotopic ossification and hip dislocation (Fig. 9). Treatment ranges from supportive care to hip arthroplasty depending on severity of disease and functional status on presentation.

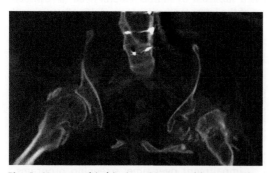

Fig. 9. Neuropathic hip in a 29-year-old man with a history of spina bifida, Chiari malformation, and paraplegia. Coronal nonenhanced bone window setting CT of the pelvis shows a left hip with a flattened dysmorphic femoral head, acetabular dysplasia, heterotopic bone formation, and a pathologic dislocation; less extensive changes are seen contralaterally.

PEARL

1. Neuropathic hip arthropathy can rarely arise secondary to *congenital abnormalities of the neuroaxis*; the consulting radiologist can play a valuable role by recommending further imaging in appropriate scenarios.

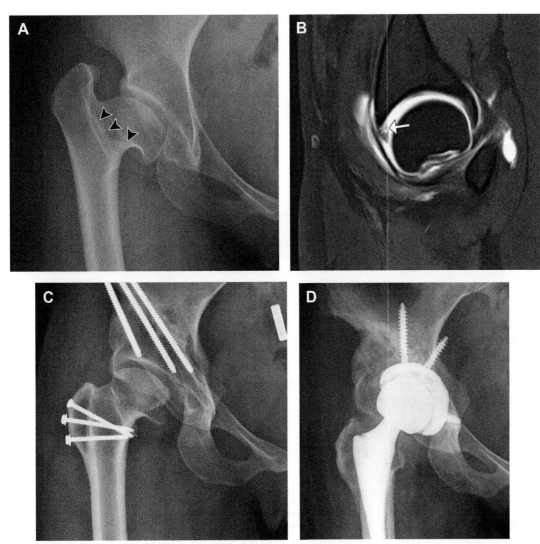

Fig. 10. LCPD in a 25-year-old woman with chronic right hip pain (serial images over 3 years of care showing disease sequela and progression of treatment) (*A*). AP radiograph of the right hip shows coxa plana, acetabular dysplasia, a shortened femoral neck, and extraarticular greater trochanter impingement. The "sagging rope" sign of Perthes disease (a sclerotic line running across the femoral neck) is also visible (*arrowheads*) (2016) (*B*). Sagittal T1-weighted MR arthrogram of the right hip shows an anterior/superior pathologic labral tear (*arrow*) (2016) (*C*). AP radiograph of the right hip shows a periacetabular osteotomy with a trochanteric osteotomy and distalization; note the relative femoral neck lengthening and decreased greater trochanter external impingement postoperatively (2017) (*D*). AP radiograph of the right hip shows a later total hip arthroplasty (2018).

Legg-Calve-Perthes Disease

Legg-Calve-Perthes disease (LCPD) is a pediatric disorder characterized by compromised blood flow to the femoral head (most frequently seen with steroid use, sickle cell disease, and trauma) leading to avascular necrosis and femoral head collapse.[29] Adult patients with sequelae of childhood LCPD may present with a range of deformities of the hip, including coxa plana, coxa magna, coxa valga, acetabular dysplasia, intraarticular or extraarticular CAM impingement from the aspheric flattened femoral head and relative trochanteric overgrowth, labral damage, and early degenerative osteoarthropathy[30] (**Fig. 10**). MR imaging and computed tomography (CT) may be used to identify cartilaginous/labral injury and aid in 3-dimensional (3D) operative reconstruction planning.[30] Corrective surgeries may include femoral and acetabular osteotomies to restore normal articular congruency and correct CAM and pincer deformities if present, and trochanteric osteotomy and distalization to lengthen the

Trochanteric Osteotomy and Distalization

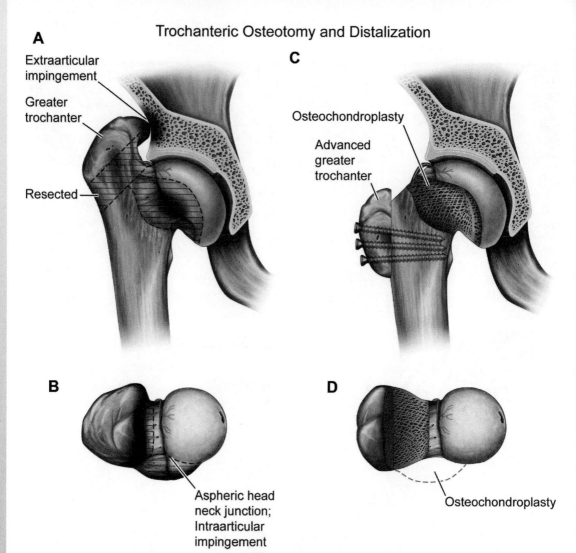

Fig. 11. The pathologic sequela of avascular necrosis with a shortened femoral neck and intraarticular and extraarticular impingement (*A, B*); surgical correction via trochanteric osteotomy and advancement followed by osteochondroplasty of the camshaft deformity leading to resolution of the intraarticular and extraarticular impingement (*C, D*). (*Courtesy of* Nadezhda Kiriyak, University of Rochester Medical Center, Rochester, NY; with permission.)

femoral neck, reduce external impingement, and improve abductor leverage[31] (**Fig. 11**). Osteochondroplasty and labral debridement are common adjuncts to the above surgeries.[31]

PEARLS

1. Pain and mechanical symptoms can occur in adults with sequelae of childhood LCPD because of abductor fatigue secondary to abductor lever insufficiency (high-riding greater trochanter), limb-length discrepancy, and osteochondritic lesions in the femoral head.

2. The "sagging rope sign," a thin sclerotic line crossing the femoral neck in LCPD, represents the margin of an enlarged overhanging femoral head projecting over the femoral neck.

Slipped Capital Femoral Epiphysis

Slipped capital femoral epiphysis (SCFE) results from pathologic physeal stress or weakness leading to anterior and lateral slippage of the femoral neck relative to the femoral head[29] (**Fig. 12**). Imaging of the adult patient with sequela of childhood SCFE may also show relative anterior/lateral CAM deformity, and acetabular dysplasia. The relative CAM deformity seen in SCFE leads to impingement upon the acetabulum with associated premature degenerative osteoarthropathy[32–34] (**Fig. 13**). Treatment of SCFE involves femoral head pinning acutely followed by femoral osteotomy and osteochondroplasty to redirect the femoral head into the acetabulum

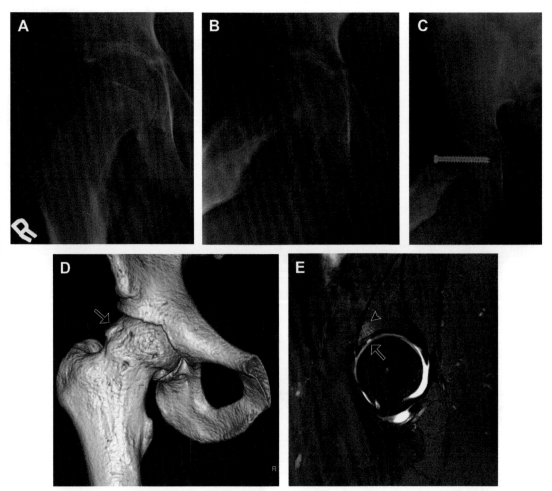

Fig. 12. SCFE in a 25-year-old man with right hip pain and a history of childhood SCFE who failed conservative therapy. The patient is currently undergoing workup for arthroscopy and intervention. (*A, B*) AP and frog-leg lateral radiographs of the right hip on presentation (age 16) show anterior slippage of the femoral neck consistent with an SCFE-type injury. (*C*) Frog-leg lateral radiograph of the right hip after a therapeutic femoral head pinning. (*D*) 3D reformatted CT of the right hip (age 25) shows the anterior lateral camshaft deformity of the femoral neck (*arrow*). (*E*) Sagittal intermediate, fat-suppressed MR arthrogram of the right hip (age 25) shows a chondral defect (*arrow*) with adjacent marrow edema (*arrowhead*).

and remove impinging bone. Total hip arthroplasty is reserved for late severe degenerative change.[33]

PEARL

1. Two types of impingement occur with SCFE injuries:

   A. Severe slip: "impaction"-type impingement: prominent femoral metaphysis strikes and damages the anterior acetabular rim/labrum and levers the femoral head out of the acetabulum with flexion, causing posterior labral and cartilage damage.

   B. Minor slip: "inclusion"-type impingement: metaphyseal protuberance slides into the acetabulum with flexion causing cartilage delamination.

Infectious/Inflammatory Arthritis

A wide spectrum of inflammatory arthritides may affect the hip. Most of these share similar morphologic features. Inflammatory arthritis may cause local hyperemia leading to early growth plate closure and limb length discrepancy. Damage to the blood supply of the hip and increased intracapsular pressure during acute infection may lead to avascular necrosis and its sequelae.[35–37] Direct erosive damage to the hip can produce early osteoarthritis and progressive destruction of the femoral head and acetabulum (**Figs. 14** and **15**). Joint ankylosis is also a sequela of several of the inflammatory arthritides, such as juvenile idiopathic arthritis (JIA).[35] Numerous corrective strategies are used to address inflammatory arthritis, including observation and

Femoroacetabular Impingement

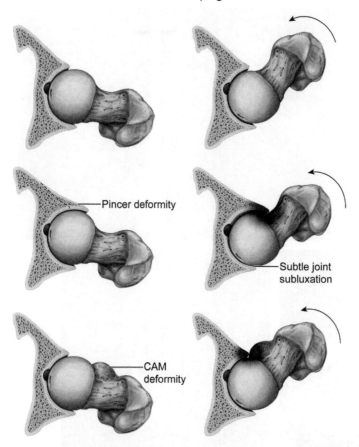

Fig. 13. Normal hip anatomy versus the sequela of a pincer or camshaft deformity, which causes impingement with flexion or internal rotation. (*Courtesy of* Nadezhda Kiriyak, University of Rochester Medical Center, Rochester, NY; with permission.)

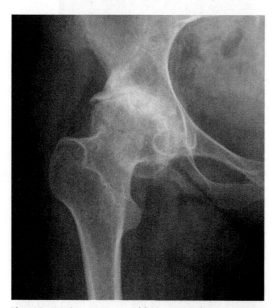

Fig. 14. JIA in a 41-year-old woman who presented with right hip pain and a history of pediatric JIA. AP radiograph of the right hip shows severe degenerative change with coxa plana, coxa magna, sclerosis, subchondral cysts, osteophytes, and joint space narrowing. The patient ultimately underwent a total hip arthroplasty.

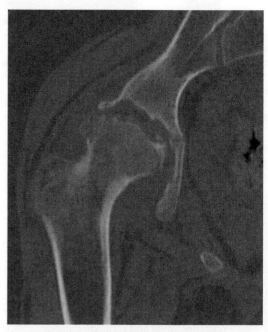

Fig. 15. Septic arthritis in a 12-year-old boy with a remote history of right septic hip. Coronal nonenhanced bone-window setting CT of the right hip shows erosion, flattening, and lateralization of the femoral head with an eroded dysmorphic acetabulum.

containment for mild cases, femoral varus/valgus osteotomies, various acetabuloplasties to improve femoral head/acetabulum congruence, and femoral lengthening and contralateral epiphysiodesis to address leg length discrepancy. Advanced disease may require trochanteric osteotomy with femoral varus osteotomy or total hip arthroplasty for adequate reconstruction.[35,37–39]

PEARLS

1. Septic hip may be complicated by premature physeal closure, avascular necrosis of the femoral head, pseudoarthrosis of the femoral neck, complete femoral head and neck destruction, and premature osteoarthritis.

2. Hip involvement occurs in approximately 35% to 63% of children with JIA and is more prevalent in the aggressive systemic subtypes; irreversible changes can occur within a few years of diagnosis.

Idiopathic Hip Chondrolysis

Idiopathic hip chondrolysis (IHC) refers to rapid progressive destruction of hip cartilage without identification of a causative factor. Long-term sequelae commonly seen in this condition include symmetric joint space narrowing, periarticular osteopenia, decrease in femoral head diameter (with preserved sphericity), acetabular protrusion, joint ankylosis, and early degenerative arthritis[39–43] (**Fig. 16**). Treatment of this condition generally consists of physiotherapy to maintain function as long as possible followed by more aggressive interventions, such as tendon release, capsulotomy, and surgical arthrodesis, with hip arthroplasty reserved for end-stage disease.[42,44]

PEARL

1. IHC is characterized by concentric joint space narrowing and *stiffness*; initial onset is most typical in *adolescent girls of African or Asian descent.*

Intraarticular Osteoid Osteoma of the Hip

Osteoid osteoma of the hip, particularly when occurring anteriorly and laterally along the intraarticular femoral neck, is known to contribute to the development of femoroacetabular impingement (FAI).[45–48] It has been proposed

that this FAI may be due to local hyperemia, synovitis, and periostitis leading to increased bone formation, provoked by the curative surgery or owing to residual nidus tissue.[46,47] Imaging workup in these patients may demonstrate shortening and widening of the femoral neck, coxa valga, femoral antetorsion, and eventually premature osteoarthritis because of the CAM impingement and subsequent damage to the acetabular labrum and articular cartilage. Treatment with osteochondroplasty to remove the bone overgrowth and treatment of residual osteoid osteoma has demonstrated good effect.[46,47]

PEARL

1. Femoral neck deformities and FAI arising secondary to intraarticular osteoid osteoma generally resolve after excision or ablation of the nidus, but *may occasionally continue to progress despite adequate nidus removal.*

Trauma/Iatrogenic Hip Disorders

Hip injuries occurring in children may be articular or periarticular. These injuries may heal without incident or lead to hip dysmorphologies, including femoroacetabular, ischiofemoral, and subspine impingement and associated abnormal hip mechanics. Although a comprehensive review of hip trauma is beyond the scope of this article, apophyseal avulsions, particularly of the anterior inferior iliac spine (AIIS), is briefly addressed here because of their onset in the young athlete and potential for causing long-term hip dysmorphology. AIIS avulsion occurs after repetitive rectus femoris strain or direct trauma, both frequently encountered in young runners and athletes participating in kicking activities, such as soccer and football.[49–54] Malunion or nonunion of the AIIS after healing or bone proliferation during the healing process can both contribute to painful external pincertype impingement as the AIIS contacts the anterior femoral neck with hip flexion.[49,50,52,53] CAM deformities of the femoral neck are frequently encountered concurrently.[49,50,52] Imaging workup demonstrates bony prominence of the AIIS on frontal and lateral radiographs and reduced femoral head neck offset with increased alpha index if CAM deformity is present (**Fig. 17**). Acetabular retroversion may also be seen. Treatment generally consists of surgical or arthroscopic debridement of the overriding AIIS with

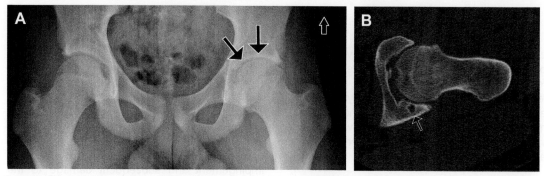

Fig. 16. Idiopathic chondrolysis of the hip in a 16-year-old male adolescent who presented with chronic right hip pain and stiffness. Patient had an extensive negative workup for other hip pathologic conditions (*A*). AP radiograph of the pelvis shows symmetric joint space narrowing (*arrows*) of the left hip (*B*). Transverse nonenhanced bone window setting CT of the left hip shows joint space loss and early degenerative change (subchondral cyst, *arrow*).

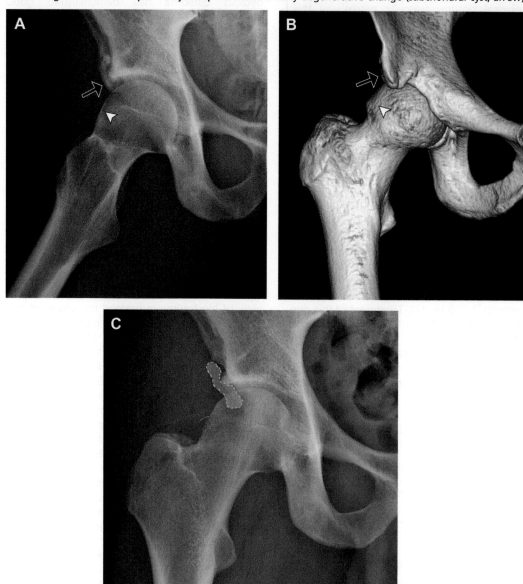

Fig. 17. AIIS impingement in a 28-year-old man with right hip pain after a deadlift; the patient participates in numerous sports. On examination, hip flexion is limited and painful (*A*). Frog-leg lateral radiograph of the right hip shows a type III AIIS (*arrow*) with a camshaft deformity of the femoral neck (*arrowhead*) (*B*). 3D reformatted CT of the right hip shows a prominent AIIS (*arrow*) with a camshaft deformity of the femoral neck (*arrowhead*); labral fraying was present on a concurrent MR imaging (*C*). AP radiograph of the right hip status post arthroscopy with decompression of the AIIS (*green shading*), femoral head-neck osteochondroplasty (*red shading*), and labral debridement.

concurrent labral repair and osteochondroplasty for femoral neck CAM deformity as necessary.[49–52] Preoperative 3D CT is useful for analysis of the precise location of impingement/contact with the femoral neck and operative planning.[49,52]

PEARL

1. Sports injuries in the young athlete can lead to both *extraarticular* and *intraarticular* *impingement* in the adult with their associated morbidity.

SUMMARY

Sequelae of pediatric hip disorders can manifest as bony dysmorphisms, chondral/labral damage, articular incongruity and destruction, and structural hip instability in the adult patient. Clear understanding of these imaging manifestations can improve diagnostic interpretations, facilitating more effective patient counseling and prompt referral when needed for general radiologists.

DISCLOSURE

The authors have nothing to disclose.

REFERENCES

1. Chang CY, Huang AJ. MR imaging of normal hip anatomy. Magn Reson Imaging Clin N Am 2013; 21(1):1–19.
2. DuBois DF, Omar IM. MR imaging of the hip: normal anatomic variants and imaging pitfalls. Magn Reson Imaging Clin N Am 2010;18(4):663–74.
3. Resnick D, Kransdorf MJ. Bone and joint imaging. 3rd edition. Philadelphia: Elsevier Saunders; 2005.
4. Wylie JD, Peters CL, Aoki SK. Natural history of structural hip abnormalities and the potential for hip preservation. J Am Acad Orthop Surg 2018; 26(15):515–25.
5. Sutter R, Zanetti M, Pfirrmann CW. New developments in hip imaging. Radiology 2012;264(3):651–67.
6. Clohisy JC, Carlisle JC, Beaulé PE, et al. A systematic approach to the plain radiographic evaluation of the young adult hip. J Bone Joint Surg Am 2008;90(Suppl 4):47–66.
7. Welton KL, Jesse MK, Kraeutler MJ, et al. The anteroposterior pelvic radiograph: acetabular and femoral measurements and relation to hip pathologies. J Bone Joint Surg Am 2018;100(1):76–85.
8. Tannast M, Siebenrock KA, Anderson SE. Femoroacetabular impingement: radiographic diagnosis–

9. what the radiologist should know. AJR Am J Roentgenol 2007;188(6):1540–52.
9. Gosvig KK, Jacobsen S, Palm H, et al. A new radiological index for assessing asphericity of the femoral head in cam impingement. J Bone Joint Surg Br 2007;89(10):1309–16.
10. Mascarenhas VV, Caetano A. Imaging the young adult hip in the future. Ann Joint 2018;3(5):47.
11. Crowe JF, Mani VJ, Ranawat CS. Total hip replacement in congenital dislocation and dysplasia of the hip. J Bone Joint Surg Am 1979;61(1):15–23.
12. Hartofilakidis G, Stamos K, Ioannidis TT. Low friction arthroplasty for old untreated congenital dislocation of the hip. J Bone Joint Surg Br 1988;70(2):182–6.
13. Beltran LS, Rosenberg ZS, Mayo JD, et al. Imaging evaluation of developmental hip dysplasia in the young adult. AJR Am J Roentgenol 2013;200(5): 1077–88.
14. Kosuge D, Yamada N, Azegami S, et al. Management of developmental dysplasia of the hip in young adults: current concepts. Bone Joint J 2013;95-b(6):732–7.
15. Bedoya MA, Chauvin NA, Jaramillo D, et al. Common patterns of congenital lower extremity shortening: diagnosis, classification, and follow-up. Radiographics 2015;35(4):1191–207.
16. Aitken GT. Proximal femoral focal deficiency: definition, classification, and management. In: Aitken GT, editor. A Symposium on Proximal Femoral Focal Deficiency: A Congenital Anomaly. Washington, DC: National Academy of Sciences; 1969. p. 1–22.
17. Dwek JR. The hip: MR imaging of uniquely pediatric disorders. Magn Reson Imaging Clin N Am 2009; 17(3):509–20, vi.
18. Biko DM, Davidson R, Pena A, et al. Proximal focal femoral deficiency: evaluation by MR imaging. Pediatr Radiol 2012;42(1):50–6.
19. Thompson RM, Foley J, Dias L, et al. Hip status and long-term functional outcomes in spina bifida. J Pediatr Orthop 2019;39(3):e168–72.
20. Asif S, Umer M, Beg R, et al. Operative treatment of bilateral hip dislocation in children with arthrogryposis multiplex congenita. J Orthop Surg (Hong Kong) 2004;12(1):4–9.
21. Huser A, Mo M, Hosseinzadeh P. Hip surveillance in children with cerebral palsy. Orthop Clin North Am 2018;49(2):181–90.
22. Davids JR. Management of neuromuscular hip dysplasia in children with cerebral palsy: lessons and challenges. J Pediatr Orthop 2018;38(Suppl 1):S21–7.
23. Cho Y, Park ES, Park HK, et al. Determinants of hip and femoral deformities in children with spastic cerebral palsy. Ann Rehabil Med 2018;42(2):277–85.
24. Dearden PM, Lowery KA, Bates J, et al. Hip dislocation following minor trauma in a patient with neurofibromatosis type 1: a case report and review of the literature. Hip Int 2015;25(2):188–90.

25. Galbraith JG, Butler JS, Harty JA. Recurrent spontaneous hip dislocation in a patient with neurofibromatosis type 1: a case report. J Med Case Rep 2011;5:106.

26. Waheed W, Diego FLDF, Nathaniel Nelms N, et al. Multifactorial pathological hip subluxation in neurofibromatosis type-1 (NF1) due to intra-articular plexiform neurofibroma, lumbar radiculopathy and neurofibromatous polyneuropathy. BMJ Case Rep 2016;2016 [pii:bcr2016217971].

27. Memarpour R, Tashtoush B, Issac L, et al. Syringomyelia with Chiari I malformation presenting as hip Charcot arthropathy: a case report and literature review. Case Rep Neurol Med 2015;2015:487931.

28. Viens NA, Watters TS, Vinson EN, et al. Case report: neuropathic arthropathy of the hip as a sequela of undiagnosed tertiary syphilis. Clin Orthop Relat Res 2010;468(11):3126–31.

29. Karkenny AJ, Tauberg BM, Otsuka NY. Pediatric hip disorders: slipped capital femoral epiphysis and Legg-Calve-Perthes disease. Pediatr Rev 2018;39(9):454–63.

30. Podeszwa DA, DeLaRocha A. Clinical and radiographic analysis of Perthes deformity in the adolescent and young adult. J Pediatr Orthop 2013; 33(Suppl 1):S56–61.

31. Novais EN, Clohisy J, Siebenrock K, et al. Treatment of the symptomatic healed Perthes hip. Orthop Clin North America 2011;42(3):401–17, viii.

32. Klit J, Gosvig K, Magnussen E, et al. Cam deformity and hip degeneration are common after fixation of a slipped capital femoral epiphysis. Acta Orthop 2014;85(6):585–91.

33. Hosalkar HS, Pandya NK, Bomar JD, et al. Hip impingement in slipped capital femoral epiphysis: a changing perspective. J Child Orthop 2012;6(3):161–72.

34. Helgesson L, Johansson PK, Aurell Y, et al. Early osteoarthritis after slipped capital femoral epiphysis. Acta Orthop 2018;89(2):222–8.

35. Choi IH, Pizzutillo PD, Bowen JR, et al. Sequelae and reconstruction after septic arthritis of the hip in infants. J Bone Joint Surg Am 1990;72(8):1150–65.

36. Baghdadi T, Saberi S, Sobhani Eraghi A, et al. Late sequelae of hip septic arthritis in children. Acta Med Iran 2012;50(7):463–7.

37. Forlin E, Milani C. Sequelae of septic arthritis of the hip in children: a new classification and a review of 41 hips. J Pediatr Orthop 2008;28(5):524–8.

38. Dobbs MB, Sheridan JJ, Gordon JE, et al. Septic arthritis of the hip in infancy: long-term follow-up. J Pediatr Orthop 2003;23(2):162–8.

39. Manzotti A, Rovetta L, Pullen C, et al. Treatment of the late sequelae of septic arthritis of the hip. Clin Orthop Relat Res 2003;(410):203–12.

40. Johnson K, Haigh SF, Ehtisham S, et al. Childhood idiopathic chondrolysis of the hip: MRI features. Pediatr Radiol 2003;33(3):194–9.

41. Sureka J, Jakkani RK, Inbaraj A, et al. Idiopathic chondrolysis of hip. Jpn J Radiol 2011;29(4):283–5.

42. Dechosilpa C, Mulpruek P, Woratanarat P, et al. Idiopathic chondrolysis of the hip (ICH): report of three cases. Malays Orthop J 2014;8(3):30–2.

43. Provencher M, Navaie M, Solomon D, et al. Current concepts review: joint chondrolysis. J Bone Joint Surg Am 2011;93:2033–44.

44. Segaren N, Abdul-Jabar HB, Segaren N, et al. Idiopathic chondrolysis of the hip: presentation, natural history and treatment options. J Pediatr Orthop B 2014;23(2):112–6.

45. Ly JA, Coleman EM, Cohen GS, et al. Unrecognized osteoid osteoma of the proximal femur with associated cam impingement. J Hip Preserv Surg 2016; 3(3):236–7.

46. Jang WY, Lee SH, Cho IY. Progressive femoroacetabular impingement after complete excision of osteoid osteoma in adolescents: a report of two cases. Skeletal Radiol 2017;46(4):553–7.

47. Song MH, Yoo WJ, Cho TJ, et al. Clinical and radiological features and skeletal sequelae in childhood intra-/juxta-articular versus extra-articular osteoid osteoma. BMC Musculoskelet Disord 2015;16:3.

48. Pianta M, Crowther S, McNally D, et al. Proximal femoral intra-capsular osteoid osteoma in a 16-year-old male with epiphyseal periostitis contributing to Cam-type deformity relating to femoro-acetabular impingement. Skeletal Radiol 2013;42(1):129–33.

49. Hetsroni I, Larson CM, Dela Torre K, et al. Anterior inferior iliac spine deformity as an extra-articular source for hip impingement: a series of 10 patients treated with arthroscopic decompression. Arthroscopy 2012;28(11):1644–53.

50. Novais EN, Riederer MF, Provance AJ. Anterior inferior iliac spine deformity as a cause for extra-articular hip impingement in young athletes after an avulsion fracture: a case report. Sports Health 2018;10(3):272–6.

51. Pan H, Kawanabe K, Akiyama H, et al. Operative treatment of hip impingement caused by hypertrophy of the anterior inferior iliac spine. J Bone Joint Surg Br 2008;90(5):677–9.

52. Larson CM, Kelly BT, Stone RM. Making a case for anterior inferior iliac spine/subspine hip impingement: three representative case reports and proposed concept. Arthroscopy 2011;27(12): 1732–7.

53. Carr JB 2nd, Conte E, Rajadhyaksha EA, et al. Operative fixation of an anterior inferior iliac spine apophyseal avulsion fracture nonunion in an adolescent soccer player: a case report. JBJS Case Connect 2017;7(2):e29.

54. Schuett DJ, Bomar JD, Pennock AT. Pelvic apophyseal avulsion fractures: a retrospective review of 228 cases. J Pediatr Orthop 2015;35(6): 617–23.

Imaging Assessment of Complications from Transplantation from Pediatric to Adult Patients
Part 1: Solid Organ Transplantation

Erin K. Romberg, MD[a], Nathan David P. Concepcion, MD[b,c,d], Bernard F. Laya, MD[c,d,e], Edward Y. Lee, MD, MPH[f], Grace S. Phillips, MD[g],*

KEYWORDS

- Lung transplantation • Liver failure • End-stage renal disease
- Posttransplant lymphoproliferative disorder

KEY POINTS

- The diseases leading to solid organ failure differ between children and adults; however, similar postoperative complications are seen after transplantation.
- Children in general have higher rates of many types of postoperative complications following solid organ transplantation.
- Differences in surgical technique in the pediatric population, including use of downsized grafts, lead to varied postoperative anatomy and imaging appearance compared with adults.
- Posttransplant malignancies are an increasingly important consideration as overall posttransplant survival rates improve and pediatric transplant patients age into adulthood.

INTRODUCTION

Solid organ transplantation is performed for end-stage organ disease in both children and adults. Overall, similar types of complications are seen between the 2 populations; however, children's small size can impact surgical methods, as well as the relative frequency of complications, particularly vascular complications. Adolescents have on average poorer outcomes posttransplant, likely due to difficulties with medication compliance.[1] In addition, the different etiologies leading to end-organ failure and transplantation between the 2 populations have some bearing on the postoperative imaging appearance. As there are relatively few transplant centers, many patients travel considerable distances to receive their transplants.[2] Travel back to these transplant centers for routine follow-up is often not feasible. Thus, the general radiologist may encounter these patients in their practice. As clinical presentations

[a] Department of Radiology, Seattle Children's Hospital, University of Washington School of Medicine, MA.7.220, 4800 Sand Point Way Northeast, Seattle, WA 98105, USA; [b] Section of Pediatric Radiology, Institute of Radiology, St. Luke's Medical Center-Global City, Rizal Drive cor. 32nd Street and 5th Avenue, Taguig City, 1634 Philippines; [c] St. Luke's Medical Center College of Medicine-William H. Quasha Memorial, Quezon City, Philippines; [d] Philippine Society for Pediatric Radiology; [e] Section of Pediatric Radiology, Institute of Radiology, St. Luke's Medical Center-Quezon City, 279 East Rodriguez Sr. Avenue, Quezon City 1112, Philippines; [f] Division of Thoracic Imaging, Department of Radiology, Boston Children's Hospital, Harvard Medical School, 300 Longwood Avenue, Boston, MA 02115, USA; [g] Department of Radiology, Seattle Children's Hospital, University of Washington School of Medicine, MA.7.220, 4800 Sand Point Way Northeast, Seattle, WA 98105, USA
* Corresponding author.
E-mail address: grace.phillips@seattlechildrens.org

Radiol Clin N Am 58 (2020) 549–568
https://doi.org/10.1016/j.rcl.2019.12.005
0033-8389/20/© 2019 Elsevier Inc. All rights reserved.

are frequently nonspecific or asymptomatic, it is essential that general radiologists recognize complications of common solid organ transplants on imaging, particularly in the intermediate to delayed time frame.

This article discusses the imaging appearance of lung, kidney, and liver transplants in children and adults, with a focus on imaging techniques, normal radiological appearance, and complications specific to graft type. In addition, this article also reviews the imaging diagnosis of postoperative fluid collections and posttransplant lymphoproliferative disease (PTLD), which may be seen with all 3 types of transplantation.

LUNG TRANSPLANTATION

Lung transplantation is relatively infrequent in children compared with adults, and is performed much less frequently in children than heart, liver, or kidney transplants.[3] However, as there are relatively few lung transplant centers, particularly for children, routine follow-up of these patients may occur in the community rather than at the transplant center.[2] Therefore, general radiologists must be familiar with findings concerning for intermediate and particularly late complications of lung transplantation.

Underlying diseases leading to lung transplantation differ between pediatric and adult populations. In children, pulmonary hypertension constitutes the most common illness requiring lung transplantation in 1-year-olds to 5-year-olds, whereas cystic fibrosis accounts for the overwhelming majority in 6-year-olds to 11-year-olds.[2,4] Combined heart-lung transplantation is now rarely performed, predominantly for idiopathic pulmonary hypertension.[5] In contrast to children, the most common underlying cause in adults is fibrotic lung disease, such as idiopathic pulmonary fibrosis, followed by obstructive disease, such as emphysema.[2]

Surgical Techniques

The chief difference in surgical technique between pediatric and adult lung transplants revolves around donor-recipient size mismatch. Size mismatch may occur in both the pulmonary parenchymal size, and the bronchial anastomotic size.[6] The relative paucity of pediatric donors leads to the use of downsized adult donor lungs in pediatric recipients. Lungs may be downsized via lobectomies or with a nonanatomic reduction using a linear stapling device (**Fig. 1**).[5] Oversized pulmonary transplants may manifest as atelectasis on postoperative radiographs. Conversely, undersized pulmonary transplants may lead to

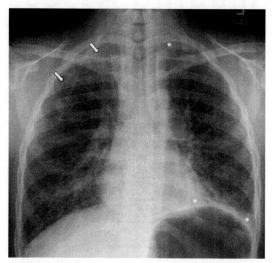

Fig. 1. A 17-year-old boy with lung transplantation due to cystic fibrosis. Frontal chest radiograph shows expected findings of lung transplantation including surgical sutures (*arrows*) to decrease the size of right lung from the donor to fit into the recipient's hemithorax, pleural thickening (*asterisks*), and horizontal sternotomy wires.

chronic pleural effusion or pneumothorax due to residual unfilled thoracic cavity (**Fig. 2**).[6]

Imaging Techniques and Normal Findings

Chest radiographs are most commonly used for the initial postoperative evaluation of lung transplants, as they are portable, fast, and low radiation. A

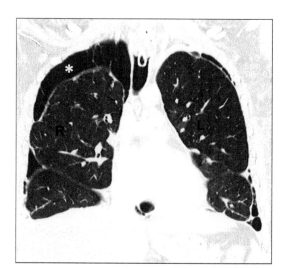

Fig. 2. A 17-year-old girl with lung transplantation due to idiopathic pulmonary hypertension. Coronal lung window CT image shows small transplanted right lung (R) due to size mismatch with chronic pneumothorax (*asterisk*). Of note, left lung (L) size is appropriate for this patient's thoracic size.

Box 1
Normal chest radiograph appearance of lung transplant

- Transverse sternotomy wires
- Pulmonary sutures from graft downsizing, particularly in children
- Pleural thickening, small pleural effusions, and pneumothoraces are common immediately after transplantation
- Nonspecific pulmonary infiltrates are expected in the first 3 days after transplantation
  - Primary graft dysfunction affects nearly all patients in the immediate postoperative period

summary of normal postoperative chest radiograph findings is summarized in **Box 1** and **Fig. 1**. Additional imaging strategies include computed tomography (CT), CT angiography, and nuclear medicine (NM) pulmonary perfusion scintigraphy as outlined in **Table 1**.

Complications

Potential complications of lung transplantation are wide ranging, vary by time period posttransplant, and are of overall similar types in children compared with adults. Early complications (<1 week posttransplant) include primary graft dysfunction, seen in nearly all transplants and manifesting as nonspecific pulmonary opacities.[3] Vascular anastomotic complications, primarily thrombosis, are relatively uncommon and may be evaluated by echocardiography or perfusion scintigraphy.[3] Intermediate complications (1 week to 2 months) include acute rejection, pulmonary thromboembolism, and bronchial anastomotic complications.[6,7]

Bronchial anastomotic complications

The bronchial anastomoses are particularly vulnerable to ischemic complications, as the bronchial arteries are typically not reconnected following transplantation.[3,8] There may be a mismatch between the donor and recipient bronchial sizes, which can be addressed surgically by downsizing via sutures, or by overlapping/telescoping anastomotic techniques.[6,8] Anastomoses are typically covered with vascularized pericardial or parabronchial tissue to minimize risk of dehiscence.[3] Airway stenosis or malacia may result in poor sputum clearance and repeated infections, requiring recurrent bronchoscopy and stenting.[9]

Bronchial anastomotic dehiscence

Anastomotic dehiscence is a rare complication (1%–10%); however, results in high morbidity and mortality.[10] Bronchoscopy is the gold standard for both clinically suspected and occult dehiscence, as affected patients are often asymptomatic with normal imaging studies.[8,11] However, radiographic findings suggestive of dehiscence include delayed presentation of pneumomediastinum or pneumothorax on chest radiograph, as well as bronchial wall irregularities and extraluminal gas on CT.[12] However, it is important to recognize that small linear air pockets may be seen adjacent to normal telescoping bronchial anastomoses.[11]

Bronchial anastomotic stenosis

Anastomotic strictures are the most common airway complication, occurring in approximately 10% of patients.[8,10] Significant stenosis is defined as focal airway narrowing of greater than 70% without improvement with inspiration or expiration.[11] Bronchial stenosis may be suggested on chest radiograph with recurrent lobar collapse or

Table 1
Imaging techniques for lung transplantation

Imaging Techniques	Indication	Imaging Pearls
Chest radiograph	• Initial screening examination	• Fast, portable, and low radiation • Low sensitivity and specificity
Contrast-enhanced CT	• Evaluation of fluid collections, infection, PTLD, and general complications	• Allows global assessment of the graft and mediastinal anastomoses
Noncontrast CT	• Standard examination for late complications of chronic lung allograft dysfunction	• Exhalation images improve sensitivity for air trapping
NM pulmonary perfusion scintigraphy and CT angiography	• Problem-solving evaluation for suspected vascular complications	• Sedation may be required for CT angiography in young children

Abbreviations: CT, computed tomography; NM, nuclear medicine; PTLD, posttransplant lymphoproliferative disease.

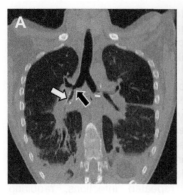 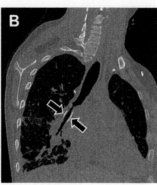

Fig. 3. A 16-year-old girl with cystic fibrosis status post lung transplantation who presented with progressively worsening shortness of breath. (*A*) Coronal bone window CT image shows a focal high grade stenosis (*black arrow*) at the bronchial surgical anastomosis. Also noted is a stent (*white arrow*) located in the bronchus intermedius. (*B*) Oblique sagittal CT image better demonstrates metallic stent (*arrows*) located in the bronchus intermedius.

post obstructive pneumonia. CT is more sensitive, and is useful for preintervention planning by demonstrating the site of focal bronchial narrowing (**Fig. 3**).[10]

Bronchomalacia

Bronchomalacia is a less common airway complication, occurring in approximately 3% of patients, frequently within the first 4 postoperative months.[10] Bronchomalacia represents dynamic airway narrowing of greater than 50% between inspiration and expiration, which may be best demonstrated on bronchoscopy.[13] Inspiration and expiration CT or dynamic CT acquisitions also may demonstrate bronchomalacia in a cooperative patient.[8] Indirect findings on chest radiograph include areas of segmental atelectasis or recurrent infiltrate.[10]

Chronic lung allograft dysfunction

Chronic lung allograft dysfunction (CLAD) remains a significant challenge in all patients with lung transplantation, but is accentuated in children due to their generally longer life expectancy. Long-term survival of pediatric patients with lung transplantation remains lower than that of other pediatric solid organ transplants, with 5-year survival for lung transplant approximately 60% compared with 85% in liver and 98% in kidney transplants.[2,14,15] CLAD is the main reason for this disparity, and eventually affects most patients with lung transplantation.[5,15] No well-proven therapy exists for CLAD.[5] Although bronchiolitis obliterans may be the most familiar form of CLAD, the term encompasses multiple variants, including obstructive and restrictive patterns. The presence of CLAD is defined clinically by spirometry values.[16] Imaging studies demonstrate poor sensitivity for initial disease detection; however, CT evaluation may help differentiate between forms of CLAD, as well as provide additional data as to disease progression.[16]

Bronchiolitis obliterans syndrome

Bronchiolitis obliterans syndrome (BOS) is the most common form of CLAD, and is characterized by progressive airflow obstruction with decreased forced expiratory volume on spirometry.[17] Chest radiographs are often normal. High-resolution CT (HRCT) demonstrates bronchiectasis, bronchial wall thickening, and mosaic air trapping on expiratory sequences (**Fig. 4**).[10]

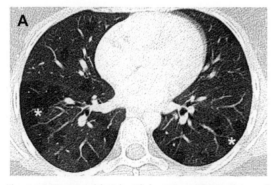 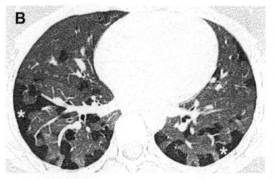

Fig. 4. A 17-year-old girl with lung transplantation and decreasing pulmonary function tests. Axial lung window CT image (*A*) obtained at end-inspiration and axial lung window CT image (*B*) obtained at end-expiration show extensive lobular air trapping (*asterisks*) in both lungs, which are accentuated and more prominent on end-expiration CT image (*B*). Subsequently obtained lung biopsy confirmed the diagnosis of posttransplant bronchiolitis obliterans.

Azithromycin-reversible allograft dysfunction

Azithromycin-reversible allograft dysfunction (ARAD) is a reversible form of allograft dysfunction characterized by improvement in spirometry and radiographic abnormalities following treatment with azithromycin.[3] Although the acute features are reversible, ARAD has been shown to correlate with impaired long-term survival.[17] HRCT findings of ARAD overlap with BOS, and include geographic air trapping, bronchial wall thickening, and bronchiectasis. However, the presence centrilobular and tree in bud micronodules may be helpful in differentiating ARAD from BOS, although acute infection must be excluded. Micronodules that are seen with ARAD on CT should resolve following azithromycin treatment.[17]

Restrictive allograft syndrome

Restrictive allograft syndrome (RAS) is a restrictive/fibrotic form of CLAD that affects approximately 30% of transplant recipients. Compared with BOS, patients with RAS have a poorer prognosis, with a median survival of less than 2 years.[18] RAS demonstrates an upper lobe predilection, with a fibrotic pattern on imaging. Chest radiograph may reveal persistent upper lobe–predominant infiltrates with signs of volume loss. HRCT may demonstrate upper lobe–predominant peripheral consolidations, septal and subpleural thickening, reticular-nodular or mosaic ground-glass opacities, peripheral predominant traction bronchiectasis, and air trapping.[7,12]

Acute fibrinoid organizing pneumonia

Acute fibrinoid organizing pneumonia (AFOP) is an additional rare form of restrictive lung injury that occurs more frequently in patients with lung transplantation. HRCT demonstrates consolidations and ground-glass opacities with interlobular septal thickening.[19] Given its rarity compared with infection, AFOP should be considered in the presence of persistent radiographic findings with absent infectious symptoms or lack of response to infectious therapies.[17]

Infections

Infection is a significant challenge following lung transplantation.[5] Multiple factors contribute to the high rate of posttransplant infection, including high level of immunosuppression, graft exposure to infectious agents via the airway, and reduced mucociliary and lymphatic clearance.[12] In addition, patients with cystic fibrosis may be colonized with atypical or resistant organisms (**Fig. 5**).[20] A full description of the varied imaging findings seen in pulmonary infections is beyond the scope of this article. However, radiologists should be familiar

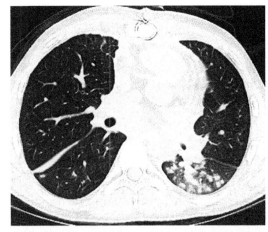

Fig. 5. A 15-year-old boy with lung transplantation secondary to cystic fibrosis. Axial lung window CT image shows multiple nodular opacities in the left lower lobe, which was found to be pseudomonas infection. Also noted is sternotomy.

with the common trends in infection etiology by time of onset posttransplantation.

Within the first month posttransplantation, bacterial and fungal infections are commonly seen. Angioinvasive aspergillus is a particularly morbid fungal infection that can occur during this period. Viral pneumonias commonly occur in the second to sixth months posttransplantation. Viral respiratory infections are particularly common following pediatric lung transplantation, and are associated with decreased 1-year survival.[21] Immunosuppression is typically lower following the sixth month, leading to fewer opportunistic infections. Late infections frequently include community-acquired viral or bacterial organisms, as well as reactivation of latent *Mycobacterium tuberculosis*.[7]

LIVER TRANSPLANTATION

Orthotopic liver transplantation (OLT) is the treatment of choice for children and adults with end-stage liver disease. In the adult population, the etiology of liver failure is frequently viral hepatitis, nonalcoholic steatosis, or alcoholic liver disease. In contrast, in children, cholestatic liver disease, particularly biliary atresia, is the most common cause of liver failure.[14] Other indications for OLT in children include acute liver failure, primary sclerosing cholangitis, and malignancy such as hepatoblastoma.[14] Pediatric OLT remains a complicated surgery with many potential complications; however, 5-year survival remains greater than 80%.[14] In contrast, overall adult OLT 5-year survival is close to 75%.[14] Intermediate and late-term complications include infection, biliary tract obstruction, vascular compromise, rejection, lymphoproliferative disease, and recurrence of the original disease.

Surgical Techniques

Surgical technique can vary widely, particularly in pediatric OLT, depending on patient and donor size as well as vascular and biliary anatomy. A full understanding of each patient's postoperative anatomy is essential for imaging evaluation. In addition to the typical whole-liver transplant performed in adult patients, children may receive split liver or segmental grafts.[22] Left lateral segment transplants may be positioned with the neo-porta hepatis at the right lateral aspect of the graft within the far right lateral peritoneal cavity, leading to a characteristic position of the biliary and vascular structures within the abdomen (**Fig. 6**).

Although hepatic arterial (HA) anastomoses are typically performed end-to-end in a fishmouth fashion, vascular conduits arising from the infrarenal aorta may be used if the recipient's hepatic artery is too small, or in the case of recurrent transplant or HA thrombosis.[23] In the presence of accessory hepatic arteries, multiple anastomoses may be performed.[23] An end-to-end anastomosis is typically performed between the main portal vein (PV) of the recipient and donor. However, interposition grafts may be used in the setting of PV thrombosis or when there is substantial caliber discrepancy between the recipient and donor PV.[22] Hepatic vein (HV) anastomosis is frequently performed in a "piggyback" technique in children, with end-to-side or side-to-side anastomosis of the donor HVs or inferior vena cava (IVC) to the preserved recipient IVC (**Fig. 7**).[22]

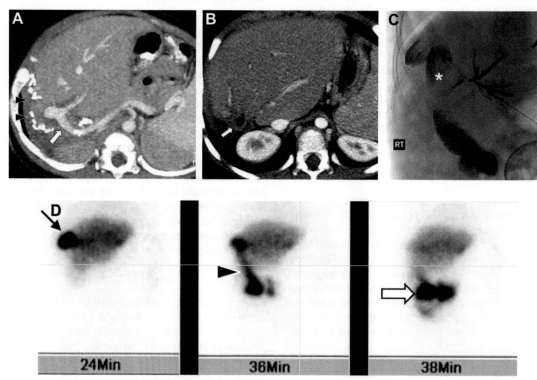

Fig. 6. A 6-month-old boy who is status post left lateral segment liver transplantation. (*A*) Axial enhanced soft tissue window setting CT image demonstrates expected position of reduced-size left lateral segment transplant. Surgical clips (*arrowheads*) are present along the cut liver edge. The extrahepatic PV (*arrow*) courses posterior to the liver before entering the liver along the lateral cut edge. (*B*) Axial enhanced soft tissue window setting CT image shows the position of the hepaticojejunostomy roux loop (*arrow*) along the right lateral liver edge, which should not be mistaken for a fluid collection. (*C*) Frontal fluoroscopic image during percutaneous transhepatic cholangiogram again shows contrast filling the hepaticojejunostomy roux loop (*asterisk*) in the far lateral right upper quadrant, which should not be mistaken for a bile leak. (*D*) Frontal planar images during NM HIDA scan demonstrate temporary accumulation of radiotracer (*black arrow*) at the hepaticojejunostomy roux loop in the right upper quadrant, followed by expected progressive drainage into the distal portions of the roux loop (*arrowhead*) along the right liver edge and downstream bowel (*white arrow*). It is important to know the position of the roux loop to avoid erroneously attributing intraluminal radiotracer to a bile leak.

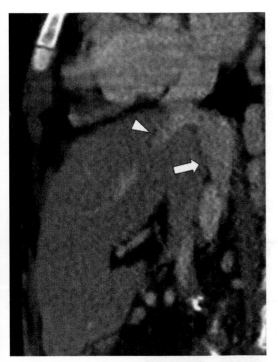

Fig. 7. A 13-year-old boy who is status post whole-liver transplantation. Sagittal enhanced soft tissue window setting CT image shows the normal appearance of piggyback IVC anastomosis. The native IVC (*arrow*) is preserved and courses posteriorly to the liver, with the donor HVs (*arrowhead*) anastomosed at the superior aspect.

Because of the high prevalence of biliary atresia in the pediatric OLT population, biliary reconstruction is frequently performed via hepaticojejunostomy in a Roux-en-Y configuration.[22] End-to-end common bile duct anastomoses may be performed in the absence of underlying biliary disease.

Imaging Techniques and Normal Findings

Sonography is rapid and easily accessible, and is therefore the first choice for the evaluation of liver transplants in the immediate and late postoperative periods (Fig. 8). A summary of normal sonographic findings following liver transplantation is listed in Box 2. Additional imaging strategies for the evaluation of complications include the use of CT, MR, and NM, as outlined in Table 2.

Vascular Complications

Hepatic artery thrombosis

Hepatic artery thrombosis (HAT) carries a high mortality and rate of graft loss. The reported incidence of HAT varies widely, occurring in 1% to 26% of children and 2% to 9% of adults.[24,25] Doppler ultrasound has high accuracy (85%–92%) in identifying HAT.[26] Sonographic findings include an absence of color flow or Doppler signal in the extrahepatic or intrahepatic arteries (Fig. 9). CT or MR angiography may be used in inconclusive cases and will show lack of normal enhancement within the hepatic artery.[22] False negatives may occur in the setting of collateral arteries, in which case the intrahepatic arteries will show parvus-tardus waveforms.[23]

Hepatic artery stenosis

Hepatic artery stenosis (HAS) is more common in pediatric OLT compared with adults,[27] and frequently occurs at the site of anastomosis.[23] Grayscale ultrasound may demonstrate focal arterial narrowing, although this may be difficult to identify, and an absence of this finding does not preclude HAS. Doppler ultrasound may demonstrate focally increased peak systolic velocity (PSV) and aliasing at the site of stenosis, with poststenotic turbulence (Fig. 10). Farther downstream from the stenosis, Doppler ultrasound reveals parvus-tardus waveforms characterized by decreased resistive indices and prolonged acceleration times.[22] However, ultrasound may not detect low-grade stenosis.[22,26] In addition, in the early postoperative period, vasospasm and edema may mimic HAS.[27] CT or MR angiography may demonstrate focal HA narrowing.[22]

Portal vein complications

PV thrombosis occurs in 1% to 2% of all OLT but is more common in children and in reduced-size transplants.[22,23] Acute thrombus may be echogenic or anechoic on ultrasound, with undetectable flow on Doppler.[23] CT or MR imaging may demonstrate a filling defect or lack of internal enhancement. PV thrombus may result in portal hypertension and eventual cavernous transformation.[26]

PV stenosis is a relatively uncommon complication, occurring in 1% to 4% of OLT, but is again more common in reduced-size transplants.[23,27] Up to 5 mm in caliber difference between the donor and recipient portal veins is normal. In the presence of stenosis, Doppler ultrasound demonstrates focally increased PSV and aliasing at the site of focal grayscale luminal narrowing (Fig. 11).[26]

Hepatic veins and inferior vena cava complications

HV and IVC complications are uncommon, occurring in fewer than 2% of patients.[23] A tight abdomen or donor-recipient size discrepancy may result in rotation and torqueing of the HV anastomosis, resulting in pseudostenosis that may resolve with changes in patient or graft position.[27,28] Piggyback IVC anastomoses, commonly used in pediatrics, are more prone to complications, such as Budd-

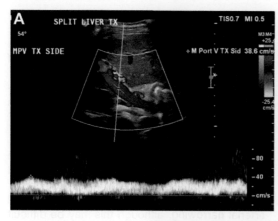
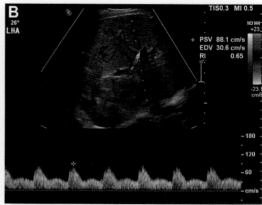
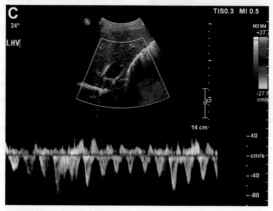

Fig. 8. A 12-year-old girl who is 5 days status post split liver transplantation, undergoing routine screening evaluation. (*A*) Transverse Doppler ultrasound image shows the normal appearance of the PV, with hepatopetal flow, monophasic waveform, and PSV of less than 40 cm/s. (*B*) Transverse Doppler ultrasound image shows the normal appearance of the hepatic artery, with sharp upstroke and RI of 0.65. A normal hepatic artery RI is typically between 0.50 and 0.80. (*C*) Transverse Doppler ultrasound image shows the normal appearance of the hepatic vein with a triphasic waveform.

Chiari syndrome.[26] Stenosis or thrombus may result in monophasic waveforms, although this finding is nonspecific. Other sonographic findings of stenosis include focal grayscale narrowing and a 3 to 4 times focal increase in interrogated velocities with color Doppler aliasing.[22]

Biliary Complications

Biliary complications are the second leading cause of graft dysfunction in OLT (behind rejection).[22,26] As the biliary tracts are perfused solely by the HA system, they are vulnerable to ischemia. Biliary complications most frequently occur within the first 3 months after transplantation, but may also occur years later.[26]

Biliary strictures are often detected due to dilated intrahepatic ducts on grayscale ultrasound or magnetic resonance cholangiopancreatography

(MRCP), although ductal dilation also may be seen with intestinal obstruction or extrinsic compression.[22] However, lack of ductal dilatation on ultrasound does not preclude a stricture.[23] If a biliary stricture is suspected clinically despite an absence of ductal dilation, further direct evaluation is needed. In the adult population, endoscopic retrograde cholangiopancreatography is frequently used for biliary assessment and therapeutic intervention. However, as pediatric liver transplants are frequently performed with a Roux-en-Y hepaticojejunostomy, percutaneous cholangiography is often required for direct biliary evaluation and treatment.

Anastomoses are the most common site of stricture, and are characterized by diffuse intrahepatic dilatation with focal anastomotic narrowing (**Fig. 12**).[26] The post-anastomotic common bile duct, if present, should be normal in caliber. Ischemia may result in multifocal biliary strictures,

---

Box 2
Normal sonographic appearance of liver transplant

- Grayscale
  - Homogeneous hepatic parenchyma
  - Small perihepatic fluid collections are common
  - Mild focal widening at hepatic arterial (HA) anastomosis is common (with fishmouth anastomosis), as is slight narrowing
  - Up to 5-mm caliber change at portal vein (PV) anastomosis is normal
- Color Doppler
  - Homogeneous flow within insonated vessels, without turbulence
- Spectral Doppler
  - HA demonstrates a sharp upstroke with peak systolic velocity (PSV) of less than 200 cm/s and resistive index (RI) of 0.5 to 0.8
  - PV demonstrates hepatopedal flow with mild phasicity and PSV between 16 and 40 cm/s
  - Hepatic veins demonstrate triphasic waveform without turbulence, aliasing, or focally increased PSV

---

typified by focal or diffuse intrahepatic biliary dilatation on grayscale ultrasound, and multifocal narrowing on MRCP or percutaneous cholangiogram (see **Fig. 9**D). The hepatic artery should be carefully evaluated in these cases. Other etiologies of multifocal biliary strictures include infection and recurrence of pretransplant diseases, such as primary sclerosing cholangitis.[27]

Biliary leaks are a common early complication following OLT.[26] Leaks may result in a perihepatic biloma, characterized by complex or simple fluid collection on grayscale sonography (**Fig. 13**). Alternatively, patients may present with diffuse peritonitis.[23] In the presence of a bile leak, NM hepatoiminodiacetic acid (HIDA) scans may demonstrate a focal extraluminal collection of radiotracer that does not dissipate on delayed imaging.[26] Small leaks may be detected only by presence of radiotracer in a surgical drain. MR imaging with a hepatocyte-specific contrast agent also may be helpful for detecting small leaks.[29]

RENAL TRANSPLANTATION

Renal transplantation is generally accepted as the optimal treatment for children and adults with end-stage renal disease. Historically, higher complication rates have been documented in pediatric renal transplant recipients when compared with their adult counterparts. The highest vascular complication rates were seen with transplanting small pediatric grafts into small pediatric recipients, which has led to the general practice of avoiding transplanting infant or young child donor kidneys into infant or young child recipients. Rather, several centers transplant adult kidneys into children above a weight threshold of 6.5 to 10.0 kg.[30] Kidneys of small children are allocated to adults and typically

---

Table 2
Imaging techniques for liver transplant evaluation

Imaging Technique	Indications	Imaging Pearls
Grayscale and Doppler sonography	• Mainstay of orthotopic liver transplantation evaluation	• Knowledge of each patient's surgical technique is essential to fully evaluate all vessels
Computed tomography angiography	• Problem-solving modality to evaluate vasculature and anastomoses, particularly when Doppler is indeterminate	• May require multiple phases
Magnetic resonance cholangiopancreatography	• Problem-solving modality to evaluate for biliary stricture and leak	• Biliary-specific contrast agents may improve visualization
Angiography and endoscopic retrograde cholangiography or percutaneous cholangiography	• Direct vascular and biliary assessment	• Provides opportunity for therapeutic intervention
Nuclear medicine hepatoiminodiacetic acid biliary scintigraphy	• Evaluate for biliary leaks	• Include surgical drains within imaging field of view to detect radiotracer within drains

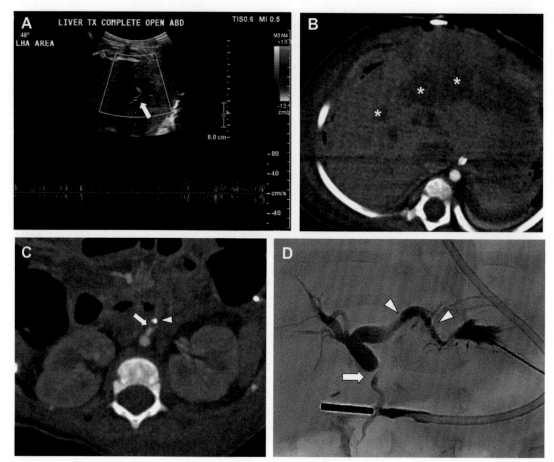

Fig. 9. An 11-month-old girl who is 8 days status post whole-liver transplantation with rising hepatic enzymes. (*A*) Transverse Doppler ultrasound image in the expected region of the left hepatic artery (HA) demonstrates lack of color or spectral Doppler flow. No arterial flow was seen throughout the transplant. The adjacent PV (*arrow*) shows normal hepatopetal flow. (*B*) Axial arterial phase enhanced CT image again demonstrates lack of arterial enhancement throughout the liver. Patchy areas of hypoattenuation (*asterisks*) likely represent infarcts. (*C*) Axial arterial phase enhanced CT image shows the infrarenal vascular graft supplying the hepatic artery, with abrupt cutoff (*arrow*) approximately 1 cm from the origin adjacent to a surgical clip (*arrowhead*). Knowledge of each patient's postsurgical anatomy is essential for accurate assessment. (*D*) Frontal fluoroscopic image during percutaneous transhepatic cholangiogram demonstrates multifocal areas of biliary irregularity and stenosis (*arrowheads*), most prominent at the biliary anastomosis (*arrow*). Multifocal biliary strictures are a common ischemic complication of HA thrombosis.

transplanted "en bloc," with both kidneys transplanted together into one adult recipient.[30] More recently, improved survival rates have been seen in renal transplant recipients younger than 5 years of age, likely reflecting refinements in surgical technique, improved donor selection, and better immunosuppression regimens.[30]

Surgical Techniques

There are several important differences in the surgical approach for pediatric patients (<30 kg) undergoing renal transplantation compared with adults, some of which relate to the higher frequency of obstructive uropathy in children.

Children with posterior urethral valves may require an open vesicostomy for urinary bladder decompression before renal transplantation, which may be left in place for months after transplantation.[30] Furthermore, children with small urinary bladder capacity may require augmentation before transplantation.[30] In children weighing less than 10 kg, the graft is most commonly placed intraperitoneally, as opposed to extraperitoneally in adults, although some centers have reported favorable results with an extraperitoneal approach for small children.[31,32] In small children, the arterial and venous anastomoses are typically to the aorta and IVC, rather than to the iliac vessels.[30]

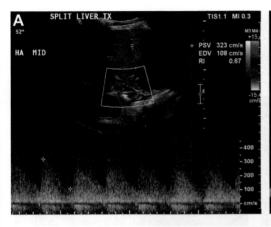

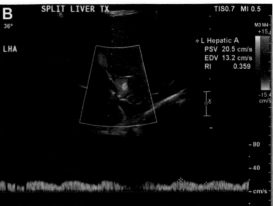

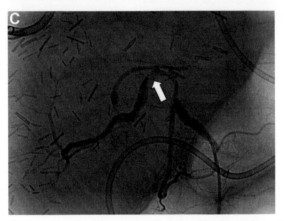

Fig. 10. A 1-year-old girl who is 2 months status post left lateral segment liver transplantation undergoing routine follow-up imaging. Interrogation of the native hepatic artery (HA) (not shown) demonstrated a normal waveform with sharp upstroke and RI of 0.74. (A) Transverse Doppler ultrasound image of the HA anastomosis shows marked increase in PSV to 323 cm/s with aliasing and turbulence. (B) Transverse Doppler ultrasound image of the intrahepatic arteries demonstrates parvus-tardus waveforms with abnormally low RI of 0.36. (C) Frontal digital subtracted angiographic image during common hepatic artery injection confirms anastomotic stenosis (arrow).

Imaging Techniques and Normal Findings

Sonography is the primary imaging tool for assessing the graft for immediate as well as late postoperative complications. A summary of normal sonographic findings is listed in Box 3 and demonstrated in Fig. 14. Other modalities, such as CT, MR, and scintigraphy have important, specific roles in the diagnosis of postoperative complications, as detailed in Table 3. Importantly, children undergoing MR or CT examinations may require sedation.

Vascular Complications

Vascular complications are relatively common, especially in young patients, and are associated with significantly decreased graft survival.[33]

Vascular complications include complete or partial occlusion of graft inflow or outflow. Both thrombosis and kinks may cause either complete or partial vascular occlusion. Vascular stenosis is an additional cause of partial occlusion.

Transplant renal artery stenosis (Fig. 15) is the most common vascular complication, with an incidence between 4.6% and 9.0% in children[34,35] and between 0.9% and 8.0% in adults.[36] Gray-scale sonography may delineate the focal luminal narrowing of renal artery stenosis with corresponding increased peak systolic velocities and aliasing on Doppler interrogation. Beyond the site of renal artery stenosis, Doppler evaluation shows poststenotic turbulence and a characteristic downstream "tardus-parvus" waveform.

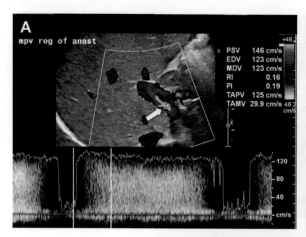
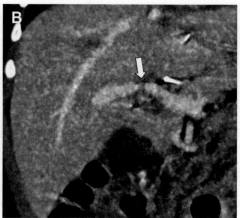
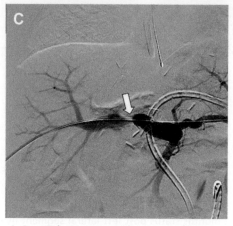

Fig. 11. A 7-month-old girl who is 2 months status post liver transplantation. Imaging evaluation for elevated liver enzymes revealed PV stenosis. Doppler interrogation of the pre-anastomotic PV (not shown) demonstrated a normal monophasic waveform and PSV of 28 cm/s. (*A*) Transverse Doppler ultrasound image of the PV anastomosis shows marked increase in PSV to 146 cm/s with color aliasing (*arrow*) and turbulence. (*B*) Coronal enhanced soft tissue window CT image demonstrates focal narrowing (*arrow*) at the site of stenosis. (*C*) Frontal digital subtracted angiographic image during PV injection confirms focal stenosis (*arrow*).

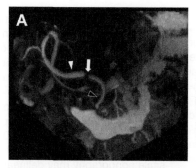
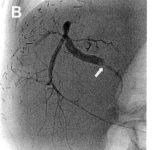

Fig. 12. A 6-month-old boy who is 1 month status post left lateral segment liver transplant. Imaging evaluation for elevated bilirubin found a biliary anastomotic stricture. Sonographic evaluation of the graft (not shown) showed no evidence of biliary ductal dilatation. (*A*) Coronal thick slab maximum intensity projection (MIP) nonenhanced T2-weighted MRCP image demonstrates mild dilation of the donor common bile duct (*white arrowhead*) with abrupt narrowing at the anastomosis (*arrow*). The distal common bile duct (CBD) is decompressed (*black arrowhead*). (*B*) Frontal fluoroscopic image during percutaneous transhepatic cholangiogram confirms the presence of anastomotic stenosis (*arrow*).

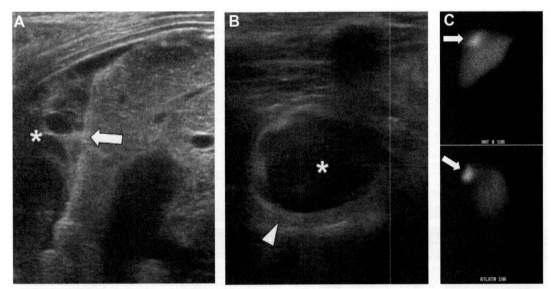

Fig. 13. A 3-year-old boy who is 5 days status post left split liver transplantation. Transverse (*A*) and longitudinal (*B*) grayscale sonographic images demonstrate a complex fluid collection (*asterisks*) adjacent to the superior cut edge of the liver (*A, arrow*) with thick organized rim (*B, arrowhead*). (*C*) Planar 1-hour delay images from NM HIDA biliary scintigraphy demonstrates a corresponding focal collection of radiotracer adjacent to the superior cut edge (*arrow*), consistent with bile leak.

Thrombosis of the transplant renal artery shows grayscale findings of luminal low-level echoes and color Doppler absent or decreased flow, depending on whether the occlusion is complete or partial, respectively. Similar to renal artery stenosis, partial arterial thrombosis shows an elevated velocity in the area of luminal narrowing, in this case related to thrombosis, with a characteristic downstream "tardus-parvus" waveform.

Urinary Complications

In children, urinary complications are more common than vascular complications, and in rare cases, may lead to graft loss. In particular, Irtan and colleagues[37] found that pediatric patients with posterior urethral valves had a significantly higher rate of urologic complications after renal transplantation. Urologic complications include vesicoureteral reflux (VUR), ureteral stricture or obstruction, and urine leak, either related to anastomotic leak or ureteral necrosis. VUR is the most common urologic complication in children (**Fig. 16**), with an incidence of 12%.[37] In adults, the 2 most common collecting system complications are urine leak and obstruction.[36] Pediatric patients with renal transplantation and VUR typically present with a urinary tract infection. Voiding cystourethrogram shows reflux of contrast into the transplant collecting system, and occasionally into the native ureter. Ureteral stricture or obstruction is suggested by increasing transplant collecting system dilation on sonography, and may be confirmed with either renal scintigraphy or MR urogram (MRU). Urine leaks may be suspected with increasing perinephric fluid collection

---

Box 3
Renal transplant: normal sonographic findings

- Grayscale sonography
  - Corticomedullary differentiation is preserved
  - Trace fullness of the central collecting system may be seen
  - Trace perinephric fluid is common
- Color or Power Doppler
  - Homogeneous perfusion of the renal transplant
- Spectral waveform analysis
  - Arcuate parenchymal arteries show brisk upstrokes and resistive index between 0.50 and 0.80
  - Main renal artery demonstrates brisk upstroke and PSV less than 200 cm/s
  - Main renal vein shows phasic waveform without focal turbulence or aliasing

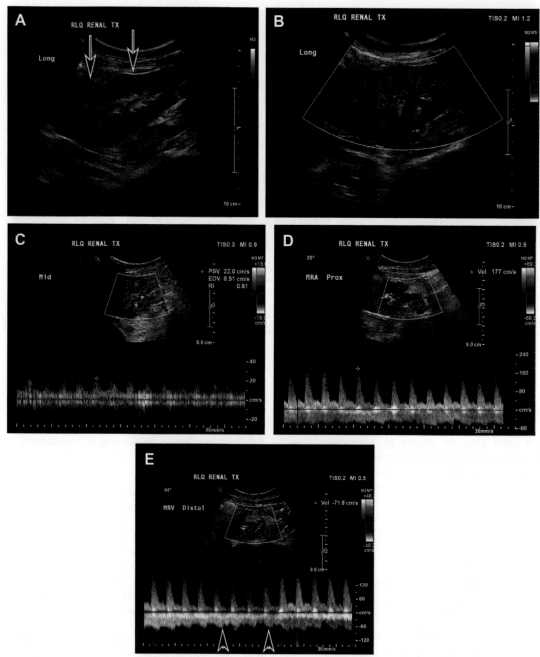

Fig. 14. An 8-year-old girl undergoing routine evaluation on postoperative day 1 after renal transplantation. (*A*) Longitudinal grayscale sonogram shows normal echogenicity and preservation of corticomedullary junction of the graft (*arrows*) in the right lower quadrant. (*B*) Longitudinal power Doppler ultrasound image shows homogeneous perfusion throughout the graft, without focal defect. (*C*) Transverse Doppler ultrasound image shows insonation of an arcuate artery in the midzone with a normal waveform and RI of 0.61. (*D*) Transverse Doppler ultrasound image shows insonation of the proximal portion of the transplant main renal artery, with a normal waveform and PSV of 177 cm/s. (*E*) Transverse Doppler ultrasound image of the main transplant renal vein shows a normal, biphasic waveform (*arrowheads*) and velocity of 71 cm/s. Small amounts of arterial contamination are noted above the baseline.

Table 3
Imaging techniques for pediatric renal transplant evaluation

Imaging Technique	Indication	Imaging Pearls
Sonography	• Grayscale, color Doppler, and spectral waveform sonography are the mainstays of screening and diagnostic evaluation	• Easily performed at the bedside • Rarely requires sedation in children • Avoids ionizing radiation
Noncontrast CT	• Evaluation of renal and bladder stones	• Dual-energy CT allows for compositional analysis of renal and bladder calculi
Contrast-enhanced CT	• Evaluation of fluid collections, PTLD, and general complications	• Allows global assessment of the graft with respect to adjacent structures, such as compression by fluid collections
Contrast-enhanced CT angiogram and MR angiogram	• Assessment of vasculature, particularly anastomoses	• Use of gadolinium contrast agents is contraindicated in patients with renal dysfunction
MRU and CTU	• Assessment of cortical scarring and collecting system complications	• Use of gadolinium contrast agents is contraindicated in patients with renal dysfunction
DMSA renal scintigraphy	• Assessment of parenchymal scarring	• Focal defects are nonspecific and may indicate scarring or infection
Diuretic technetium^{99m} MAG3 renography	• Physiologic assessment of function, scarring, and collecting system complications	• Renal scintigraphy and MRU are preferred over CTU for the assessment of collecting system obstruction and leak
Voiding cystourethrogram (VCUG)	• Detection of vesicoureteral reflux	• Vesicoureteral reflux is a relatively common complication in children after renal transplantation

Abbreviations: CT, computed tomography; CTU, CT urogram; DMSA, dimercaptosuccinic acid; MRU, MR urogram; NM, nuclear medicine; PTLD, posttransplant lymphoproliferative disease.

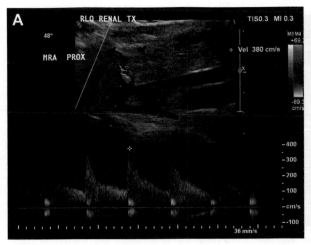
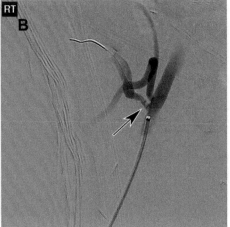

Fig. 15. A 16-year-old girl who was status post renal transplantation 8 months prior, with suspected recurrent transplant renal artery stenosis. (*A*) Longitudinal Doppler ultrasound image demonstrates insonation of the transplant renal artery with an elevated velocity of 380 cm/s and spectral broadening. (*B*) Frontal conventional arteriography shows narrowing of the proximal aspect of the inferiormost (*arrow*) of 2 transplant renal arteries.

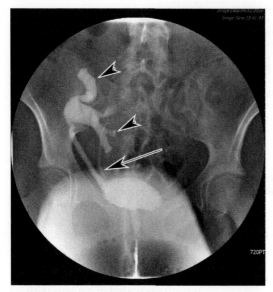

Fig. 16. A 15-year-old girl with a urinary tract infection 1 year after renal transplantation. Frontal fluoroscopic image from a voiding cystourethrogram shows vesicoureteral reflux into the transplant kidney collecting system (*arrowheads*), as well as into the native distal right ureter (*arrow*).

or urine ascites. Renal scintigraphy or MRU is used to confirm the diagnosis, and demonstrates extraluminal activity or excreted extraluminal contrast, respectively.

Post Biopsy Complications

Biopsies of the renal graft are an important method of diagnosing rejection, as well as other causes of graft dysfunction that may be radiologically or clinically occult. Percutaneous biopsy of the renal graft confers a lower complication rate than biopsy of the native kidney, with a major complication rate of 1.9% to 4.0%.[38] The most common biopsy-related complication is bleeding, which may manifest as macroscopic hematuria or a perinephric hematoma.[39] Arteriovenous fistula (AVF) is also a common complication (**Fig. 17**), and when large, can impair graft function or cause hypertension, requiring embolization. AVF demonstrates high-velocity flow, systolic pulsatility, and a low resistive index (<0.50) on Doppler interrogation. Pseudoaneurysm is a relatively rare complication of biopsy, related to arterial injury and constituting a contained arterial rupture. On sonographic evaluation, pseudoaneurysms are anechoic on grayscale sonography and have a characteristic "yin and yang" sign on color Doppler, representing multidirectional, swirling vascular flow. Symptomatic pseudoaneurysms occasionally also require surgical treatment or embolization.[39]

POSTOPERATIVE FLUID COLLECTIONS

Postoperative fluid collections are a common occurrence after the various types of organ transplantations, including lung, liver, and renal transplantation.[40–42] Postoperative fluid collections can be further characterized as hematomas, lymphoceles, and abscesses. In liver transplantation, the differential diagnosis also would include a bile leak, whereas after renal transplantation, urinoma also may be considered.

Following lung transplantation, postoperative fluid collections are typically confined to the pleural

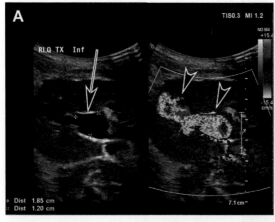
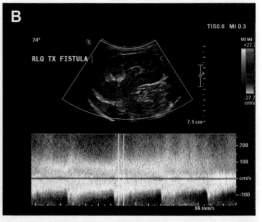

Fig. 17. A 15-year-old boy with decreasing renal function after renal transplantation. (*A*) Transverse color-compare grayscale and color Doppler sonogram shows an anechoic structure (*arrow*) within the inferior pole of the graft with turbulent color flow (*arrowheads*). (*B*) Longitudinal Doppler ultrasound image shows turbulent, high-velocity arterial flow, consistent with an arteriovenous fistula, which was subsequently embolized by interventional radiology (not shown).

spaces, as in the case hemothorax, chylothorax, and empyema, with the exception of fluid collections associated with the wound. After liver transplantation, postoperative fluid collections are typically perihepatic, although they may extend into the intraperitoneal space with increasing size. Fluid collections after renal transplantation are typically perinephric in location, although fluid may expand further into either the intraperitoneal or retroperitoneal spaces, depending on the location of the graft. Lymphoceles in the setting of renal transplants are typically located between the graft and the bladder.[43]

Fluid collections can to some extent be differentiated based on their clinical course. Hemothorax is suspected when there is increasing bloody pleural drain output. Hematomas and seromas are most commonly seen in the immediate postoperative period, although lymphoceles may also present later in the postoperative period.[44] Fluid collections in general can become symptomatic when large (**Fig. 18**). Abscesses are most common 1 to 3 weeks after transplantation.[43] Due to immunosuppression, transplant recipients may have a blunted clinical response to an abscess, and sampling of fluid collections may be necessary for definitive diagnosis.

Imaging plays an important role in both the detection and characterization of fluid collections. On sonography, hematomas demonstrate internal echoes (see **Fig. 18**) and sometimes septations as they organize. Abscesses also show internal complexity on sonography and are typically loculated collections with a defined hyperemic wall. Seromas are usually anechoic collections. In the setting of liver or renal transplants, sonography may be used to assess compromised graft inflow and outflow related to the collection. CT and MR also may be used to characterize postoperative fluid collections. Internal attenuation of 30 to 40 Hounsfield units (HU) is suggestive of hematoma, abscess, or empyema, whereas the attenuation of lymphoceles and chylothorax is closer to 0 HU. Gas within a collection is suggestive of abscess[45] or empyema. MR can help to distinguish hematoma from other fluid collections with the demonstration of blooming on gradient echo sequences.

POSTTRANSPLANT LYMPHOPROLIFERATIVE DISEASE AND OTHER POSTTRANSPLANT MALIGNANCIES

Patients with hematopoietic stem cell (HSCT) and solid organ transplantation are at increased risk for malignancy, with PTLD being the most common malignant complication. Most cases of PTLD are associated with the Epstein-Barr virus (EBV). Children who are EBV seronegative are at increased risk for PTLD when they receive a graft from an EBV seropositive donor.[46] The risk of PTLD in HSCT is 4%, although can be as high as 10% to 20% in patients with HSCT with multiple risk factors.[47] The risk of PTLD in patients with solid organ transplantation varies with degree and type of immunosuppression. Overall, PTLD occurs in 2% to 10% of patients with lung transplantation, and 1% to 3% of patients with liver or renal transplantation.[46] There is a bimodal temporal distribution of PTLD, with a peak in the first year after transplantation and a second peak 4 to 5 years after transplantation.[46]

PTLD constitutes a diverse group of entities that range from somewhat benign lymphoid

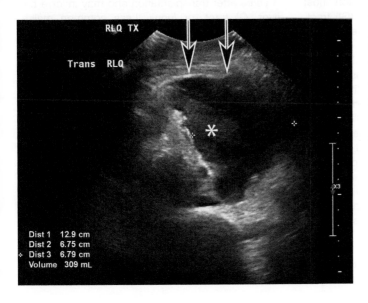

Fig. 18. A 17-year-old boy on postoperative day 1 after renal transplantation who presented with increasing incisional pain and fullness. Reexploration revealed a perinephric hematoma. Transverse grayscale sonogram demonstrates a perinephric fluid collection (*arrows, and demarcated by cursors*) inferior to the graft with low-level internal echoes (*asterisk*).

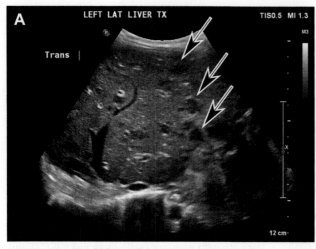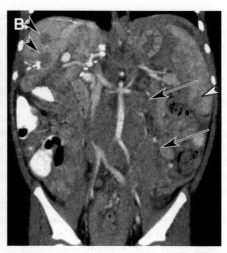

Fig. 19. A 3-year-old boy who presented 2 years after liver transplantation for surveillance ultrasound. Subsequent biopsy was consistent with posttransplant lymphoproliferative disorder. (*A*) Transverse grayscale sonogram shows multiple hypoechoic lesions (*arrows*) throughout the graft. (*B*) Coronal contrast-enhanced CT image shows multiple hypodense lesions (*black arrowheads*) within the transplanted liver, as well as bulky retroperitoneal lymphadenopathy (*arrows*) and subtle hypodense splenic lesions (*white arrowhead*). Hypodense renal lesions (not shown) also were present.

hyperplasia to poorly differentiated lymphoma. Children are at increased risk of PTLD-associated lymphoma compared with adults.[48] Importantly, tissue sampling is essential for establishing a diagnosis. Imaging allows for delineating extent of disease, and monitoring response to treatment and progression. PTLD can be nodal or extranodal. Nodal disease typically involves either the mediastinum or retroperitoneum. In contrast, extranodal PTLD may involve the gastrointestinal tract, solid organs, or central nervous system. PTLD most commonly involves the allografts after liver and lung transplantation. In contrast, PTLD after renal transplantation most frequently involves the gastrointestinal (GI) tract, followed by the central nervous system (CNS) and kidneys.[46]

Although ultrasound may detect PTLD on surveillance imaging, CT or FDG-PET CT is typically used both for staging as well as for identifying suitable targets for tissue sampling.[49] Importantly, fludeoxyglucose (FDG) PET CT is superior to CT for evaluating suspected PTLD, with the potential to both detect occult disease and upstage extent.[50,51] At imaging, nodal PTLD is characterized by enlarged, hypoenhancing lymphadenopathy on CT, which demonstrates avidity on FDG-PET. Extranodal disease involving the GI tract can manifest as nodules or infiltrating soft tissue density within the peritoneum, as well as bowel wall thickening, aneurysmal dilation, polypoid masses, or ulceration of bowel segments.[46] Solid organ involvement may be present as solitary or

multiple hypoenhancing masses on CT (**Fig. 19**), which are avid on FDG-PET and demonstrate low T1-weighted and T2-weighted signal on MR.[46] CNS involvement is typically evaluated by MR, and usually presents as multiple, low T1-weighted and high T2-weighted signal intensity, homogeneously or rim-enhancing lesions with surrounding edema.[46] Most common sites of CNS involvement of PTLD include the basal ganglia and subcortical white matter.[46]

Posttransplant smooth muscle spindle cell tumors are also associated with EBV, but are exceedingly rare. On average, these tumors occur 4 years after transplantation and may involve the liver, GI tract, or lungs. Less common malignancies after HSCT and solid organ transplantation include nonmelanomatous skin cancer and Kaposi sarcoma.[52–54] Of note, Kaposi sarcoma can mimic PTLD involvement of the lungs, and should be included in the differential diagnosis of posttransplant patients with multiple lung lesions on imaging.

SUMMARY

Lung, liver, and renal transplantation offers definitive treatment for patients with the respective end-organ failure. Although survival rates in general are high, familiarity with the normal postoperative appearance as well as the imaging appearance of complications is essential to ensure best outcomes. Delayed complications, such as PTLD, may occur years after transplantation, and therefore, it is important that the radiologist maintains a high level of suspicion in this population.

DISCLOSURE

The authors have nothing to disclose.

REFERENCES

1. Sweet SC, Wong H-H, Webber SA, et al. Pediatric transplantation in the United States, 1995–2004. Am J Transplant 2006;6(5p2):1132–52.
2. Valapour M, Lehr CJ, Skeans MA, et al. OPTN/SRTR 2017 annual data report: lung. Am J Transplant 2019;19(S2):404–84.
3. Sweet SC. Pediatric lung transplantation. Respir Care 2017;62(6):776–98.
4. Goldfarb SB, Hayes D, Levvey BJ, et al. The International Thoracic Organ Transplant Registry of the International Society for Heart and Lung Transplantation: Twenty-first Pediatric Lung and Heart–Lung Transplantation Report—2018; focus theme: multiorgan transplantation. J Heart Lung Transplant 2018; 37(10):1196–206.
5. Benden C. Pediatric lung transplantation. J Thorac Dis 2017;9(8):2675–83.
6. Madan R, Chansakul T, Goldberg H. Imaging in lung transplants: checklist for the radiologist. Indian J Radiol Imaging 2014;24(4):318.
7. Habre C, Soccal PM, Triponez F, et al. Radiological findings of complications after lung transplantation. Insights Imaging 2018;9(5):709–19.
8. Crespo MM, McCarthy DP, Hopkins PM, et al. ISHLT Consensus Statement on adult and pediatric airway complications after lung transplantation: definitions, grading system, and therapeutics. J Heart Lung Transplant 2018;37(5):548–63.
9. Olland A, Reeb J, Puyraveau M, et al. Bronchial complications after lung transplant are associated with primary lung graft dysfunction and surgical technique. J Heart Lung Transplant 2017;36(2):157–65.
10. Tejwani V, Panchabhai TS, Kotloff RM, et al. Complications of lung transplantation. Chest 2016;149(6):1535–45.
11. Luecke K, Trujillo C, Ford J, et al. Anastomotic airway complications after lung transplant: clinical, bronchoscopic and CT correlation. J Thorac Imaging 2016;31(5):W62–71.
12. Chia E, Babawale SN. Imaging features of intrathoracic complications of lung transplantation: what the radiologists need to know. World J Radiol 2017;9(12):438–47.
13. Jokerst C, Sirajuddin A, Mohammed T-LH. Imaging the complications of lung transplantation. Radiol Clin North Am 2016;54(2):355–73.
14. Kim WR, Lake JR, Smith JM, et al. OPTN/SRTR 2017 annual data report: liver. Am J Transplant 2019; 19(S2):184–283.
15. Valapour M, Skeans MA, Smith JM, et al. Lung. Am J Transplant 2016;16(S2):141–68.
16. Verleden SE, Vos R, Verleden GM. Chronic lung allograft dysfunction: light at the end of the tunnel? Curr Opin Organ Transplant 2019;24(3):318–23.
17. Hota P, Dass C, Kumaran M, et al. High-resolution CT findings of obstructive and restrictive phenotypes of chronic lung allograft dysfunction: more than just bronchiolitis obliterans syndrome. Am J Roentgenol 2018;211(1):W13–21.
18. Sato M, Waddell TK, Wagnetz U, et al. Restrictive allograft syndrome (RAS): a novel form of chronic lung allograft dysfunction. J Heart Lung Transplant 2011;30(7):735–42.
19. Paraskeva M, McLean C, Ellis S, et al. Acute fibrinoid organizing pneumonia after lung transplantation. Am J Respir Crit Care Med 2013;187(12): 1360–8.
20. Liu M, Worley S, Mallory GB, et al. Fungal infections in pediatric lung transplant recipients: colonization and invasive disease. J Heart Lung Transplant 2009;28(11):1226–30.
21. Respiratory viral infections within one year after pediatric lung transplantâ"Liuâ"2009â"Transplant Infectious Diseaseâ"Wiley Online Library. Available at: https://onlinelibrary-wiley-com.offcampus. lib.washington.edu/doi/full/10.1111/j.1399-3062.2009. 00397.x. Accessed July 18, 2019.
22. Horvat N, Marcelino ASZ, Horvat JV, et al. Pediatric liver transplant: techniques and complications. Radiographics 2017;37(6):1612–31.
23. Berrocal T, Parrón M, Álvarez-Luque A, et al. Pediatric liver transplantation: a pictorial essay of early and late complications. RadioGraphics 2006;26(4): 1187–209.
24. Seda-Neto J, Antunes da Fonseca E, Pugliese R, et al. Twenty years of experience in pediatric living donor liver transplantation: focus on hepatic artery reconstruction, complications, and outcomes. Transplantation 2016;100(5):1066–72.
25. Algarni AA, Mourad MM, Bramhall SR. Anticoagulation and antiplatelets as prophylaxis for hepatic artery thrombosis after liver transplantation. World J Hepatol 2015;7(9):1238–43.
26. Baheti AD, Sanyal R, Heller MT, et al. Surgical techniques and imaging complications of liver transplant. Radiol Clin North Am 2016;54(2):199–215.
27. Caiado AHM, Blasbalg R, Marcelino ASZ, et al. Complications of liver transplantation: multimodality imaging approach. RadioGraphics 2007;27(5):1401–17.
28. Sannananja B, Seyal AR, Baheti AD, et al. Tricky findings in liver transplant imaging: a review of pitfalls with solutions. Curr Probl Diagn Radiol 2018; 47(3):179–88.

29. Akin E, Vitellas K, Rajab A, et al. Magnetic resonance cholangiography with Mangafodipir Trisodium (Teslascan) to evaluate bile duct leaks after T-Tube removal in liver transplantation. J Comput Assist Tomogr 2004;28(5):613–6.

30. Dharnidharka VR, Fiorina P, Harmon WE. Kidney transplantation in children. N Engl J Med 2014; 371(6):549–58.

31. Heap SL, Webb NJA, Kirkman MA, et al. Extraperitoneal renal transplantation in small children results in a transient improvement in early graft function. Pediatr Transplant 2011;15(4):362–6.

32. Vitola SP, Gnatta D, Garcia VD, et al. Kidney transplantation in children weighing less than 15 kg: extraperitoneal surgical access—experience with 62 cases. Pediatr Transplant 2013;17(5):445–53.

33. Rodricks N, Chanchlani R, Banh T, et al. Incidence and risk factors of early surgical complications in young renal transplant recipients: a persistent challenge. Pediatr Transplant 2017;21(7). https://doi.org/10.1111/petr.13006.

34. Fontaine E, Barthelemy Y, Gagnadoux MF, et al. A review of 72 renal artery stenoses in a series of 715 kidney transplantations in children. Prog Urol 1994;4(2):193–205 [in French].

35. Roberts JP, Ascher NL, Fryd DS, et al. Transplant renal artery stenosis. Transplantation 1989;48(4):580–3.

36. Moreno CC, Mittal PK, Ghonge NP, et al. Imaging complications of renal transplantation. Radiol Clin North Am 2016;54(2):235–49.

37. Irtan S, Maisin A, Baudouin V, et al. Renal transplantation in children: critical analysis of age related surgical complications. Pediatr Transplant 2010;14(4):512–9.

38. Morgan TA, Chandran S, Burger IM, et al. Complications of ultrasound-guided renal transplant biopsies. Am J Transplant 2016;16(4):1298–305.

39. Oates A, Ahuja S, Lee MM, et al. Pediatric renal transplant biopsy with ultrasound guidance: the "core" essentials. Pediatr Radiol 2017;47(12):1572–9.

40. Brody MB, Rodgers SK, Horrow MM. Spectrum of normal or near-normal sonographic findings after orthotopic liver transplantation. Ultrasound Q 2008; 24(4):257–65.

41. Kuczynska M, Piasek E, Swiatlowski L, et al. Sonographic assessment of the prevalence and evolution of fluid collections as a complication of kidney transplantation. J Ultrason 2018;18(73):126–32.

42. Chang PT, Frost J, Stanescu AL, et al. Pediatric thoracic organ transplantation: current indications, techniques, and imaging findings. Radiol Clin North Am 2016;54(2):321–38.

43. Erbas B. Peri- and postsurgical evaluations of renal transplant. Semin Nucl Med 2017;47(6):647–59.

44. Gander R, Asensio M, Royo GF, et al. Treatment of post-transplant lymphocele in children. Urology 2017;103:218–23.

45. Boraschi P, Della Pina MC, Donati F. Graft complications following orthotopic liver transplantation: role of non-invasive cross-sectional imaging techniques. Eur J Radiol 2016;85(7):1271–83.

46. Camacho JC, Moreno CC, Harri PA, et al. Posttransplantation lymphoproliferative disease: proposed imaging classification. Radiographics 2014;34(7):2025–38.

47. Ru Y, Chen J, Wu D. Epstein-Barr virus post-transplant lymphoproliferative disease (PTLD) after hematopoietic stem cell transplantation. Eur J Haematol 2018;101(3):283–90.

48. Opelz G, Dohler B. Lymphomas after solid organ transplantation: a collaborative transplant study report. Am J Transplant 2004;4(2):222–30.

49. Absalon MJ, Khoury RA, Phillips CL. Post-transplant lymphoproliferative disorder after solid-organ transplant in children. Semin Pediatr Surg 2017;26(4):257–66.

50. Metser U, Lo G. FDG-PET/CT in abdominal post-transplant lymphoproliferative disease. Br J Radiol 2016;89(1057):20150844.

51. Bianchi E, Pascual M, Nicod M, et al. Clinical usefulness of FDG-PET/CT scan imaging in the management of posttransplant lymphoproliferative disease. Transplantation 2008;85(5):707–12.

52. Mynarek M, Hussein K, Kreipe HH, et al. Malignancies after pediatric kidney transplantation: more than PTLD? Pediatr Nephrol 2014;29(9):1517–28.

53. Karakoyun M, Onen S, Baran M, et al. Post-transplant malignancies in pediatric liver transplant recipients: experience of two centers in Turkey. Turk J Gastroenterol 2018;29(1):89–93.

54. Fogel AL, Miyar M, Teng JMC. Cutaneous malignancies in pediatric solid organ transplant recipients. Pediatr Dermatol 2016;33(6):585–93.

Imaging Assessment of Complications from Transplantation from Pediatric to Adult Patients

Part 2: Hematopoietic Stem Cell Transplantation

Nathan David P. Concepcion, MD[a,b,c,]*, Erin K. Romberg, MD[d], Grace S. Phillips, MD[e], Edward Y. Lee, MD, MPH[f], Bernard F. Laya, MD, DO[b,c,g]

KEYWORDS

- Hematopoietic stem cell transplantation • Bone marrow transplantation • Complications
- Graft-versus-host disease

KEY POINTS

- Hematopoietic stem cell transplantation is transfusion of pluripotent stem cells harvested from the bone marrow, peripheral blood, or fetal cord blood into a recipient to repopulate the marrow and restore hematologic and immunologic competence.
- Various complications are common and may be classified according to time frames following transplantation where the patient's immune status is unique.
- There is predominance of specific infectious pathogens and disease patterns in each phase.
- Imaging appearances of cerebral infections differ from that in immunocompetent hosts but cerebrovascular complications are similar to those seen in the general population.
- Imaging appearances are nonspecific and require microbiologic and/or histopathologic correlation.

INTRODUCTION

Hematopoietic stem cell transplantation (HSCT) is an intravenous transfusion of pluripotent stem cells to repopulate the marrow and restore immunocompetence. However, before transplantation, the patient undergoes a conditioning regimen to eradicate the underlying disease, subsequently resulting in an immunocompromised state. Serious and some life-threatening complications involving any organ can occur. Currently, with advances in HSCT techniques and posttransplant management, more and

[a] Section of Pediatric Radiology, Institute of Radiology, St. Luke's Medical Center-Global City, Rizal Drive cor. 32nd Street and 5th Avenue, Taguig City 1634, Philippines; [b] St. Luke's Medical Center College of Medicine-William H. Quasha Memorial, Quezon City, Philippines; [c] Philippine Society for Pediatric Radiology; [d] Department of Radiology, Seattle Children's Hospital, University of Washington School of Medicine, MA.7. 220, 4800 Sand Point Way Northeast, Seattle, WA 98105, USA; [e] Department of Radiology, Seattle Children's Hospital, University of Washington School of Medicine, MA.7.220, 4800 Sand Point Way Northeast, Seattle, WA 98105, USA; [f] Division of Thoracic Imaging, Department of Radiology, Boston Children's Hospital, Harvard Medical School, 300 Longwood Avenue, Boston, MA 02115, USA; [g] Section of Pediatric Radiology, Institute of Radiology, St. Luke's Medical Center-Quezon City, 279 East Rodriguez Sr. Avenue, Quezon City 1112, Philippines
* Corresponding author.
E-mail address: npconcepcion@stluke.com.ph

Radiol Clin N Am 58 (2020) 569–582
https://doi.org/10.1016/j.rcl.2019.12.006
0033-8389/20/© 2019 Elsevier Inc. All rights reserved.

more pediatric patients are now living longer and into their adulthood.

The goal of this review article is to discuss the common neurologic, pulmonary, and abdominal complications associated with HSCT with emphasis on their imaging characteristics as pediatric patients transition into their adulthood.

BACKGROUND INFORMATION: HEMATOPOIETIC STEM CELL TRANSPLANTATION

HSCT is a procedure where pluripotent stem cells are intravenously transfused into a recipient to repopulate the marrow and restore hematologic and immunologic competence.[1–7] Stem cells can be harvested from the bone marrow, peripheral blood, or fetal cord blood. It is said to be *autologous* when the cells come from the same patient, *syngenic* when from an identical twin, and *allogenic* when from another donor.[1,6–8]

Common clinical indications for HSCT for both children and adults include hematologic malignancies such as leukemia, lymphoma, myelodysplastic syndrome, and multiple myeloma; nonmalignant hematologic disorders such as thalassemia and anemia, specifically sickle cell and aplastic types; solid malignancies; and immunodeficiencies.[1–7,9]

Before transfusion, the patient undergoes a conditioning regimen that involves total-body irradiation and/or high-dose chemotherapy to eradicate the underlying disease and to suppress the immune system, decreasing the risk of rejection. However, this results in an immunocompromised state.[5]

Various serious and life-threatening complications can occur even with advances of medications including immunosuppressants and antibiotic agents. Complications may be classified according to time frames following transplantation where there is a unique immune status of the patient.[1,7,8]

First is the *preengraftment phase*, which includes the time of pretransplant conditioning and up to 30 days posttransplantation. This is characterized by severe bone marrow suppression with pancytopenia particularly neutropenia, disruption of mucosal barrier, cellular and humoral immunodeficiency, and functional asplenia.[1,6–8]

The second phase begins after successful engraftment of the stem cells. This is the *early posttransplantation* or *early postengraftment phase*, which is about 30 to 100 days. In this phase, there is recovery of the neutrophils and mucosal injury, but the delay in the lymphocyte counts results in persistent cellular and humoral deficiency, as well as functional asplenia.[1,6–8] The first and second phases may also be called the *peri-engraftment period*, which is up to 100 days posttransplantation.

After 100 days, the *late posttransplantation* or *late postengraftment phase* ensues. There is relative immune reconstitution with recovery of the lymphocyte counts, but depending on clinical circumstances, the cellular and humoral immune function will recover after a year.[1,6–8]

Posttransplant complications may occur in any organ system,[1] but this review article only focuses on the more common neurologic, pulmonary, and abdominal complications with their imaging characteristics that are encountered in clinical practice.

COMPLICATIONS ASSOCIATED WITH HEMATOPOIETIC STEM CELL TRANSPLANTATION
Neurologic Complications

Neurologic complications occur in 11% to 59% of patients undergoing HSCT.[6,8] Complications could be infectious and noninfectious in nature.

Infectious complications

Preengraftment phase (up to 30 days) The most common neurologic complication is infection.[1] Imaging appearance of cerebral infections differs from that in immunocompetent hosts. The classic imaging findings of infection may be absent due to impaired inflammatory response. There is less or no rim enhancement, mass effect, or edema around the cerebral lesions.[4,6,8,9]

The most common central nervous system (CNS) infections (30%–50%) are caused by invasive *Aspergillus*.[1,6,8,10] Invasive aspergillosis initially develops in the paranasal sinuses and lungs. Extension into the brain occurs by 2 main possible mechanisms. One is via hematogenous spread from the lungs, which causes either infectious vasculopathy leading to multiple randomly distributed infarctions or hemorrhages in 25% of cases or extension into surrounding tissue resulting in cerebritis or abscesses.[8] Secondly, it can also spread contiguously through the paranasal sinuses, where it can cause brain abscesses, cavernous sinus thrombosis, or carotid artery pseudoaneurysms.[2,6,8]

More than 90% of cerebral abscesses following HSCT are caused by *Aspergillus*. Lesions are usually multiple and located in the basal ganglia, thalamus, and subcortical white matter (**Fig. 1**).[2,3,8]

Computed tomography (CT) typically demonstrates multiple low-attenuation foci, with minimal mass effect and negligible contrast enhancement.

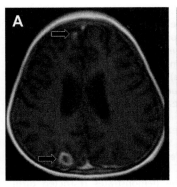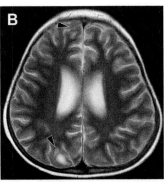

Fig. 1. A 3-year-old boy with acute lymphoblastic leukemia, post–bone marrow transplantation, who presented with neutropenic fever and convulsion on day 29 of induction chemotherapy. Laboratory workup revealed *Aspergillus* infection. (*A*) Axial enhanced T1-weighted MR image shows presence of multiple rim-enhancing lesions (*arrows*) on the right. (*B*) Axial unenhanced T2-weighted MR image demonstrates minimal surrounding vasogenic edema (*arrowheads*). (Case Courtesy of Dr. Winnie Chu, Hong Kong, China.)

MR imaging can detect more lesions than CT when evaluating intracranial extension of the disease. Increased signal on T1-weighted images may be due to hemorrhage or the manganese content of the fungus. On T2-weighted images, lesions may have peripheral low signal intensity, better appreciated on gradient recall echo sequence or susceptibility-weighted images, likely from surrounding hemorrhage. The lesions can also have a peripheral ring of restricted diffusion corresponding to infarction from angioinvasion. Ringlike enhancement may be absent.[1,6,8,9]

Early postengraftment period (days 31–100)
Viral infections The herpes group of viruses is the most likely cause of neurologic complications, although routine prophylaxis has greatly reduced the incidence of encephalitis due to herpes simplex virus, varicella zoster virus (VZV), and cytomegalovirus (CMV).[6,8,9]

Human herpes virus 6 (HHV-6) encephalitis after allogenic HSCT is a serious complication occurring in up to 78% of patients, usually during either early or late posttransplant phases. It causes posttransplant acute limbic encephalitis (PALE).[6,8,11–13] PALE manifests with anterograde amnesia, changes in mental state, headache, fever, and drowsiness.[8] MR imaging typically shows symmetric, bilateral T2-weighted and fluid-attenuated inversion recovery (FLAIR) hyperintense lesions in the limbic system particularly at the medial temporal lobe, hippocampus, and amygdala.[6,8,12,13]

Toxoplasma infection Parasitic CNS infections due to *Toxoplasma gondii*[3,6] are almost always fatal,[8] with a frequency of 0.3% to 13%.[4,6] Clinical symptoms are nonspecific, usually presenting with fever, seizure, headache, or altered mental status.[8] MR imaging shows multiple lesions in the basal ganglia,[3,6,8] posterior fossa, or at the gray-white matter junction. On T2-weighted

images, lesions can be hyperintense due to necrotizing encephalitis or isointense from organizing abscess.[8]

Imaging appearance of toxoplasmosis after HSCT is different from those in the human immunodeficiency virus (HIV)-infected population. Lesions are initially hemorrhagic following HSCT, whereas in HIV infection, hemorrhages are only seen after initiating antitoxoplasma therapy. Edema and contrast enhancement may also be absent unlike in HIV infection. The lesions may have peripheral diffusion restriction due to hemorrhage within the walls but not within the center as seen in pyogenic abscesses.[8]

Bacterial infections Gram-positive bacterial infections also frequently occur in this period.[2,6,8] Methicillin-resistant *Staphylococcus aureus* and *Staphylococcus epidermidis* as well as *Listeria monocytogenes* may cause severe meningitis and ventriculitis.[2,8]

Meningitis presents with hyperintense extra-axial spaces with leptomeningeal enhancement on the postcontrast FLAIR images. Contrast-enhanced FLAIR sequence is more sensitive and specific than contrast-enhanced T1. For pyogenic ventriculitis, the typical MR imaging findings are hydrocephalus, abnormal ependymal enhancement, and intraventricular debris with diffusion restriction, which is highly sensitive.[2,8]

Late postengraftment period (more than 100 days)
CNS aspergillosis is common and tends to present in a median of 131 days after HSCT.[6,9] The most important risk factor is prolonged neutropenia.[4,6] It may manifest as meningitis, abscess formation, or vascular invasion, leading to thrombosis, infarction, hemorrhage, or mycotic aneurysms. Imaging reveals isointense to low signal intensity lesions on T2-weighted images in the cerebral hemispheres, basal ganglia, thalami, corpus callosum, cerebellum, or brainstem.

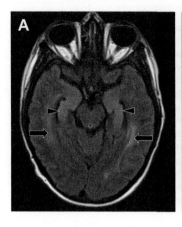 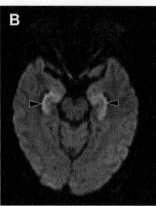

Fig. 2. An 18-year-old woman, after 2 bone marrow transplants for multiple-relapse acute lymphocytic leukemia, presented with fever and confusion, ultimately diagnosed with herpes (varicella) zoster encephalitis. (*A*) Axial unenhanced FLAIR MR image shows increased signal (*arrowheads*) in the mesial temporal lobes. Abnormal increased signal (*arrows*) in the posterior temporal lobes was thought to represent treatment-related changes. (*B*) Axial diffusion-weighted MR image demonstrates restricted diffusion (*arrowheads*) in the mesial temporal lobes.

Diffusion-weighted imaging may show restriction suggesting early ischemic changes caused by fungal embolism.[6]

Because of antiviral prophylaxis, VZV infection emerges later and continues beyond the first 6 months. This may cause vasculitis, which may lead to thrombosis, resulting in cerebral infarction and rarely hemorrhage. MR imaging demonstrates multiple infarctions in the cortices, gray-white matter junctions, deep central gray and white matter, and brainstem. Although the aforementioned are typical features, it may also present with nonspecific manifestations and can mimic HHV-6 encephalitis (Fig. 2). Conventional or MR angiography may reveal stenosis or occlusion of the major arteries in the circle of Willis.[8]

Noninfectious central nervous system complications

Peri-engraftment period (up to 100 days)

Cerebrovascular complications Cerebrovascular complications most often manifest in the preengraftment or in the early postengraftment period, occurring in 3.8% to 8.8% of patients following HSCT.[2,8]

The most common hemorrhagic complication during bone marrow depletion is a subdural hematoma. It is usually associated with underlying acute leukemia and persistent thrombocytopenia.[2–4,6,8,9]

Intraparenchymal hemorrhages (Fig. 3) are more common in allogenic HSCT particularly when accompanied by severe graft-versus-host disease (GVHD). This is probably related to microvascular endothelial injury or vasculitis.[3,4,6,8]

Infarctions may also occur in this phase and may be the result of using dimethylsulfoxide in autologous HSCT, fungal emboli, or with prolonged neutropenia. According to a retrospective study by Coplin and colleagues,[14] nearly one-third of strokes were caused by *Aspergillus fumigatus*,

Staphylococcus endocarditis (5.6%), and noninfectious endocarditis (2.8%).[6,8]

Subdural hematomas, infarctions, and intraparenchymal hemorrhages are common complications, and imaging characteristics are similar to those seen in the general population.[1]

Posterior reversible encephalopathy syndrome Posterior reversible encephalopathy syndrome (PRES), also known as posterior reversible leukoencephalopathy syndrome, is the most commonly reported neurologic complication after

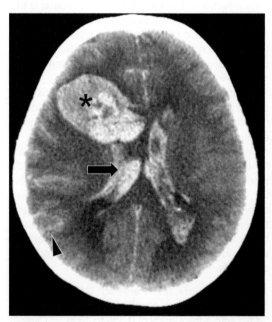

Fig. 3. An 11-year-old boy with acute myelogenous leukemia, post–bone marrow transplantation. Axial nonenhanced soft tissue window setting CT image shows a large right frontal lobe intraparenchymal hematoma (*asterisk*), with intraventricular (*arrow*) and subarachnoid (*arrowhead*) extension.

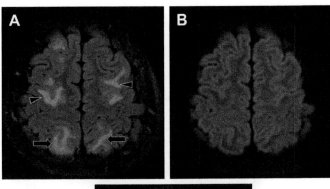

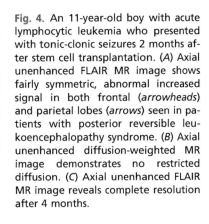

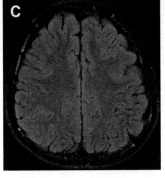

Fig. 4. An 11-year-old boy with acute lymphocytic leukemia who presented with tonic-clonic seizures 2 months after stem cell transplantation. (A) Axial unenhanced FLAIR MR image shows fairly symmetric, abnormal increased signal in both frontal (arrowheads) and parietal lobes (arrows) seen in patients with posterior reversible leukoencephalopathy syndrome. (B) Axial unenhanced diffusion-weighted MR image demonstrates no restricted diffusion. (C) Axial unenhanced FLAIR MR image reveals complete resolution after 4 months.

pediatric allogenic HSCT. The incidence is 1.1% to 20%.[6,8] It is most common during the early posttransplant period but can occur in any stage.[4,6] PRES is also a known complication of pretransplant steroids and calcineurin inhibitors such as tacrolimus and cyclosporine A, used as GVHD prophylaxis.[1,2,4,6,8,9,15] PRES manifests with rapid onset of seizures primarily, but hypertension, cortical blindness, headache, vomiting, and altered mental status may follow.[6,8,16] The pathophysiology remains unclear, but theories entail a breakdown of the blood-brain barrier leading to vasogenic edema (6.8).

CT is the first-line imaging modality, mainly used to exclude hemorrhages,[8,15,16] but MR imaging is the current imaging modality of choice. The characteristic imaging appearance consists of fairly symmetric (Fig. 4A), bilateral vasogenic edema without diffusion restriction (Fig. 4B) in the cortical-subcortical gray and white matter of the parietooccipital lobes in 50% to 99%.[6,8,16,17] Atypical PRES may involve the frontal and temporal lobes, cortical watershed zones, basal ganglia, brainstem, and cerebellum.[1,6,8,16,17] Other findings may include contrast enhancement (20%); restricted diffusion (11%–26%); and hemorrhages (5%–19%) including petechial hemorrhage (<5 mm), subarachnoid hemorrhage, and intraparenchymal hematoma.[8,16]

Most of the patients with PRES resolve completely with no detectable residual abnormalities (Fig. 4C), but residual gliosis may happen when infarcts or hemorrhages do occur.[6,8,9,16,17] Complete clinical recovery usually precedes neuroimaging resolution.[8,16]

Wernicke encephalopathy Metabolic encephalopathies are also common but occur less frequently than other CNS complications. They usually occur in the preengraftment or early postengraftment period.[2,8] Prolonged fasting, hyperemesis, and prolonged total parenteral nutrition may result in Wernicke encephalopathy.[6,8,9] The most frequent manifestation is a change in mental status.[8] MR imaging may reveal symmetric, hyperintense T2 and FLAIR signal in the mammillary bodies, medial thalami, around the aqueduct of Sylvius and in the tectal plate. Contrast enhancement is most common in the mammillary bodies.[6,8,9]

Late posttransplantation stage (more than 100 days) In the late phase after HSCT, malignancies can develop in either of the following forms: CNS relapse and therapy-induced neoplasms.[2]

Relapse of the underlying CNS disease can also occur, especially with leukemia or lymphoma. The clinical presentation can mimic the late neurologic sequelae of HSCT.[8]

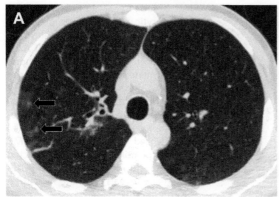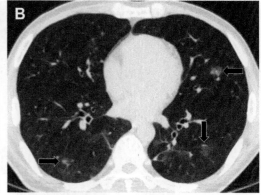

Fig. 5. A 34-year-old man with progressive non-Hodgkin lymphoma presented with cough about 1 month after bone marrow transplantation. (*A, B*) Axial unenhanced lung window setting CT images show multiple nodular densities (*arrows*) scattered in both lungs with surrounding ground-glass haziness ("halo" sign). Serum galactomannan was positive, reflective of invasive pulmonary aspergillosis.

Patients who undergo treatment of hematopoietic malignant disease, especially with high doses of total-body irradiation, are at high risk for developing a solid malignant tumor within 10 years or more. CNS tumors such as glioblastoma, astrocytoma, lymphoma, and meningioma can occur.[6,8] The risk of malignant brain tumors is 4.3 times higher in allogenic HSCT.[3,6,8]

Thoracic Complications

Pulmonary complications occur because of the toxicity of the pretransplantation medications and the effects of pancytopenia, with a frequency of 40% to 60%. However, noninfectious pulmonary complications are more common due to the increasing use of prophylactic antibiotics. The imaging modality of choice following transplantation is CT.[1]

Preengraftment phase (up to 30 days)
Infectious complications Fungal infections account for 25% to 50% of all pneumonias in allogenic transplant recipients. The most frequent fungal pathogen is *Aspergillus*, followed by *Mucor* and *Candida*.[1,7]

Aspergillus pneumonia can occur at any time following transplantation. It happens mostly but not exclusively in allogenic recipients, with a prevalence of 10% to 15%. Two forms have been described, namely angioinvasive aspergillosis, which is more common, and airway-invasive (tracheobronchial) aspergillosis.[1,7]

Angioinvasive aspergillosis manifests as multiple pulmonary nodules or masses, parenchymal opacification, or a combination of these, with upper lobe predominance. On CT, the nodules may be surrounded by ground-glass haziness ("halo" sign) (**Fig. 5**), which is a common, but not specific,

sign because it may also be seen in other infectious causes including *Candida*, *Pseudomonas*, CMV, and *Actinomycosis* infections. The halo represents hemorrhage around an area of infarction and necrosis secondary to invasion and blockage of the venules by the fungus. This may be seen within 2 weeks of infection. The "air crescent" sign may also be seen, which is a crescent-shaped lucency within a nodule or area of consolidation. This is a good prognostic sign because it reflects neutrophil recovery, thus observed later in the disease process.[1,7] Detection of galactomannan, a cell wall antigen, in the blood or bronchoalveolar lavage fluid is highly sensitive and specific (>90%) for invasive pulmonary aspergillosis.[1]

Tracheobronchial aspergillosis presents with cough, wheeze, and stridor, due to invasion of the central and peripheral airways. On CT, findings are nonspecific and include thickening of the tracheal and bronchial walls, debris-filled lumen, small (<5 mm) centrilobular nodules, and patchy peribronchial or lobar consolidation.[1,7]

Mucormycosis is a life-threatening infection caused by most commonly *Rhizopus* species followed by *Mucor*. The pulmonary form is the second most common manifestation after rhinocerebral disease and occurs after inhalation of fungal spores or via hematogenous spread from a distant focus of infection. These infections are also angioinvasive leading to tissue infarction and necrosis.[7] The common radiographic findings include lobar consolidations (66%), cavitary disease (41%), solitary or multiple masses (25%), solitary or multiple nodules (16%), and "air-crescent" sign (13%). The "halo" sign is observed in 78% of nodules. Mucormycosis may also be associated with pulmonary artery pseudoaneurysms and

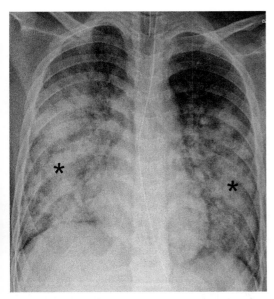

Fig. 6. A 14-year-old boy with acute myelogenous leukemia who presented with bloody sputum. Frontal supine chest radiograph shows diffuse bilateral airspace opacities (*asterisks*) in the mid- to lower lung zones. This is reflective of alveolar hemorrhage.

invasion of contiguous structures such as the chest wall, spine, aorta, pericardium, and diaphragm.[7]

Aspergillosis and mucormycosis have similar CT findings. Features that favor mucormycosis over aspergillosis include more than 10 nodules, presence of pleural effusions, "reversed halo" sign, underlying diabetes mellitus, and presence of sinusitis. The "reversed halo" sign appears as a focal, round, ground-glass opacity surrounded by a crescent or ring of consolidation.[7]

Candidiasis Candida is a commensal organism of mucocutaneous surfaces of the respiratory and

gastrointestinal tracts.[7] Affected patients present with a rapid onset of fever, respiratory distress, productive cough, and chest pain.[1] *Candida* can enter the lungs either by hematogenous dissemination or from aspiration of contaminated oropharyngeal secretions. Hematogenous spread of infection is more common and manifests as nodules measuring 3 to 30 mm, without or with a halo. In contrast, in aspiration, a bronchopneumonia pattern predominates in about one-third of cases.[7]

Noninfectious complications Pulmonary edema, diffuse alveolar hemorrhage, engraftment syndrome, and drug-induced pulmonary toxicity are the 4 most common noninfectious pulmonary complications.[1,7]

Pulmonary edema Pulmonary edema is the most common noninfectious complication in the neutropenic phase following HSCT.[7] It is multifactorial and can be due to increased hydrostatic pressure from intravenous fluids, chemotherapy, and radiation-induced cardiac or renal dysfunction, or due to abnormal capillary permeability from drug-induced pulmonary toxicity, sepsis, or transfusion reactions. It is almost always diagnosed clinically and with chest radiography. Radiographic findings include Kerley B lines, indistinct pulmonary vessels, rapid-onset pulmonary infiltrates, and pleural effusions. If CT is performed, diffuse but predominantly dependent ground-glass attenuation, engorgement of the pulmonary vessels, peribronchial cuffing, and interlobular septal thickening are seen.[1,7]

Diffuse alveolar hemorrhage Diffuse alveolar hemorrhage is a potentially life-threatening complication, with prevalence of 2% to 20% and is seen more commonly following allogenic

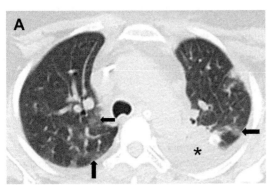
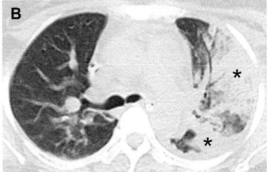

Fig. 7. A 24-year-old woman with acute myelogenous leukemia presenting with fever and cough 50 days after post–bone marrow transplantation. (*A, B*) Axial enhanced lung window setting CT images show ground-glass opacities (*arrows*) in both upper lobes and areas of consolidation (*asterisks*) in the left lung. Plasma polymerase chain reaction reveals positive CMV DNA.

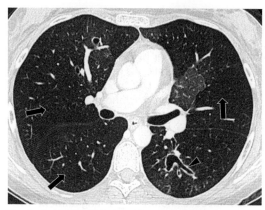

Fig. 8. A 17-year-old girl with acute myelogenous leukemia, post–bone marrow transplantation, complicated by chronic lung GVHD, who presented with exertional dyspnea and obstructive lung function pattern. Axial high-resolution lung setting CT image shows mosaic pattern with multiple areas of air trapping (*arrows*) and bronchiectasis (*arrowhead*) compatible with bronchiolitis obliterans. (Case Courtesy of Dr. Winnie Chu, Hong Kong, China.)

transplantation.[1] It occurs from 12 to 19 days after HSCT; however the pathogenesis is not well known.[7] Patients present with acute-onset fever, dyspnea, and nonproductive cough. On imaging, hemorrhage resembles pulmonary edema with diffuse air-space opacities (**Fig. 6**) and interlobular as well as intralobular septal thickening.[1,7] Pleural effusions are uncommonly seen in this condition.[7] CT may also show bilateral consolidation or ground-glass attenuation predominantly in the

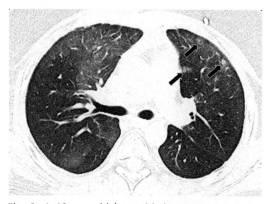

Fig. 9. A 10-year-old boy with bone marrow transplant due to aplastic anemia who presented with dyspnea, cough, and low-grade fevers. Axial lung window setting CT image shows multifocal nodular (*arrows*) and ground glass opacities in subpleural and peribronchial distribution compatible with cryptogenic organizing pneumonia. No definite features of infection on laboratory examination were noted.

perihilar and lower lung zones. Radiographic appearances may worsen rapidly despite minimal change in clinical signs.[1]

Engraftment syndrome Engraftment syndrome manifests with fever, erythematous rash, and noncardiogenic pulmonary edema. It can occur in about 7% to 11% of recipients.[1] This syndrome usually happens within 5 days of engraftment or 7 to 21 days after HSCT.[7] Imaging studies may be normal or may reveal bilateral ground-glass opacification, airspace consolidation predominantly in the hilar and peribronchial regions, interlobular septal thickening, and small pleural effusions.[1,7]

Drug-induced lung toxicity Drug-induced lung toxicity occurs in up to 10% after chemotherapy with bleomycin, methotrexate, and busulfan. Concomitant radiotherapy increases the risk up to 30%. Imaging findings are varied, reflecting different histologic patterns; thus, diagnosis is made by exclusion. Most common patterns include diffuse alveolar damage, hypersensitivity pneumonitis, eosinophilic pneumonia, and organizing pneumonia. On CT, there may be bilateral ground-glass attenuation, intralobular and interlobular interstitial thickening, centrilobular nodules, and peribronchial or subpleural areas of consolidation.[1,7]

Early posttransplantation phase (days 31–100)
Infectious causes
Cytomegalovirus Although allogenic transplant recipients are at increased risk of CMV pneumonia due to delayed reconstitution of cellular immunity and immunosuppression for GVHD prophylaxis, the use of CMV-negative marrow and blood products and early use of antivirals have significantly decreased the incidence of CMV infection.[1] Radiographic findings include bilateral interstitial opacities, focal or diffuse consolidation, and nodular opacities predominantly in the mid- and lower lung zones. CT usually demonstrates a mixed pattern of ground-glass opacities, small (1–5 mm) centrilobular nodules, and air-space consolidation (**Fig. 7**).[1,7]

Pneumocystis jiroveci The frequency of *Pneumocystis jiroveci* (previously called *Pneumocystis carinii*) pneumonia is decreased in the presence of trimethoprim-sulfamethoxazole prophylaxis. The median onset of the disease is after 60 days. Radiographs may be normal or show reticulonodular infiltrates progressing to air-space consolidation. On CT, ground-glass attenuation, diffuse or perihilar in distribution or in mosaic pattern, with

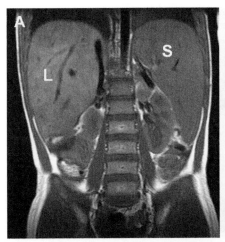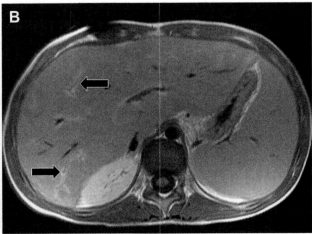

Fig. 10. A 6-year-old girl with acute lymphocytic leukemia undergoing therapy develops myelosuppression and abdominal distention. (*A*) Coronal unenhanced T1-weighted MR image demonstrates hepatosplenomegaly (*L, S*) with heterogenous signal. (*B*) Axial enhanced T1-weighted MR image shows prominent periportal enhancement (*arrows*), which corresponds to periportal fibrosis in this patient with sinusoidal obstruction.

sparing of secondary pulmonary lobules is most characteristic.[1,7]

Noninfectious causes
Idiopathic pneumonia syndrome Idiopathic pneumonia syndrome (IPS) is also called idiopathic syndrome of pneumopathy with diffuse alveolar injury. It can have a delayed onset from 30 to 180 days after HSCT. This is the most common cause of diffuse radiographic abnormalities in this phase, although it remains a diagnosis by exclusion after infectious and noninfectious causes have been ruled out.[1,7] IPS is a result of human leukocyte antigen (HLA) mismatch, thus does not occur in autologous recipients.[7] Radiographic findings are nonspecific and include bilateral, multilobar air-space opacification. CT reveals progressive air-space consolidation predominantly in both lung bases with or without pleural effusion, similar to noncardiogenic pulmonary edema.[1,7]

Acute radiation pneumonitis Acute radiation pneumonitis has been reported in patients 6 weeks to 6 months following HSCT in the setting of radiation therapy for mediastinal lymphoma. On imaging, symmetric ground-glass opacities and consolidation in the paramediastinal regions are usually observed.[7]

Late posttransplantation phase (more than 100 days)
Chronic graft-versus-host disease Chronic GVHD is the most common complication in this phase but occurs solely in allogenic recipients. As a result, bronchiolitis obliterans or less commonly cryptogenic organizing pneumonia may occur.[1,7]

Bronchiolitis obliterans Bronchiolitis obliterans (BO) is characterized by nonreversible obstruction of the small airways by intraluminal fibrosis, with prevalence of 6% to 20%, most commonly between 7 to 15 months following allogenic transplantation.[1,7] Patients present with progressive nonproductive cough, dyspnea, and wheezing with deterioration of pulmonary function. There is absence of fever and pulmonary infiltrates on imaging, distinguishing it from cryptogenic organizing pneumonia and infections.[1] Chest radiograph may be normal or may show hyperinflation. CT with inspiratory and expiratory scans may show bronchial and bronchiolar dilatation, mosaic attenuation (**Fig. 8**), and expiratory air-trapping.[1,7]

Cryptogenic organizing pneumonia Cryptogenic organizing pneumonia (previously called bronchiolitis obliterans organizing pneumonia) is characterized by intraluminal polypoid granulation tissue of bronchioles and alveolar ducts with interstitial and air-space mononuclear cell infiltration. It has a median onset of 3 months after HSCT.[7] On CT, there are bilateral patchy areas of air-space consolidation, predominantly peripheral subpleural or peribronchial in location, randomly distributed ground-glass opacities, and nodules or masses (**Fig. 9**).[1]

Abdominal Complications

Peri-engraftment period (up to 100 days)
Both infectious and noninfectious complications have been reported in this period. Common complications include hepatic veno-occlusive

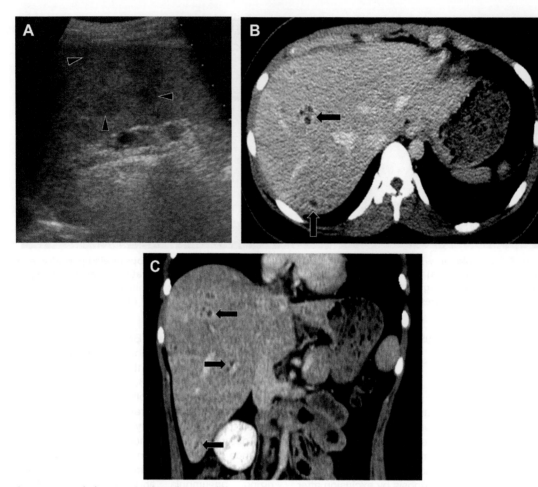

Fig. 11. Fungal abscesses in the spleen and liver as shown on ultrasound and CT scan in 2 patients. (*A*) Longitudinal gray-scale ultrasound image in a 6-year-old boy with acute myelogenous leukemia, post–bone marrow transplant, shows multiple hypoechoic nodules (*arrowheads*) in the spleen. (*B*, *C*) Axial (*B*) and coronal (*C*) enhanced liver window setting CT images in an 18-year-old girl with acute myelogenous leukemia, posttransplantation, show multiple small peripherally enhancing lesions (*arrows*) in the liver. Laboratory workup revealed Candida infection.

disease (VOD), acute GVHD, infections, neutropenic typhlitis, pneumatosis intestinalis, and hemorrhagic cystitis.[1]

Hepatic veno-occlusive disease Hepatic VOD may occur within the first 20 days but typically in the first 4 weeks. It affects 10% to 60% of patients, more commonly in allogenic transplantation.[1] Metabolite-induced endothelial damage of the hepatic sinusoids causes venous congestion, hepatic necrosis, and eventual fibrosis, which results in subsequent occlusion of hepatic outflow similar to Budd-Chiari syndrome. Affected patients present with painful hepatomegaly, jaundice, and ascites or unexplained weight gain.[1,5]

Common imaging findings include hepatomegaly (**Fig. 10**A), ascites, and marked gallbladder wall thickening of more than 6 mm.[1,5] Doppler

ultrasound is more specific and may reveal pulsatile or hepatofugal flow in the portal vein, increased resistive index (>0.8) in the hepatic artery, and loss of triphasic flow pattern in the hepatic veins. Splenomegaly, ascites, and flow in the paraumbilical vein correlate with more severe disease.[1]

Periportal edema or fibrosis (**Fig. 10**B), ascites, and narrowed right hepatic vein on CT may be used to distinguish VOD from hepatic GVHD. However, the distinction cannot be reliably made on the imaging findings alone. Biopsy is the gold standard for the diagnosis.[1,5]

Graft-versus-host disease GVHD is an immune-mediated reaction when donor T lymphocytes damage the organ epithelium, particularly in allogenic transplantation. HLA-mismatched recipients are most at risk.[1] GVHD has 2 distinct forms

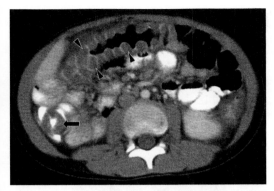

Fig. 12. A 6-year-old boy with leukemia, post-HSCT, who presented with diffuse abdominal pain and bloody stool. Axial enhanced soft tissue setting CT image demonstrates wall thickening in the ascending colon (*arrow*) with edema of the haustral folds ("accordion" sign) in the transverse colon (*arrowheads*) characteristic for pseudomembranous colitis.

based on the time of occurrence and clinical manifestations: acute (within 100 days) and chronic (100 days or more).[1,5]

The acute form presents with skin symptoms such as maculopapular rash and pruritus, after which liver and gastrointestinal problems follow.[1] Any segment of the gastrointestinal tract can be involved but most commonly in the small bowel with or without colonic lesions. CT may reveal dilated bowel loops with diffuse wall thickening and mucosal enhancement. This may progress to stricture formation causing obstruction.[1,5] "Target" sign may be apparent if there is also abnormal serosal enhancement.[5] Associated findings may include perienteric stranding, engorgement of the vasa recta, and ascites.[1,5]

Hepatic graft-versus-host disease The liver is the most commonly involved organ in GVHD after the skin. Hepatic GVHD is characterized by damage of the bile duct epithelium and sloughing of epithelial cells into the bile duct lumens. Patients may manifest cholestatic jaundice, nausea, vomiting, and abdominal pain. The clinical picture may mimic hepatitis due to injury to hepatocytes. Liver biopsy may differentiate VOD and hepatic GVHD. Periportal edema and ascites are more common in VOD, whereas concomitant small bowel wall thickening favors hepatic GVHD.[5]

Infections involving abdominal organs Hepatic and splenic infections can occur in this phase, most commonly in the form of microabscesses (**Fig. 11**) caused by fungal infections, although these can also be bacterial in nature.[1,5]

Ultrasound findings in fungal infections correspond to different stages in evolution. In the active phase, "bull's eye" lesions are seen, and in the late phases, echogenic foci correspond with healing.[1] CT and MR imaging are superior to ultrasound in the detection of fungal microabscesses. CT findings include multiple, small, hypoattenuating "target" lesions with peripheral enhancement[1,5] or uniformly hyperattenuating foci. Fungal lesions in the liver or spleen, however, may not be visible in the presence of neutropenia. Repeat imaging may be done within 2 weeks in patients with strong clinical suspicion.[1]

Intestinal tract involvement
Pseudomembranous colitis Pseudomembranous colitis (PMC), also called *Clostridium difficile* colitis, usually occurs as a result of broad-spectrum antimicrobials or chemotherapy agents with antibacterial properties used in the conditioning regimen.[1,5] PMC commonly involves the entire colon. Typical CT findings include diffuse, marked colonic wall thickening that is more pronounced when compared with GVHD or other colitides. The "accordion" sign (**Fig. 12**) that represents edema of the haustral folds is characteristic. Associated findings may include ascites and mesenteric stranding.[5]

Neutropenic enterocolitis Neutropenic enterocolitis or typhlitis (from *typhlon*, Greek word for cecum) is a complication more commonly seen in children and is potentially life-threatening. Affected patients present with the clinical triad of fever, right

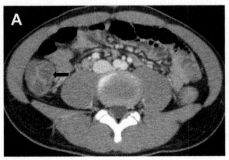
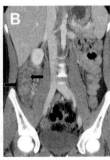

Fig. 13. A 14-year-old boy with acute myelogenous leukemia, post–bone marrow transplant, presented with fever and diarrhea. All cultures and microbiological studies were negative. Neutrophil count was decreased. (*A, B*) Axial (*A*) and coronal (*B*) enhanced soft tissue setting CT images show bowel thickening and edema (*arrows*) in the cecum and proximal ascending colon reflective of typhlitis.

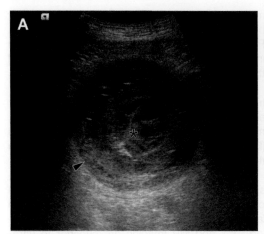 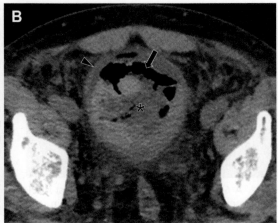

Fig. 14. A 58-year-old man with acute lymphocytic leukemia who presented with gross hematuria. (*A*) Transverse gray-scale image of the urinary bladder shows markedly diffuse wall thickening (*arrowhead*) with heterogenous intravesical echogenicities (*asterisk*). (*B*) Axial nonenhanced soft tissue window setting CT image after cystoscopy shows mixed but predominantly hyperdense material (*asterisk*) representing blood and air locules (*arrow*) within the inflamed urinary bladder (*arrowhead*) in this patient with hemorrhagic cystitis.

lower quadrant pain, and bloody or watery diarrhea. CT demonstrates bowel wall thickening and edema in any bowel segment but most commonly in the cecum, ascending colon (**Fig. 13**), and occasionally the terminal ileum. In 50% of recipients, pericolic fat stranding and ascites may be appreciated. Small bowel involvement may differentiate neutropenic enterocolitis from PMC.[1,5]

Cytomegalovirus colitis Colitis caused by CMV is similar to PMC and can manifest as pancolitis; however, the cecum is the most common site showing extensive wall thickening and nodularity.[1,5]

Benign pneumatosis intestinalis Benign pneumatosis intestinalis (BPI) occurs in asymptomatic patients following transplantation. A possible pathogenesis is steroid-induced hypertrophy of Peyer patches causing mucosal defects through which air can enter. BPI usually involves the ascending colon and is often observed incidentally. Associated mesenteric and portal venous gas and pneumoperitoneum may also be seen. These do not warrant surgical intervention and could resolve after conservative management. However, pneumatosis in patients with neutropenic typhlitis or CMV enteritis implies imminent bowel perforation.[1,5] Imaging findings are nonspecific and usually overlap with infectious, inflammatory, and radiation enteritis. Biopsy is often necessary for diagnosis.[1]

Pneumatosis, mesenteric stranding, and ascites are more frequent with neutropenic colitis than GVHD,[1] but the mucosal enhancement and bowel dilatation is greater with acute GVHD than with neutropenic colitis or PMC.[5]

Hemorrhagic cystitis Hemorrhagic cystitis may occur in up to 76% of patients after HSCT. Affected patients typically present with suprapubic pain and hematuria. This is often due to cyclophosphamide treatment or may be related to GVHD.[5] There are 2 forms. The preengraftment form is mild, brief, and responds to supportive therapy, whereas post-engraftment cystitis that occurs 40 to 80 days following transplantation is protracted, associated with GVHD, and usually requires surgical management.[1] Ultrasound and CT in both forms demonstrate bladder-wall thickening sometimes with intravesical material that represents blood clots or sloughed mucosa (**Fig. 14**).[1,5]

Late posttransplantation phase (more than 100 days)

Chronic graft-versus-host disease The most common complication is chronic GVHD, seen in 60% to 80% of patients with allogenic transplantation. Clinical manifestations resemble autoimmune collagen vascular disorders such as esophagitis and stricture, scleroderma, and myositis. The liver may be involved, frequently manifesting as cholestasis. In severe cases, vanishing bile duct syndrome with multiple biliary strictures resembling sclerosing cholangitis has been reported.[1]

Posttransplant lymphoproliferative disorders Posttransplant lymphoproliferative disorders (PTLD) are lymphoma-like conditions characterized by proliferation of lymphoid cells due to immunosuppression after transplantation, typically caused by Epstein-Barr virus in up to 80% of recipients. PTLD

Table 1
Summary of the various phases of transplantation and most common complications

Phase of Transplantation	Neurologic Complications	Thoracic Complications	Abdominal Complications
Preengraftment (from pretransplant up to 30 d posttransplant)	Infectious: Aspergillus Noninfectious: 1. Subdural hematoma 2. Intraparenchymal hemorrhage 3. Infarctions 4. PRES 5. Wernicke encephalopathy	Infectious: Fungal (aspergillosis, mucormycosis, and candidiasis) Noninfectious: 1. Pulmonary edema 2. Diffuse alveolar hemorrhage 3. Engraftment syndrome 4. Drug-induced lung toxicity	Infectious: 1. Microabscesses in liver and spleen (fungal or bacterial) 2. Pseudomembranous colitis 3. CMV colitis Noninfectious: 1. Hepatic veno-occlusive disease 2. Acute GVHD 3. Neutropenic enterocolitis 4. Benign pneumatosis intestinalis 5. Hemorrhagic cystitis
Early posttransplantation or early postengraftment (30–100 d posttransplant)	Infectious: 1. Viral 2. *Toxoplasma* 3. Bacterial Noninfectious: 1. Subdural hematoma 2. Intraparenchymal hemorrhage 3. Infarctions 4. PRES 5. Wernicke encephalopathy	Infectious: CMV, *Pneumocystis jiroveci* Noninfectious: 1. Idiopathic pneumonia syndrome 2. Acute radiation pneumonitis	
Late posttransplantation or late postengraftment (100 d posttransplant)	Infectious: Aspergillus, varicella zoster Noninfectious: Relapse or therapy-induced neoplasms	Noninfectious: 1. Chronic GVHD 2. Bronchiolitis obliterans (BO) 3. Cryptogenic organizing pneumonia (COP)	Noninfectious: 1. Chronic GVHD 2. Posttransplant lymphoproliferative disorders

are potentially fatal complications following HSCT. Frequency is however lowest in HSCT among the transplant population,[6,18–20] but majority (>80%) occurs within the first year posttransplant.[20]

PTLD could present with extranodal and less commonly nodal masses, most frequently within the abdomen involving the gastrointestinal tract and liver.[18,20] Radiologic evidence of masses with increased serum lactate dehydrogenase levels in the proper clinical setting suggest PTLD. A tissue biopsy is required to confirm the diagnosis.[6,19,20] PTLD is also discussed in Part 1: Solid Organ Transplantation.

Table 1 is a summary of the various phases of HSCT and the common infectious and noninfectious complications.

SUMMARY

Various complications may occur after HSCT. These are an important cause of morbidity and mortality in recipients. Imaging is important for early and accurate diagnosis, which is crucial for prompt treatment and a optimal prognosis. Because of the unique immune status of the recipient during these various stages, there is predominance of specific pathogens and disease patterns in each phase. Therefore, it is important for radiologists to be aware of the different time frames after HSCT. The recognition of the common imaging patterns of disease in every stage will help narrow the differential diagnosis, if not suggest a specific diagnosis.

DISCLOSURE

E.Y. Lee received traveling and honorarium support from the Guebert Group as an invited speaker at an international meeting (AOSPR). The other authors have nothing to disclose.

REFERENCES

1. Jagannathan JP, Ramaiya N, Gill RR, et al. Imaging of complications of hematopoietic stem cell transplantation. Radiol Clin North Am 2008;46:397–417.

2. Yoshida S, Hayakawa K, Yamamoto A, et al. The central nervous system complications of bone marrow transplantation in children. Eur Radiol 2008;18(10):2048–59.

3. Saiz A, Graus F. Neurologic complications of hematopoietic cell transplantation. Semin Neurol 2010;30:287–95.

4. Pruitt AA, Graus F, Rosenfeld MR. Neurological complications of transplantation: part I: hematopoietic cell transplantation. Neurohospitalist 2013;3:24–38.

5. Vlachou PA, O'Malley ME. Imaging of abdominal complications associated with hematopoietic stem cell transplantation. Can Assoc Radiol J 2014;65: 35–41.

6. Server A, Bargalló N, Fløisand Y, et al. Imaging spectrum of central nervous system complications of hematopoietic stem cell and solid organ transplantation. Neuroradiology 2017;59(2): 105–26.

7. Shroff GS, Marom EM, Wu CC, et al. Imaging of pneumonias and other thoracic complications after hematopoietic stem cell transplantation. Curr Probl Diagn Radiol 2019;48(4):393–401.

8. Bonardi M, Turpini E, Sanfilippo G, et al. Brain imaging findings and neurologic complications after allogenic hematopoietic stem cell transplantation in children. Radiographics 2018;38:1223–38.

9. Stone TJ, Misra SP, McKinstry RC, et al. Imaging of central nervous system complications of hematopoietic stem cell transplant: a chronologic approach to pathology and implications for management. Neurographics 2015;5:133–44.

10. Rodriguez TE. Neurologic complications of bone marrow transplantation. Handb Clin Neurol 2014; 121:1295–304.

11. Sadighi Z, Sabin ND, Hayden R, et al. Diagnostic clues to human herpesvirus 6 encephalitis and Wernicke encephalopathy after pediatric hematopoietic cell transplantation. J Child Neurol 2015;30: 1307–14.

12. Ogata M, Fukuda T, Teshima T. Human herpesvirus-6 encephalitis after allogenic hematopoietic cell transplantation: what we do and do not know. Bone Marrow Transplant 2015;50:1030–6.

13. Seeley WW, Marty FM, Holmes TM, et al. Post-transplant acute limbic encephalitis: clinical features and relationship to HHV6. Neurology 2007;69:156–65.

14. Coplin WM, Cochran MS, Levine SR, et al. Stroke after bone marrow transplantation: frequency, aetiology and outcome. Brain 2001;124:1043–51.

15. Dandoy CE, Linscott LL, Davies SM, et al. Clinical utility of computed tomography and magnetic resonance imaging for diagnosis of posterior reversible encephalopathy syndrome after stem cell transplantation in children and adolescents. Biol Blood Marrow Transplant 2015;21(11):2028–32.

16. Masetti R, Cordelli DM, Zama D, et al. PRES in children undergoing hematopoietic stem cell or solid organ transplantation. Pediatrics 2015;135:890–901.

17. Osborn A, editor. Hydrocephalus and CSF disorders. Osborn's brain: imaging, pathology and anatomy. Philadelphia: Amirsys Inc; 2013. p. 1005–44.

18. Jeon TY, Kim JH, Eo H, et al. Post-transplantation lymphoproliferative disorder in children: manifestations in hematopoietic cell recipients in comparison with liver recipients. Radiology 2010;257:490–7.

19. Dharnidharka VR, Webster AC, Martinez OM, et al. Post-transplant lymphoproliferative disorders. Nat Rev Dis Primers 2016;28(2):15088.

20. Friedberg JW, Aster JC. Epidemiology, clinical manifestations, and diagnosis of post-transplant lymphoproliferative disorders. Waltham (MA): Up To Date; 2018. Available at: https://www.uptodate.com/contents/epidemiology-clinical-manifestations-and-diagnosis-of-post-transplant-lymphoproliferative-disorders/print. Accessed July 30, 2019.

Spectrum of Imaging Manifestations of Vascular Malformations and Tumors Beyond Childhood
What General Radiologists Need to Know

Jared R. Green, MD[a], Scott A. Resnick, MD[b], Ricardo Restrepo, MD[c],
Edward Y. Lee, MD, MPH[d],*

KEYWORDS

- Vascular malformation • Vascular tumor • Vascular anomaly
- ISSVA (International Society for the Study of Vascular Anomalies)

KEY POINTS

- Clinical history and physical examination findings are often helpful when interpreting imaging of vascular anomalies in both pediatric and adult patients.
- The International Society for the Study of Vascular Anomalies classification provides a framework for diagnosis and management of vascular anomalies.
- Imaging features of vascular anomalies carry considerable overlap, and biopsy may be required in cases that remain indeterminate after diagnostic imaging.

INTRODUCTION

Vascular anomalies encompass a wide range of diagnoses that differ in terms of clinical presentation, natural history, imaging findings, and management. Vascular anomalies are typically diagnosed in the first 2 decades of life.[1] Clinical history and physical examination alone may allow for correct diagnosis in some cases, but diagnostic imaging is often necessary to make an accurate imaging diagnosis. Radiologists can help establish a diagnosis in clinically indeterminate cases, as well as recommend additional imaging in cases of suspected syndromic association or multiorgan involvement.[2] Evaluation by a multidisciplinary vascular anomaly clinic can provide valuable insight into the diagnosis and management of vascular anomalies.

Mulliken and Glowacki[3] devised a cell-oriented classification of vascular anomalies in 1982, delineating entities based on pathophysiology, namely endothelial cell characteristics. Vascular tumors, such as hemangiomas, being true neoplasms, exhibit endothelial proliferation and hyperplasia, whereas vascular malformations do not. Vascular malformations are categorized by predominant channel type, including capillary, venous, lymphatic, arterial, and combinations thereof. This classification was adopted by the International Society for the Study of Vascular Anomalies (ISSVA) in 1996 and last revised in 2018.[4]

[a] Department of Medical Imaging, Ann and Robert H. Lurie Children's Hospital, 225 East Chicago Avenue, Medical Imaging, Box 9, Chicago, IL 60611, USA; [b] Division of Vascular and Interventional Radiology, Northwestern University Feinberg School of Medicine, 225 East Chicago Avenue, Medical Imaging, Box 9, Chicago, IL 60611, USA; [c] MR Body and Interventional Radiology, Department of Radiology, Nicklaus Children's Hospital, 3100 SW 62nd Avenue, Miami, FL 33155, USA; [d] Division of Thoracic Imaging, Department of Radiology, Boston Children's Hospital, 300 Longwood Avenue, Boston, MA 02115, USA
* Corresponding author.
E-mail address: edward.lee@childrens.harvard.edu

Radiol Clin N Am 58 (2020) 583–601
https://doi.org/10.1016/j.rcl.2020.01.004
0033-8389/20/© 2020 Elsevier Inc. All rights reserved.

ISSVA is a multispecialty group that created the most widely accepted classification system for vascular anomalies. The ISSVA classification provides a standardized nomenclature that takes into account imaging findings, clinical presentation, lesion histology, natural history, and management. Radiologists should use accurate ISSVA terminology when evaluating vascular anomalies, because the use of improper or nonuniform terminology may lead to diagnostic confusion and preclude appropriate clinical management.

The overarching goal of this article is to provide an imaging-focused overview of noncentral nervous system (CNS) vascular anomalies beyond childhood to heighten the understanding of the often challenging diagnosis of vascular anomalies particularly for general practicing radiologists. Vascular anomalies seen in childhood only, including infantile hemangioma, are therefore not discussed in this review.

IMAGING TECHNIQUES

There is considerable overlap of imaging features of various vascular malformations, vascular tumors, and other diagnoses. Doppler ultrasound (US) and magnetic resonance (MR) imaging are the current primary diagnostic imaging modalities used to evaluate vascular anomalies, which are frequently complimentary in establishing a diagnosis and treatment plan. Invasive imaging, including arteriography and venography, is beyond the scope of this article, and is not discussed.

Radiography and Computed Tomography

Radiography and computed tomography (CT) provide limited value in evaluation of vascular anomalies due to poor lesion conspicuity relative to US and MR imaging, as well as exposure of the patient to ionizing radiation. Recent publications have proposed use of multiphasic 4D computed tomography angiography (CTA) performed at 70 kVp with dual source CT as a low-radiation alternative to contrast-enhanced MR imaging, although this technique is likely best suited to patients unable to undergo MR imaging.[5]

Ultrasound

US is often the first-line imaging modality for suspected vascular anomalies in both pediatric and adult patients. Grayscale US allows for evaluation of lesion architecture and Doppler imaging with spectral tracings allows for characterization of lesion flow dynamics. US is widely available, inexpensive, does not use ionizing radiation, does not require sedation, and allows for real-time evaluation with dynamic maneuvers. Limitations of US include operator dependency, a smaller field-of-view, difficulty evaluating deeper and extensive lesions, and inability to penetrate bone and air. US can also be used to monitor response to therapy, when applicable.

MR Imaging

MR imaging plays a key role in the diagnosis of vascular anomalies via multiplanar imaging with superior soft tissue discrimination. Noncontrast MR imaging delineates lesion characteristics, cellularity, extent, and relationship to surrounding structures, such as neurovascular bundles. Contrast-enhanced MR imaging, including time-resolved MR angiography, allows for assessment of lesion dynamics and enhancement patterns. Similar to US, MR imaging can be used to monitor response to therapy when US is not a reasonable alternative.

Optimal MR imaging protocols vary by institution. Vascular anomaly MR imaging evaluation should include multiplanar T1-weighted sequences, with and without fat suppression, for an anatomic overview, fat-suppressed T2-weighted sequences or short tau inversion recovery sequences for lesion extent, and early and delayed contrast-enhanced T1-weighted fat-suppressed sequences for enhancement characteristics. Optional noncontrast sequences, such as T2 gradient recalled echo (GRE) may help identify the presence of hemosiderin, calcification, and high-flow vessels, and diffusion-weighted imaging allows for evaluation of lesion cellularity. MR angiography often proves extremely helpful, particularly dynamic time-resolved MR angiography, as this sequence demonstrates lesion blood flow patterns previously only possible via conventional angiography.

SPECTRUM OF IMAGING MANIFESTATIONS OF VASCULAR MALFORMATIONS AND TUMORS BEYOND CHILDHOOD
Vascular Malformations

Vascular malformations arise via errors in vascular morphogenesis, and lack the increased mitotic activity and cellular proliferation that characterizes vascular tumors. Vascular malformations are always present at birth; however, they may be inconspicuous at that time. Vascular malformations grow commensurate with the patient until puberty, and never involute. Vascular malformations can be considered as "high flow" or "low flow" according to the presence or absence of an arterial component, respectively, and this distinction often

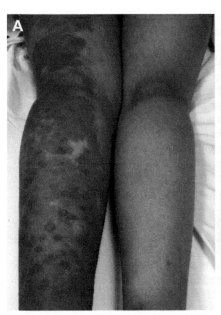
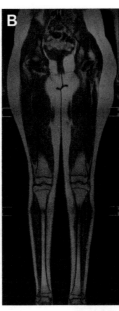

Fig. 1. A 24-year-old woman with extensive lower extremity capillary malformation. (*A*) Clinical photo demonstrates a geographic red skin stain extending from the left upper thigh to the ankle. (*B*) Coronal T1-weighted nonenhanced MR scanogram image demonstrates slight asymmetric increased subcutaneous fat in the left thigh, with no subcutaneous or deep abnormality otherwise.

guides therapeutic decisions. The low-flow category includes capillary, venous, and lymphatic malformation, whereas the high-flow category includes arteriovenous malformation and arteriovenous fistulas.[6]

Low-Flow Vascular Malformations

Capillary malformation

Capillary malformation (CM) presents as a red or pink discoloration of the skin (Fig. 1), and is primarily a clinical diagnosis. Diagnostic imaging of isolated CM is usually not required, although may be performed to evaluate for the presence of a soft tissue component, limb hypertrophy, or a concomitant high-flow component. US and MR imaging may show thickening of the skin and subcutaneous plane, with hyperemia manifested as increased color Doppler flow or contrast enhancement, respectively.[7]

CMs may be seen as part of multiple syndromes, including Sturge-Weber, Klippel-Trénaunay, and Parkes Weber, among others. Therefore, it is important to be familiar with entities associated with CMs to guide imaging investigations in possible syndromic patients.[8]

Venous Malformation

Common venous malformation

Venous malformations (VMs) are the most common vascular anomaly, with an estimated prevalence of 1%; however, this prevalence is likely underestimated due to misdiagnosis and variability of terminology used in the literature.[9,10] VMs comprise abnormal tortuous and dilated veins lined by a thin endothelium. VMs are found in the head and neck in 40% of patients, the extremities in 40%, and the trunk in 20%, although they may also be present in the viscera.[1,9]

As with all vascular malformations, VMs are present at birth; however, because they grow commensurate to the patient, they may escape detection until later in life. Likewise, VMs in deep locations, including intramuscular and visceral, may not become symptomatic until the hormonal influence of puberty. VMs are expected to have reached full size in the adult patient, although increases in size can be seen in the setting of hormonal influences, such as menstrual cycling, pregnancy, and with spontaneous intralesional thrombosis.

Morphologic imaging patterns of VMs may include focal dilation of a vein, multiple dilated tortuous dysplastic veins, and multiple mass-like cavitary or spongiform venous channels.[10] Various imaging classification systems for VMs have been proposed, although they are not commonly used in diagnostic practice, as management options are similar throughout.[9]

Radiography and CT have limited value in the diagnosis of VMs, with the exception of phleboliths, which are considered nearly pathognomonic (Fig. 2).[10] Bony distortion, including organized periosteal reaction or hypoplasia, may occur due to the presence of an adjacent VM, although this finding is nonspecific.[9]

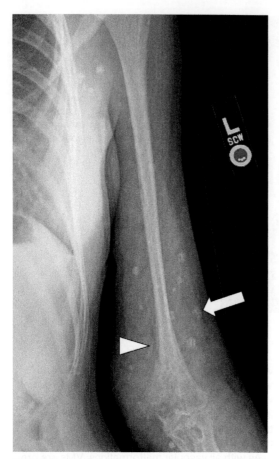

Fig. 2. A 13-year-old boy with extensive chest wall and upper extremity venous malformation (VM). Frontal radiograph of the left humerus demonstrates numerous phleboliths (*arrow*). Left humerus distal metaphysis periosteal reaction (*arrowhead*) is present at the site of a healing pathologic fracture related to intraosseous extension of the VM.

US is often used as first-line imaging in cases of suspected VMs. Up to 98% of VMs appear heterogeneous on grayscale US, with 82% appearing hypoechoic relative to adjacent structures, 10% hyperechoic, and 8% isoechoic.[11] Evidence of a solid component on US should suggest a diagnosis other than VMs, although care must be taken to differentiate intralesional thrombosis from a solid component. Phleboliths, although nearly pathognomonic, are seen in only 16% of cases on US.[11] Dynamic maneuvers, such as application of a tourniquet, can be performed during an US examination and may provide additional information. A superficial VM is expected to be compressible during US examination, although it may be noncompressible in the presence of an intralesional thrombus (Fig. 3). VMs may show engorgement dependent on positioning, Valsalva, or placement of a tourniquet (Fig. 4).[1]

Doppler US of VMs is expected to demonstrate internal flow in 84% of patients, monophasic in 78%, with absence of Doppler flow being the second most common appearance.[2,11] Fluid-fluid levels may be present in VMs due to its low-flow nature, although they are not specific for this diagnosis.[1] The presence of arterial flow can be seen due to adjacent and crossing arteries, as well as in cases of complex malformation with a capillary component, although a true arterial component should not be present with VMs.[2]

VMs on MR imaging may be trans-spatial, and can involve subcutaneous and deep tissues, muscle, bone, solid organs, and joint spaces. VMs are commonly iso- to hypointense on T1-weighted imaging and hyperintense of T2-weighted imaging. Fat-suppressed T2-weighted imaging most accurately depicts lesion extent (Fig. 5).[9] Hyperintense T1-weighted foci can be seen in the presence of intralesional thrombus, whereas T1-weighted and T2-weighted hypointense foci may correspond to thrombi, phleboliths, and areas of previous treatment or vascular septa (Fig. 6). Hypointense foci within a VM on spin echo imaging may mimic flow voids, although GRE imaging can help to differentiate as flow voids appear hyperintense.[7] The presence of intralesional flow voids would indicate high-flow vessels, and should therefore suggest an alternate diagnosis.

Postcontrast imaging of VMs demonstrates variable enhancement depending on timing of image acquisition, ranging from early homogenous enhancement to delayed heterogenous enhancement.[1,12] Dynamic time-resolved MR angiography is valuable to establish lesion flow characteristics. Perilesional edema or presence of an enhancing soft tissue component should prompt consideration of biopsy to evaluate for malignancy.[7] Post-treatment change may manifest as regional T1-weighted and T2-weighted hypointense signals, with corresponding lack of enhancement (Fig. 7).

Venous malformation associated with blue rubber bleb nevus syndrome

Blue rubber bleb nevus syndrome (BRBNS) is a rare, sporadic entity comprising multifocal VMs, involving the skin in all patients, and commonly the gastrointestinal (GI) tract.[13,14] Cutaneous VMs in BRBNS are typically small, on the order of 1 to 3 cm diameter, and may be painful.[14] VMs in BRBNS may be located anywhere along the gastrointestinal tract, most commonly in the small bowel.[14] GI VMs may manifest as unexplained anemia or GI bleeding, although they may also be the lead point for an intussusception.[14,15]

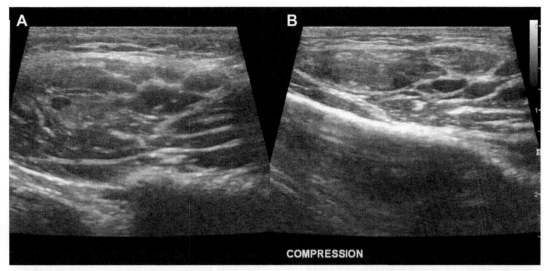

Fig. 3. A 15-year-old girl with lower leg intramuscular venous malformation. (*A*) Grayscale ultrasound (US) image demonstrates an intramuscular circumscribed hypoechoic lesion with thin septations and no soft tissue component. (*B*) Grayscale US image during US-guided compression demonstrates compressibility of the lesion.

VMs in BRBNS demonstrate the same imaging features expected in common VMs. Nuclear medicine-tagged red blood cell scan has been described as the most sensitive imaging modality for detection of GI lesions, and may demonstrate focal or multifocal avid radiotracer uptake.[14] Fluoroscopic upper and lower GI examinations may demonstrate multiple polypoid filling defects anywhere along the GI tract, mimicking a polyposis syndrome.[15] CT and MR imaging may not identify GI tract lesions, and therefore may be most helpful to evaluate for the presence of cutaneous and solid organ involvement.[13,14]

Glomuvenous malformation

Glomuvenous malformation (GVM) is a developmental hamartoma of glomus body origin, previously referred to as glomangioma, and is categorized as a VM subtype by the 2018 ISSVA classification.[4,16] GVMs may be sporadic or demonstrate autosomal dominant inheritance.[17]

GVMs present as clustered blue or purple tender vascular nodules in the cutaneous and subcutaneous plane. Lesions may be solitary, or multifocal and plaque-like, demonstrating a "pebbly" or cobblestone appearance, which helps to differentiate this entity from common VMs.[16,17]

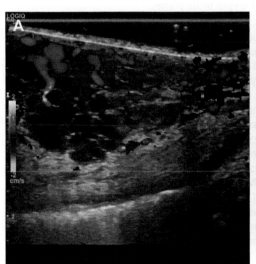
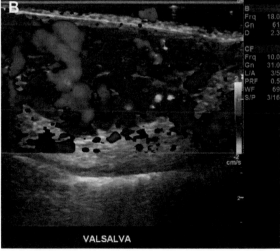

Fig. 4. A 17-year-old girl with tongue venous malformation (VM). (*A*) Color Doppler ultrasound (US) image demonstrates internal low level color flow within the VM at rest. (*B*) Color Doppler US image demonstrates substantially increased internal color flow within the VM during Valsalva maneuver.

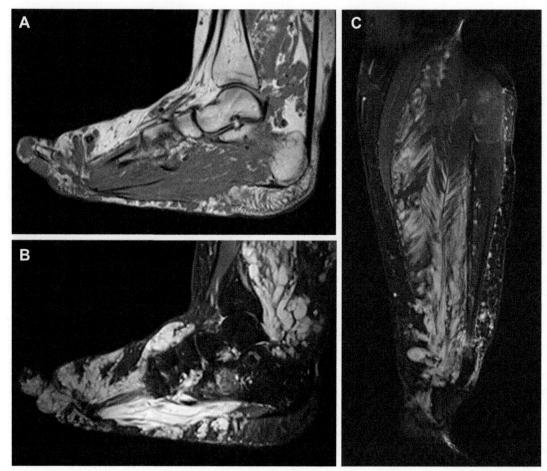

Fig. 5. A 68-year-old woman with diffuse lower extremity venous malformation (VM). (*A*) Sagittal T1-weighted MR image of the foot demonstrates hypointense dysplastic, ectatic VM involving the cutaneous, subcutaneous, and intramuscular planes. (*B*) Sagittal T2-weighted fat-suppressed MR image of the foot at the same level demonstrates nearly uniform hyperintensity of the VM. (*C*) Sagittal T2-weighted fat-suppressed MR image of the thigh clearly delineates lesion extent, with involvement of multiple tissue planes.

US of GVMs may reveal decreased compressibility compared with common VMs, and phleboliths are not expected.[10,18] MR imaging demonstrates a T1-weighted hypointense to isointense, T2-weighted hyperintense cutaneous or subcutaneous multilobulated, septated lesion with low-signal thin septa[16] (Fig. 8). Dynamic time-resolved MR angiography demonstrates patchy arterial phase enhancement. Early venous shunting may be present, although lack of dilated feeding arteries or draining veins help to distinguish this entity from arteriovenous malformation (AVM).

Lymphatic Malformation

Common lymphatic malformation

Lymphatic malformations (LMs) are benign vascular malformations arising from abnormal development of the lymphatic system, and are the second most common type of vascular malformation after VMs.[19] LMs may be microcystic, macrocystic, or mixed, according to the size of the cysts, with microcystic lesions containing cysts smaller than 1 cm.

LMs can occur anywhere throughout the body, most commonly in the head and neck, with approximately 50% occurring in this area.[20] LMs commonly involve the subcutaneous tissues, and are often trans-spatial, involving multiple additional tissue planes.[21] Sudden increased size of LMs in adult patients can be seen in the setting of bleeding secondary to trauma or infection, hence the commonly seen physical examination findings of bluish discoloration of the skin or erythema, respectively.

Radiography has a limited role in the evaluation of LMs, although it may demonstrate foci lucent areas with bone involvement. CT of macrocystic LMs may demonstrate a circumscribed,

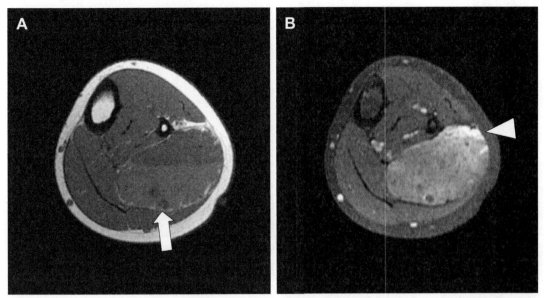

Fig. 6. A 16-year-old girl with a calf intramuscular venous malformation (VM). (*A*) Axial T1-weighted MR imaging image demonstrates a spongiform morphology VM with internal fluid level and hypointense phleboliths (*arrow*). (*B*) Axial T1-weighted fat-suppressed contrast-enhanced MR image demonstrates pooling of contrast in the nondependent portion of the VM (*arrowhead*), with no solid enhancing component.

multiseptated lesion with large locules and internal simple fluid density, although fluid density may be increased in the setting of hemorrhage or protein-aceous fluid. CT of microcystic LMs demonstrates nonspecific ill-defined fat stranding and infiltration, with no visible cystic spaces or discrete mass, often involving the subcutaneous plane.

Grayscale US of macrocystic LMs demon-strates multiple anechoic cystic spaces separated by thin septa (**Fig. 9**). Grayscale US of microcystic LMs demonstrates an ill-defined hyperechoic area with or without visible tiny cystic spaces, with the hyperechoic appearance owing to the numerous wall interfaces within the lesion (**Fig. 10**).[2] The presence of millimetric cutaneous or subcutane-ous fluid-filled spaces within the area of concern during an US examination suggests a diagnosis of LM. Doppler US may show septal flow, although

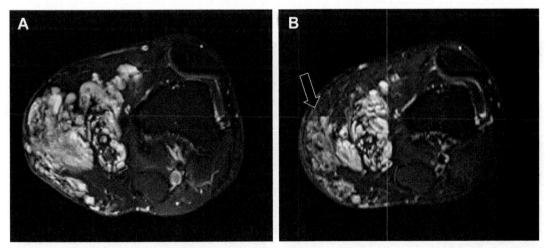

Fig. 7. A 29-year-old man with medial left knee venous malformation (VM). (*A*) Axial T2-weighted fat-suppressed MR image demonstrates the hyperintense spongiform configuration VM, with multiple hypointense septa, before treatment. (*B*) Axial T2-weighted fat-suppressed MR image demonstrates decreased size and hyperinten-sity of the subcutaneous component medially (*arrow*), consistent with treatment response after sclerotherapy.

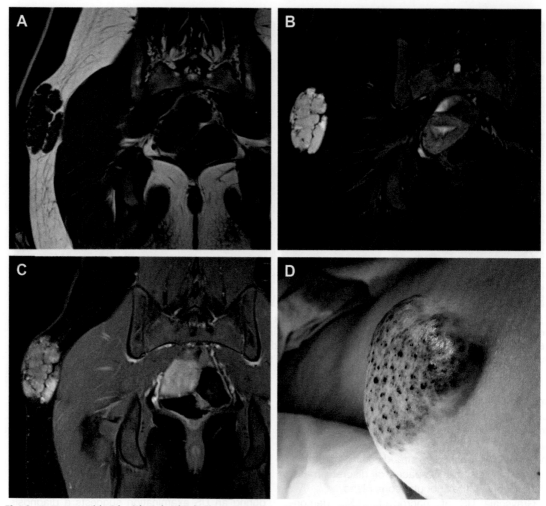

Fig. 8. A 14-year-old girl with right thigh glomuvenous malformation (GVM). (*A*) Coronal T1-weighted MR image demonstrates hypointense lesion with a lobulated "pebbly" appearance involving the cutaneous and subcutaneous planes. (*B*) Coronal T2-weighted fat-suppressed MR image demonstrates lesion hyperintensity, with hypointense thin septa present. (*C*) Coronal T1-weighted fat-suppressed contrast-enhanced MR image demonstrates patchy enhancement. (*D*) Clinical photo depicts the "cobblestone" or pebbly appearance characteristic of this entity.

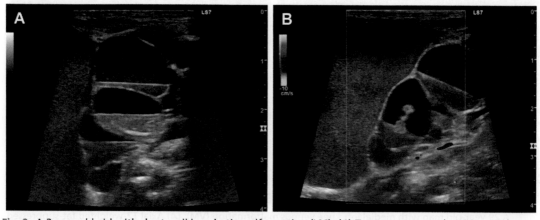

Fig. 9. A 3-year-old girl with chest wall lymphatic malformation (LM). (*A*) Transverse grayscale US image demonstrates multiple macrocysts of varying sizes within the LM, some of which demonstrate fluid-fluid levels. (*B*) Transverse color Doppler US image demonstrates absence of flow within the cystic spaces, although flow is present within a vessel adjacent to the LM.

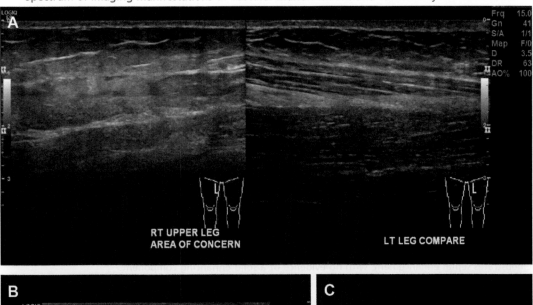

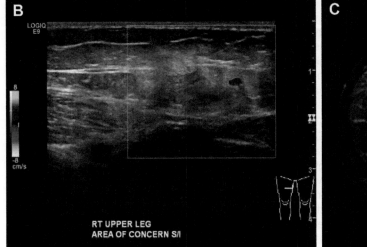

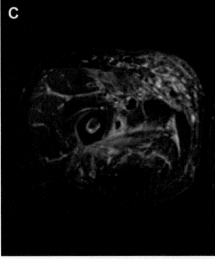

Fig. 10. An 11-year-old girl with right thigh microcystic lymphatic malformation (LM). (*A*) Longitudinal grayscale ultrasound (US) image of the involved area demonstrates diffuse, trans-spatial hyperechoic appearance of the subcutaneous and deep soft tissues, with loss of normal tissue planes; comparison image of the left thigh demonstrates preservation of the normal tissue planes and architecture. (*B*) Transverse color Doppler US image of the involved area demonstrates no evidence of hyperemia or abnormal vascular flow otherwise. (*C*) Axial T2-weighted fat-suppressed MR image of the right thigh demonstrates the trans-spatial nature of the hyperintense microcystic LM, and better delineates lesion extent.

arterial or venous flow should not be present within the cystic spaces. Peripheral hyperemia can be seen in the presence of infection or inflammation of the LM, although it should otherwise be absent. Fluid-fluid levels may be present within the cystic spaces, although this feature is not specific for LM, and is also seen in VM.[21] Dynamic maneuvers during an US examination can help to differentiate LMs from VMs; in distinction from VMs, valsalva should not lead to engorgement of an LM, and compression should only deform, not collapse, the LM cystic spaces. The presence of millimetric cutaneous fluid-filled vesicles within the area of concern at the time of a US examination suggests a diagnosis of LM.

MR imaging best delineates LM extent and internal architecture. LMs most commonly demonstrate multiple cystic spaces with hypointense to isointense appearance on T1-weighted images, although they can appear hyperintense in the presence of internal hemorrhage or proteinaceous debris. Cystic spaces most commonly demonstrate marked T2-weighted hyperintensity, although this appearance similarly varies depending on the cyst contents (**Fig. 11**). LMs tend to be trans-spatial, most commonly involving the subcutaneous plane, and isolated intramuscular involvement is uncommon. Contrast enhancement of the cystic spaces should not be seen with cystic LMs, a key

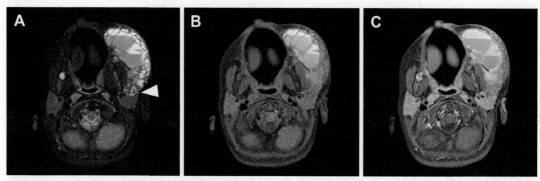

Fig. 11. A 3-year-old girl with a facial lymphatic malformation (LM). (*A*) Axial T2-weighted fat-suppressed MR image demonstrates mixed macrocystic and microcystic LM, with trans-spatial extension into the left parotid gland (*arrowhead*). (*B*) Axial T1-weighted fat-suppressed MR image demonstrates mixed iso- to hyperintense contents of the cysts, with numerous fluid levels present. (*C*) Axial T1-weighted fat-suppressed postcontrast MR image demonstrates septal enhancement, with no evidence of a solid enhancing component.

feature to differentiate LMs from VMs. Contrast-enhanced MR imaging of microcystic LMs may mimic a solid enhancing mass, although this appearance is due to the aggregate enhancement of the cyst walls and septations that are in close proximity.[8]

Complex lymphatic anomalies: Gorham-Stout disease and generalized lymphatic anomaly

Gorham-Stout disease (GSD) is a rare entity of disordered lymphangiogenesis that drives a course of progressive osteolysis.[22,23] Generalized lymphatic anomaly (GLA) is a rare entity with similarities to GSD, namely presence of bone lesions, although it carries a higher incidence of soft tissue and visceral abnormalities.

Radiographic and CT findings of GSD include discrete intramedullary lucencies, cortical lucencies, and bone resorption. Intramedullary and cortical lucencies may coalesce and result in bone loss, including tapering of long bones; bone loss is not expected to regenerate in GSD.[23] In distinction to GSD, intramedullary bone lesions of GLA are expected to spare the cortex. Both GSD and GLA bone lesions involve the axial and appendicular skeleton, with the ribs reported as the most common site in both groups (**Fig. 12**). The presence of appendicular skeletal lesions favors a diagnosis of GLA over GSD.[22] Patterns of osseous involvement can help to differentiate these entities, with appendicular lesions often continuous across joints in GSD, whereas appendicular lesions involve a greater number of bones and are often noncontiguous in GLA.[24]

In distinction to GSD, GLA patients are more likely to demonstrate visceral abnormalities, including splenic or hepatic cysts.[22] The presence of macrocystic lymphatic malformation has also

been shown to occur in GLA patients significantly more than in patients with GSD, and the presence of macrocystic LMs in patients with bone lesions should suggest the diagnosis of GLA.[22]

MR imaging helps to confirm distribution and extent of bone lesions, with whole-body survey MR imaging most helpful for this endeavor. The presence of an infiltrative soft tissue abnormality adjacent to bone lesions, marked by a T1-weighted hypointense signal, a T2-weighted hyperintense signal, and an intense contrast enhancement, is significantly associated with GSD, and can help to differentiate from GSD from GLA.[22]

HIGH-FLOW VASCULAR MALFORMATIONS
Arteriovenous Malformation

Sporadic arteriovenous malformation/arteriovenous fistula

Arteriovenous fistula (AVF) is a single abnormal connection between an artery and a vein, lacking an intervening capillary bed, and AVM is an abnormal connection of arteries and veins via a high-flow vascular nidus. The nidus, or tangle of dysmorphic vessels at the level of the artery to vein connection, is the distinguishing feature of an AVM relative to an AVF.[8,25] As diagnostic imaging techniques are similar for AVMs and AVFs, these lesions are considered as one for the purpose of this review.

Non-CNS AVMs can be found anywhere in the body, may be focal or diffuse, deep or superficial, and in any combination thereof.[26] Most AVMs are of unclear origin, although a genetic basis of some AVMs has been elucidated. Although most AVM growth is expected to occur in pediatric patients, sudden accelerated AVM growth may be seen in

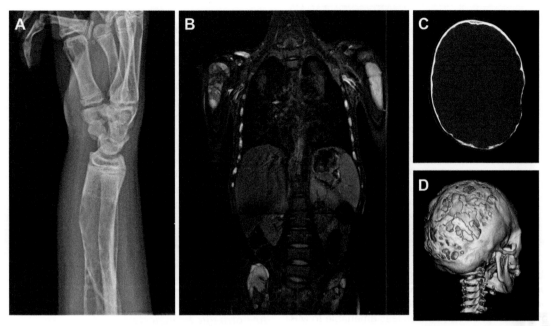

Fig. 12. A 14-year-old boy with Gorham-Stout disease (GSD). (A) Lateral radiograph of the right wrist demonstrates intramedullary lucent, expansile lesions with cortical erosions and no periostitis. (B) Coronal short tau inversion recovery (STIR) MR composite image demonstrates numerous hyperintense cystic lesions of the axial and appendicular skeleton, with no visceral or soft tissue involvement. (C) Axial contrast-enhanced CT head image bone algorithm demonstrates multiple lytic lesions of the calvarium. (D) 3-D volume rendered CT reconstruction image of the calvarium best delineates lytic lesion extent.

adults due to trauma or hormonal influence, such as pregnancy.[27]

Grayscale US of AVMs should demonstrate dilated feeding arteries and draining veins, with an intervening nidus of tortuous anechoic vessels. There should be no discernible soft tissue mass, although adjacent fat hypertrophy may be present. Doppler US demonstrates low resistance, monophasic arterial flow within feeder arteries and portions of the nidus, which may also contain turbulent multidirectional flow, and pulsatile high flow within draining veins (Fig. 13). At the time of

imaging, the radiologist may detect pulsatility, warmth, and a vascular stain in the involved area on physical examination. Imaging findings can be interpreted in the context of the clinical scenario, aided by the Schobinger clinical staging system for AVMs (Table 1). Care must be taken when performing US examinations of Schobinger stage 3 and 4 AMVs, as tissue destruction may increase risk for bleeding complications related to transducer pressure.

With advances in MR imaging spatial and temporal resolution, CTA has limited value in the

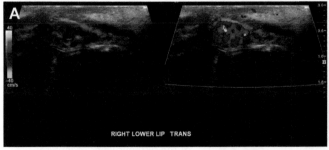
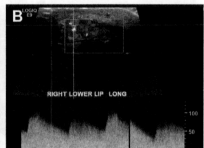

Fig. 13. A 12-year-old boy with lower lip arteriovenous malformation (AVM). (A) Transverse grayscale ultrasound (US) demonstrates a hypoechoic nidus of vessels with no soft tissue mass, with color Doppler imaging demonstrating multidirectional avid internal vascularity. (B) Longitudinal spectral Doppler US image within the AVM nidus demonstrates pulsatile low-resistance waveforms.

Table 1
Schobinger staging system for arteriovenous malformation

Stage	Clinical Findings
1 (Quiescence)	Blue or pink skin discoloration, warmth, shunting on Doppler US
2 (Expansion)	Stage 1 + engorgement, pulsatility, thrill, tortuous veins
3 (Destruction)	Dystrophic skin changes, pain, ulceration, bleeding
4 (Decompensation)	Cardiac failure

diagnosis of AVM, although CT may be needed in patients unable to undergo MR imaging, to evaluate acute bleeding complications of AVMs, or for evaluation of certain entities less amenable to MR imaging, such as pulmonary AVMs.

MR imaging is the preferred modality to determine the extent of AVM and the relationship to adjacent structures, as well as the presence of complications, such as ischemia, bleeding, thrombosis, and infection. Attempts should be made to characterize AVM complexity, via identification of inflow arteries and outflow veins. Bony involvement may manifest as flow voids and decreased T1-weighted marrow signal.[8,25] T1-weighted hyperintense fibrofatty proliferation and T2-weighted hyperintense edema may present adjacent to the AVM, with no associated soft tissue mass. High-flow vessels appear as flow voids on spin echo sequences and hyperintense foci on GRE sequences.[7]

Contrast-enhanced MR imaging should not demonstrate an enhancing soft tissue mass, although the surrounding soft tissues may show enhancement in the setting of complications, such as infection, hemorrhage, or ischemia. As mentioned above, in the presence of a discrete mass, an alternative diagnosis from AVM should be considered. Multicompartmental AVMs may demonstrate tumor-like abnormalities, including extravascular enhancement and mass-effect on surrounding tissues.[28]

Dynamic time-resolved MR angiography delineates flow dynamics via high temporal resolution (**Fig. 14**). Hallmarks of AVMs on dynamic postcontrast MR imaging include identification of a vascular nidus and early opacification of the draining veins before the normal expected venous phase of enhancement.[29] Conventional arteriography is beyond the scope of this review, although is valuable in the assessment of AVM architecture and dynamics, and is typically performed before intervention.

Arteriovenous malformation in hereditary hemorrhagic telangiectasia

Hereditary hemorrhagic telangiectasia (HHT), previously known as Rendu-Osler-Weber disease, is a rare disorder with autosomal dominant inheritance. HHT is characterized by scattered telangiectasias and AVMs, which may be present in the skin, mucous membranes, and viscera, including the lungs.[30,31] Right to left shunt physiology of a pulmonary AVM creates a risk for paradoxic embolization and associated CNS injury. Pulmonary AVM also carries a risk of rupture, although this dreaded complication is rarely encountered.

The lungs are the most common visceral site of AVMs in HHT, characterized by direct connections between pulmonary artery and vein. Pulmonary AVM in HHT is most often multiple, bilateral, and basilar predominant.[30] AVMs with a single feeding pulmonary artery, seen in approximately 80% of cases, are considered "simple," and those with

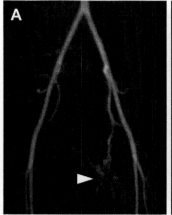
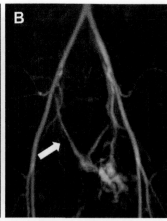

Fig. 14. A 10-year-old boy with pelvic arteriovenous malformation (AVM). (*A*) Coronal maximum intensity projection dynamic time-resolved contrast-enhanced MR angiography (MRA) image in the early arterial phase demonstrates enhancement of the nidus (*arrowhead*) via the left internal iliac artery. (*B*) Subsequent arterial phase image demonstrates early drainage of the AVM via the bilateral internal iliac veins (*arrow*), without opacification of the systemic veins otherwise.

multiple feeding arteries are considered "complex."[30] An intervening aneurysmal sac between the artery and vein can show variable morphology, including a single dilated sac or a network of abnormal serpentine vessels (Fig. 15).

CTA is the optimal modality for evaluation of pulmonary AVMs, as its short acquisition time limits respiratory motion artifact.[25] A developing pulmonary AVM on CT may appear as a ground-glass nodular opacity, with discrete vascular structures becoming evident with AVM progression. Imaging description of pulmonary AVMs must include lung segmental anatomy and delineation of the feeding artery morphology, including number of inflow vessels and inflow vessel diameter, as this important information guides therapeutic decision making. Consideration should be made for inclusion of the upper abdomen to evaluate for abdominal visceral involvement.

Vascular Malformations Associated with Other Anomalies

Klippel-Trénaunay syndrome

Klippel-Trénaunay syndrome (KTS) is defined by the presence of CM and VM with limb overgrowth, with or without LM.[4] KTS is now considered part of the spectrum of PIK3CA-related overgrowth syndromes (PROS), based on somatic mutations found involving the PIK3CA gene.[32,33] KTS is unilateral in at least 75% of patients, and may involve more than one limb on the affected side in 10% to 15% of cases.[9,34] Marked enlargement of the involved limb is primarily due to soft tissue and

bone hypertrophy rather than vascular malformation.

Venous anomalies, including persistence of embryonic veins, varicosities, and deep vein abnormalities are commonly seen. The marginal vein of Servelle, present within the lateral subcutaneous tissues the calf and thigh, is considered nearly pathognomonic, and may communicate with the deep venous system (Fig. 16). Complications that may be seen on imaging include superficial and deep vein thrombosis, as well as pulmonary emboli. Doppler US of the deep venous system may therefore be helpful, although it may be difficult to differentiate patent collateral veins from ectatic vessels of the VM.[10] Systemic deep veins may be hypoplastic or absent, which may create diagnostic difficulty and affect therapeutic approach in these patients with widely variable venous drainage of the affected limb. T1-weighted MR imaging best delineates subcutaneous fat hypertrophy of the affected limb, with T2-weighted imaging best demonstrating the location and extent of CMs, VMs, and possibly LMs.

Parkes Weber syndrome

Parkes Weber syndrome (PWS) is characterized by extensive CMs, AVMs, and overgrowth of bone and soft tissue. The presence of a high-flow arterial component most easily distinguishes this syndrome from KTS.[32] A hallmark of PWS on CTA and contrast-enhanced MR imaging is the presence of periarticular AVF-like vascular enhancement.[34]

Benign Vascular Tumor

Congenital hemangioma

The term "hemangioma" is often mistakenly applied to other vascular lesions, leading to confusion and inappropriate management.[8] There are two main categories of hemangioma: infantile hemangioma (IH) and congenital hemangioma (CH). CHs are fully developed at birth, and are divided into 3 subtypes by the ISSVA classification: rapidly involuting congenital hemangioma (RICH), noninvoluting congenital hemangioma (NICH), and partially involuting congenital hemangioma (PICH).[4] IH and RICH involute in childhood, and therefore they are not discussed further here.

PICH and NICH are rare, and there is no sex predilection.[35] PICHs appear similar to NICHs, although PICHs carry an associated history of partial involution during childhood.[36] Clinical history plays a pivotal role in diagnosing CH, as these lesions should be present and fully developed at birth. Physical examination also plays

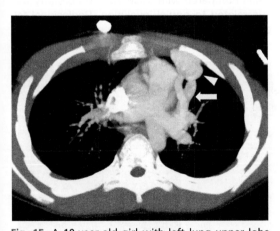

Fig. 15. A 10-year-old girl with left lung upper lobe pulmonary arteriovenous malformation (AVM) in the setting of hereditary hemorrhagic telangiectasia. Axial contrast-enhanced maximum intensity projection CT image shows that the AVM demonstrating "simple" morphology with a single feeding artery to the aneurysmal sac (*arrowhead*) and single draining pulmonary vein (*arrow*).

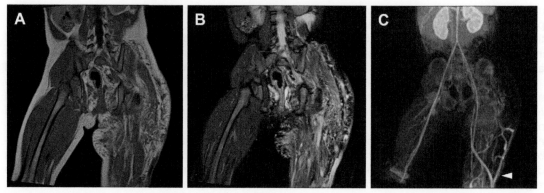

Fig. 16. A 3-year-old girl with Klippel–Trénaunay syndrome (KTS). (*A*) Coronal T1-weighted MR image demonstrates overgrowth of the left leg soft tissues, with trans-spatial involvement of the subcutaneous and deep intramuscular planes with mixed capillary, venous, and lymphatic malformation components. (*B*) Coronal T2-weighted fat-suppressed MR image demonstrates extent of the hyperintense vascular malformation. (*C*) Coronal maximum intensity projection dynamic time-resolved contrast-enhanced MRA image demonstrates numerous ectatic abnormal veins, including the Marginal Vein of Servelle (*arrowhead*).

an important role in the diagnosis of CH. These lesions typically present as a blue or purple superficial nodule or mass, often located close to a joint or in the head and neck, with central telangiectasia and a peripheral blanched "halo" or pale rim. NICHs are expected to grow proportionately with patients throughout life, reaching full size in adulthood. In distinction to IHs, biopsy of CH is expected to be negative for the Glut-1 marker, and may be helpful in clinically indeterminate cases.

Imaging of CHs may be required in certain scenarios, such as when treatment planning is necessary, including evaluation of lesion extent and relationship to adjacent structures.[37] US and MR imaging are preferred modalities. On US, CHs can appear as a circumscribed, heterogeneous

solid mass with visible vessels and high vascular density, involving the dermis and superficial subcutaneous soft tissues. Calcification can be seen with CH, with a reported incidence of up to 17% in NICH.[35] Spectral Doppler US in PICH and NICH demonstrates low-resistance arterial waveforms.[36]

MR imaging of CH demonstrates a circumscribed soft tissue mass with T1-weighted intermediate signal intensity and hyperintensity on T2-weighted imaging. Flow voids are often present within the lesion, and avid enhancement is expected postcontrast (**Fig. 17**). PICH may demonstrate a greater degree of heterogeneity when compared with NICH due to fibrofatty tissue related to partial involution. Perilesional fat stranding, without peripheral edema, may be

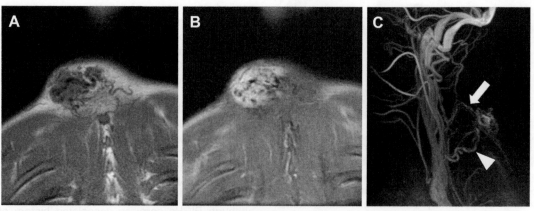

Fig. 17. A 10-year-old girl with upper back noninvoluting congenital hemangioma (NICH). (*A*) Coronal T1-weighted MR image demonstrates a soft tissue mass with isointense signal to muscle and presence of numerous flow voids. (*B*) Coronal T1-weighted fat-suppressed contrast-enhanced MR image demonstrates avid enhancement of the mass. (*C*) Sagittal 3D volume rendered reconstructed contrast-enhanced MRA image demonstrates arterial supply (*arrowhead*) and venous drainage (*arrow*) of the mass.

present in up to approximately one-third of CHs.[35]

Locally Aggressive or Borderline Vascular Tumor

Kaposiform hemangioendothelioma

Kaposiform hemangioendothelioma (KHE) is a rare vascular tumor that demonstrates locally aggressive features, and is considered a "borderline" vascular tumor by the ISSVA classification.[4] KHE most commonly presents in infancy and childhood, with continued growth of the tumor into adulthood. KHE has been reported to occur throughout the body, including in the viscera, and is often multicompartmental.[38] Metastatic disease is not expected with KHE.[39] KHE is often accompanied by the Kasabach-Meritt phenomenon, a complication described in up to 71% of patients, which comprises thrombocytopenia, coagulopathy, and hemolytic anemia.[40]

Imaging appearance of KHE varies, with the main presentations being: a solitary solid mass, a solid mass with surrounding reticular infiltrative regions, or reticular infiltrative lesions alone, with no identifiable solid mass.[38] An infiltrative morphology is relatively unique to KHE, likely representing lymphedema, and should raise the possibility of this rare diagnosis.

US of KHE most commonly demonstrates a heterogenous hyperechoic solid mass with avid internal vascularity on Doppler US.[36] CT can be helpful to identify osseous changes of KHE when present, including bony destruction and remodeling. MR imaging of KHE demonstrates T1-weighted iso- to hyperintensity and T2-weighted iso- to hyperintensity of the mass and possible infiltrative surrounding edema, with postcontrast imaging demonstrating intense heterogeneous enhancement.[38,39] Prominent vessels and flow voids related to robust arterial supply and venous drainage may be present in, and about, the mass (Fig. 18).

Malignant Vascular Tumor

Angiosarcoma

Angiosarcoma is a very rare malignant vascular tumor with aggressive behavior marked by poor prognosis, with a high rate of metastatic disease and local recurrence.[41,42] Angiosarcoma can present anywhere throughout the body, with a cutaneous location most common, and at any age, although it most commonly occurs in adult patients. Metastatic disease is most commonly found in the lungs, although it has also been described in the liver, bones, soft tissues, and lymph nodes.[41]

MR is the preferred imaging modality for evaluation of angiosarcoma, and is expected to demonstrate a soft tissue mass with T1-weighted isointensity, although hyperintense areas may be present in the presence of hemorrhage, and T2-weighted hyperintensity. Similar to KHE, angiosarcoma may demonstrate an infiltrative pattern of spread into the surrounding tissues (Fig. 19). Flow voids should be present on spin echo images, indicative of high-flow arterial vessels. Contrast-enhanced images demonstrate brisk, homogenous enhancement of the soft tissue mass, with nonenhancing areas indicative of necrosis.[41] A wide range of apparent diffusion coefficient values and map have been described, likely related to the heterogenous composition of

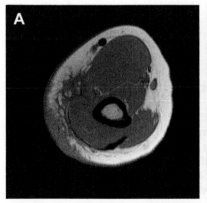
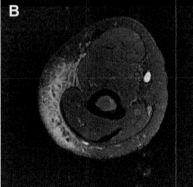
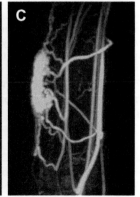

Fig. 18. A 12-year-old boy with right upper arm kaposiform hemangioendothelioma (KHE). (*A*) Axial T1-weighted MR image demonstrates a cutaneous and subcutaneous hypointense solid mass with infiltrative extension. (*B*) Axial STIR MR image demonstrates hyperintense signal throughout the mass. (*C*) Coronal maximum intensity projection time-resolved contrast-enhanced MRA image in the venous phase demonstrates avid enhancement of the mass, with multiple prominent feeding arteries and draining veins.

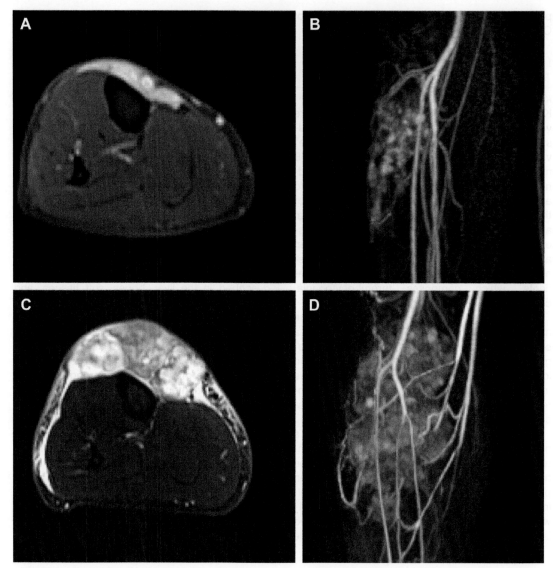

Fig. 19. A 48-year-old woman with right knee angiosarcoma. (*A*) Axial T1-weighted fat-suppressed postcontrast MR image demonstrates an enhancing soft tissue mass in the right lower leg subcutaneous plane. (*B*) Coronal maximum intensity projection time-resolved contrast-enhanced MRA image demonstrates solid enhancement with enlarged arterial supply. (*C, D*) Follow-up MR images 3 months later demonstrate interval enlargement and infiltrative extension of the mass.

this entity.[41] Because of the nonspecific imaging findings of this lesion, biopsy is required for diagnosis.

Provisionally Unclassified Vascular Anomalies

Fibroadipose vascular anomaly

Fibroadipose vascular anomaly (FAVA) was first described in a 2014 series, and is recognized as a "provisionally unclassified" entity by the ISSVA classification.[4,43] More recently, FAVA has been considered part of the PROS due to mutations involving the PIK3CA gene.[44] FAVA is an intramuscular vascular anomaly, involving a single muscle or a muscle group, most commonly located in the calf, but has also been reported in the forearm, thigh, and trunk. FAVA is distinguished by phlebectasia and a dominant solid fibrofatty infiltration or mass.[43,45] FAVA often presents clinically with pain that is constant and severe, and affected patients may present with an associated contracture.

US of FAVA demonstrates a solid-appearing lesion with indistinct borders, heterogeneous, predominantly hyperechoic fibrofatty tissue, with interspersed hypoechoic dilated venous channels

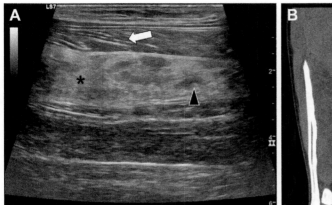
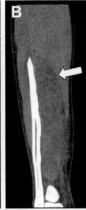
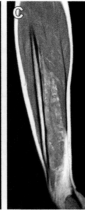
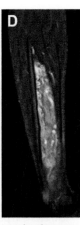

Fig. 20. An 18-year-old man with right calf fibroadipose vascular anomaly. (*A*) Longitudinal grayscale ultrasound image demonstrates an intramuscular heterogeneous, solid-appearing lesion with dominant hyperechoic fibro-fatty tissue (*asterisk*) containing interspersed hypoechoic dilated venous channels (*arrowhead*). The lesion replaces the normal fibrillary pattern of the gastrocnemius muscle, as compared with the preserved fibrillary pattern of the adjacent soleus muscle (*arrow*). (*B*) Sagittal noncontrast CT image demonstrates low-density fatty infiltration (*arrow*) related to the lesion within the gastrocnemius muscle. (*C*) Sagittal T1-weighted MR image demonstrates heterogeneous hyperintense lesion within the gastrocnemius muscle, with the hyperintensity related to fatty infiltration. (*D*) Sagittal T2-weighted MR image demonstrates heterogeneous hyperintense lesion, with multiple dilated vascular channels present.

replacing the muscle's normal fibrillary pattern.[43] The lesion is intramuscular, oriented longitudinally along the affected muscle or muscular compartment, and can cross fascial planes. Doppler imaging may demonstrate venous flow, although arterial flow within the lesion should not be present.[43]

MR imaging of FAVA typically demonstrates an intramuscular lesion with T1-weighted heterogeneous hyperintensity, likely due to the presence of solid fibrofatty tissue, as well as heterogeneous T2-weighted hyperintensity (**Fig. 20**). Osseous changes and phleboliths are present in a minority of patients. Postcontrast MR imaging demonstrates heterogeneous enhancement, with enhancement patterns ranging moderate to strong.[43]

SUMMARY

Vascular anomalies encompass a wide-ranging, heterogeneous group of entities, and they are often challenging diagnoses for general radiologists. Although clinical diagnosis is possible in many cases, imaging can facilitate a diagnosis in clinically indeterminate cases, establish lesion extent, evaluate for syndromic associations, and monitor therapy when applicable. Ideally, vascular malformations and vascular tumors should be referred to a center of excellence with experience with the diagnosis and management of vascular anomalies. Relevant clinical history and physical appearance of the lesion should be included as part of the radiology report, as these findings are

helpful in reaching a correct diagnosis. Furthermore, familiarity with the ISSVA classification terminology and its appropriate use in diagnostic imaging reports is recommended.

REFERENCES

1. Olivieri B, White CL, Restrepo R, et al. Low-flow vascular malformation pitfalls: from clinical examination to practical imaging evaluation—part 2, venous malformation mimickers. Am J Roentgenol 2016; 206(5):952–62.
2. Dubois J, Alison M. Vascular anomalies: what a radiologist needs to know. Pediatr Radiol 2010;40(6): 895–905.
3. Mulliken JB, Glowacki J. Hemangiomas and vascular malformations in infants and children: a classification based on endothelial characteristics. Plast Reconstr Surg 1982;69(3):412–22.
4. ISSVA Classification of Vascular Anomalies ©2018 International Society for the study of vascular anomalies. Available at: "issva.org/classification". Accessed February 15, 2020.
5. Henzler T, Vogler N, Lange B, et al. Low dose time-resolved CT-angiography in pediatric patients with venous malformations using 3rd generation dual-source CT: Initial experience. Eur J Radiol Open 2016;3:216–22.
6. Restrepo R. Multimodality imaging of vascular anomalies. Pediatr Radiol 2013;43(S1):141–54.
7. Flors L, Leiva-Salinas C, Norton PT, et al. Ten frequently asked questions about MRI evaluation of

soft-tissue vascular anomalies. Am J Roentgenol 2013;201(4):W554–62.

8. Flors L, Leiva-Salinas C, Maged IM, et al. MR imaging of soft-tissue vascular malformations: diagnosis, classification, and therapy follow-up. Radiographics 2011;31(5):1321–40.

9. Legiehn GM, Heran MKS. Venous malformations: classification, development, diagnosis, and interventional radiologic management. Radiol Clin North Am 2008;46(3):545–97.

10. Behr GG, Johnson CM. Vascular anomalies: hemangiomas and beyond—part 2, slow-flow lesions. Am J Roentgenol 2013;200(2):423–36.

11. Trop I, Dubois J, Guibaud L, et al. Soft-tissue venous malformations in pediatric and young adult patients: diagnosis with doppler US. Radiology 1999;212(3):841–5.

12. Dubois J, Soulez G, Oliva VL, et al. Soft-tissue venous malformations in adult patients: imaging and therapeutic issues. RadioGraphics 2001;21(6):1519–31.

13. Senturk S, Bilici A, Miroglu TC, et al. Blue rubber bleb nevus syndrome: imaging of small bowel lesions with peroral CT enterography. Abdom Imaging 2011;36(5):520–3.

14. Kassarjian A, Fishman SJ, Fox VL, et al. Imaging characteristics of blue rubber bleb nevus syndrome. Am J Roentgenol 2003;181(4):1041–8.

15. McCauley RGK, Leonidas JC, Bartoshesky LE. Blue rubber bleb nevus syndrome. Radiology 1979;133(2):375–7.

16. Flors L, Norton PT, Hagspiel KD. Glomuvenous malformation: magnetic resonance imaging findings. Pediatr Radiol 2015;45(2):286–90.

17. Myers RS, Lo AKM, Pawel BR. The glomangioma in the differential diagnosis of vascular malformations. Ann Plast Surg 2006;57(4):443–6.

18. Boon LM, Mulliken JB, Enjolras O, et al. Glomuvenous malformation (glomangioma) and venous malformation: distinct clinicopathologic and genetic entities. Arch Dermatol 2004;140(8):971–6.

19. Mamlouk MD, Danial C, McCullough WP. Vascular anomaly imaging mimics and differential diagnoses. Pediatr Radiol 2019;49(8):1088–103.

20. Elluru RG, Balakrishnan K, Padua HM. Lymphatic malformations: diagnosis and management. Semin Pediatr Surg 2014;23(4):178–85.

21. White CL, Olivieri B, Restrepo R, et al. Low-flow vascular malformation pitfalls: from clinical examination to practical imaging evaluation—part 1, lymphatic malformation mimickers. Am J Roentgenol 2016;206(5):940–51.

22. Lala S, Mulliken JB, Alomari AI, et al. Gorham-Stout disease and generalized lymphatic anomaly—clinical, radiologic, and histologic differentiation. Skeletal Radiol 2013;42(7):917–24.

23. Ruggieri P, Montalti M, Angelini A, et al. Gorham-Stout disease: the experience of the Rizzoli Institute

and review of the literature. Skeletal Radiol 2011; 40(11):1391–7.

24. Trenor CC, Chaudry G. Complex lymphatic anomalies. Semin Pediatr Surg 2014;23(4):186–90.

25. Dunham GM, Ingraham CR, Maki JH, et al. Finding the Nidus: detection and workup of non–central nervous system arteriovenous malformations. RadioGraphics 2016;36(3):891–903.

26. Uller W, Alomari AI, Richter GT. Arteriovenous malformations. Semin Pediatr Surg 2014;23(4):203–7.

27. Liu AS, Mulliken JB, Zurakowski D, et al. Extracranial arteriovenous malformations: natural progression and recurrenceafter treatment. Plast Reconstr Surg 2010;125(4):1185–94.

28. Patel AS, Schulman JM, Ruben BS, et al. Atypical MRI features in soft-tissue arteriovenous malformation: a novel imaging appearance with radiologic-pathologic correlation. Pediatr Radiol 2015;45(10):1515–21.

29. Behr GG, Johnson C. Vascular anomalies: hemangiomas and beyond—part 1, fast-flow lesions. Am J Roentgenol 2013;200(2):414–22.

30. Lacombe P, Lacout A, Marcy P-Y, et al. Diagnosis and treatment of pulmonary arteriovenous malformations in hereditary hemorrhagic telangiectasia: an overview. Diagn Interv Imaging 2013;94(9):835–48.

31. Shovlin CL, Guttmacher AE, Buscarini E, et al. Diagnostic criteria for hereditary hemorrhagic telangiectasia (Rendu-Osler-Weber syndrome). Am J Med Genet 2000;91(1):66–7.

32. Bertino F, Braithwaite KA, Hawkins CM, et al. Congenital limb overgrowth syndromes associated with vascular anomalies. Radiographics 2019; 39(2):491–515.

33. Nguyen H-L, Boon L, Vikkula M. Vascular anomalies caused by abnormal signaling within endothelial cells: targets for novel therapies. Semin Intervent Radiol 2017;34(03):233–8.

34. Nozaki T, Nosaka S, Miyazaki O, et al. Syndromes associated with vascular tumors and malformations: a pictorial review. Radiographics 2013;33(1):175–95.

35. Gorincour G, Kokta V, Rypens F, et al. Imaging characteristics of two subtypes of congenital hemangiomas: rapidly involuting congenital hemangiomas and non-involuting congenital hemangiomas. Pediatr Radiol 2005;35(12):1178–85.

36. Nasseri E, Piram M, McCuaig CC, et al. Partially involuting congenital hemangiomas: a report of 8 cases and review of the literature. J Am Acad Dermatol 2014;70(1):75–9.

37. Restrepo R, Palani R, Cervantes LF, et al. Hemangiomas revisited: the useful, the unusual and the new: part 1: overview and clinical and imaging characteristics. Pediatr Radiol 2011;41(7):895–904.

38. Ryu YJ, Choi YH, Cheon J-E, et al. Imaging findings of Kaposiform hemangioendothelioma in children. Eur J Radiol 2017;86:198–205.

39. Hu P, Zhou Z. Clinical and imaging features of Kaposiform hemangioendothelioma. Br J Radiol 2018; 91(1086):20170798.

40. Croteau SE, Liang MG, Kozakewich HP, et al. Kaposiform hemangioendothelioma: atypical features and risks of Kasabach-Merritt phenomenon in 107 referrals. J Pediatr 2013;162(1):142–7.

41. Gaballah AH, Jensen CT, Palmquist S, et al. Angiosarcoma: clinical and imaging features from head to toe. Br J Radiol 2017;90(1075): 20170039.

42. Adams DM, Hammill A. Other vascular tumors. Semin Pediatr Surg 2014;23(4):173–7.

43. Alomari AI, Spencer SA, Arnold RW, et al. Fibro-adipose vascular anomaly: clinical-radiologic-pathologic features of a newly delineated disorder of the extremity. J Pediatr Orthop 2014;34(1): 109–17.

44. Luks VL, Kamitaki N, Vivero MP, et al. Lymphatic and other vascular malformative/overgrowth disorders are caused by somatic mutations in PIK3CA. J Pediatr 2015;166(4):1048–54.e5.

45. Wang KK, Glenn RL, Adams DM, et al. Surgical management of fibroadipose vascular anomaly of the lower extremities. J Pediatr Orthop 2019;1. https://doi.org/10.1097/BPO.0000000000001406.

Three Distinct Vascular Anomalies Involving Skeletal Muscle
Simplifying the Approach for the General Radiologist

Ricardo Restrepo, MD[a], Rachel Pevsner, DO[a], Liset Pelaez, MD[b], Domen Plut, MD, PhD[c], Edward Y. Lee, MD, MPH[d],*

KEYWORDS

• Intramuscular venous malformation • Intramuscular capillary-type hemangioma
• Vascular malformation • Pediatric soft tissue mass • Sclerotherapy • Hemangioma
• Fibroadipose vascular anomaly

KEY POINTS

• Venous malformations (VM) and hemangiomas of the skeletal muscle are now recognized as 2 separate entities with different clinical presentation, histology, and imaging findings.
• Both entities have been lumped together in the literature based on the original description by Allen and Enzinger in 1972.
• Recent advances in the field of vascular anomalies and current efforts in the unification of terminology by the International Society for the Study of Vascular Anomalies are pivotal in the understanding and differentiation of these 2 distinct entities: intramuscular VM and intramuscular capillary-type hemangioma.
• Fibroadipose vascular anomaly is another recently defined vascular anomaly also affecting the skeletal muscle, particularly the calf muscles, with a distinct clinical presentation, histology, and imaging appearance.
• Confined to muscle, these 3 entities are less apparent at birth and more likely to be diagnosed during adolescence and early adulthood.

INTRODUCTION

According to the classification by the International Society for the Study of Vascular Anomalies (ISSVA), venous malformations (VMs) are not neoplasms but rather congenital structural anomalies resulting from an error in venous morphogenesis. VMs are categorized as slow-flow type, which also includes capillary and lymphatic malformations. Intramuscular VMs or VMs of the skeletal muscle (IMVMs) are a subset of VM confined to a muscle or muscle group with occasional minimal extension into the adjacent subcutaneous soft tissues. Conversely, hemangiomas are benign neoplasms, and as such undergo mitotic activity and increased endothelial cell turnover.[1–3]

[a] Department of Pediatric Radiology, Nicklaus Children's Hospital, 3100 SW 62nd Avenue, Miami, FL 33155, USA; [b] Department of Pathology, Nicklaus Children's Hospital, 3100 SW 62nd Avenue, Miami, FL 33155, USA; [c] Department of Pediatric Radiology, Clinical Radiology Institute, University Medical Centre, Ljubljana, Zaloska cesta 7, Ljubljana 1000, Slovenia; [d] Department of Radiology, Boston Children's Hospital, Harvard Medical School, 300 Longwood Avenue, Boston, MA 02115, USA
* Corresponding author.
E-mail address: Edward.Lee@childrens.harvard.edu

Radiol Clin N Am 58 (2020) 603–618
https://doi.org/10.1016/j.rcl.2020.01.005
0033-8389/20/© 2020 Elsevier Inc. All rights reserved.

VMs have been classified by their morphology and drainage pattern on phlebography by Dubois and colleagues[4] and Puig and colleagues[5,6] as spongiform, cavitary, or dysmorphic. Spongiform VMs consist of dilated blood-filled spaces with a compact, "masslike" arrangement and little to no in-line normal venous outflow to systemic veins (Fig. 1). In contrast, the phlebectatic VMs are composed of dilated vascular lakes as well as tubular and tortuous veins arranged in a haphazard fashion.[4–6] Purely IMVMs are mainly of the spongiform type and, therefore, are almost entirely isolated with almost no systemic venous drainage.[7,8] This morphologic classification that was originally described to assess the therapeutic outcomes of sclerotherapy is also useful for understanding certain aspects of the pathophysiology and imaging features of IMVMs on various modalities (ie, ultrasound and MR imaging). Due to this predominant spongiform morphology, IMVMs are often misdiagnosed on imaging as either benign or malignant neoplasms and are referred to our vascular anomaly clinic for biopsy.

In the literature, IMVMs have been lumped together with intramuscular hemangioma based on the seminal work by Allen and Enzinger almost 50 years ago.[9–11] In 2002, Hein and colleagues[1] introduced the term "VM of the skeletal muscle" based on the ISSVA classification.[3] In the same study, the existence of a hemangioma of the skeletal muscle was suggested; a term that was adopted by Yilmaz and colleagues[12] in 2014. An intramuscular capillary–type hemangioma (ICTH) is a true vascular neoplasm with unique imaging features that is considered in the provisionally unclassified category by ISSVA.[2,12] The use of different terminology in the literature has made an accurate calculation of IMVM incidence difficult. In a study by Vogel and colleagues[7] that included 115 patients with VMs, 40% were found to be confined to the skeletal muscle. In 2014, Alomari and colleagues[13] coined the term fibroadipose vascular anomaly (FAVA) to describe a new entity characterized by fibrofatty infiltration of the skeletal muscle most commonly in the calf, painful phlebectasia, and focal contracture that more frequently affects adolescent girls and young women. These lesions can potentially be confused with IMVM or even neoplasms and are currently in the provisionally unclassified category by ISSVA.[2]

In this article, these 3 distinct vascular anomalies involving skeletal muscle, based on the terminology proposed by ISSVA, are reviewed, and their histologic features, clinical presentation, imaging appearance, and treatment are discussed for general radiologists.

INTRAMUSCULAR VENOUS MALFORMATIONS

IMVMs, like all VMs, exhibit a normal rate of endothelial cell turnover and do not involute but instead grow proportional to the patient. The suffix "oma" implies cellular proliferation and neoplasia; hence, the term hemangi"oma" of the skeletal muscle, which is commonly used in the literature to refer to IMVMs, should be avoided.[1,3,14] Despite the effort pioneered by Mulliken and Glowasky,[15] the loose and imprecise use of terminology in the medical literature still poses a challenge with regard to vascular anomalies, and IMVMs are not spared.[3,14–16]

In accordance with the article by Hein and colleagues[1] published in 2002 and adhering to the ISSVA classification, it is now felt that the large vessel hemangioma–type lesions described by Allen and Enzinger[9] in 1972 represent IMVMs.

Histologic Appearance

Because IMVMs are low-flow vascular malformations, they appear clearly benign histologically. IMVMs are composed of a conglomerate of thin- to thick-walled vessels with variable amounts of smooth muscle and large gaping spaces that lack proliferative features infiltrating the skeletal muscle (Fig. 2). The nuclei of the endothelial cells are flattened and small with no mitotic figures. Intravascular thrombi at various stages and hemosiderin deposition are common, a typical feature of

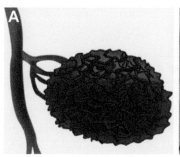
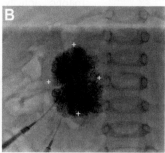

Fig. 1. (A) Spongiform venous malformation shows a masslike lesion with minimal venous drainage into systemic circulation. (B) Venogram of a spongiform venous malformation of the paraspinal musculature shows the masslike lesion (*calipers*) with no venous drainage into systemic circulation. ([A] *Adapted from* Legiehn GM, Heran MK. Classification, diagnosis, and interventional radiologic management of vascular malformations. Orthop Clin North Am 2006;37(3):435–74; with permission.)

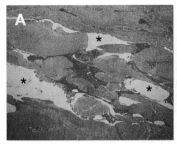
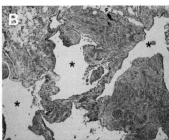

Fig. 2. (A) Histology of an intramuscular venous malformation of the gastrocnemius muscle. Abnormal large interconnecting vascular channels (asterisks) with attenuated endothelium and variable amount of disorganized smooth muscle in walls, filled with blood (hematoxylin-eosin, original magnification ×40). (B) Abnormal interconnecting vascular channels (asterisks) with attenuated endothelium and variable amount of disorganized smooth muscle in walls. Fat elements are present (F) (hematoxylin-eosin, original magnification ×100).

all VMs (Fig. 3). Fibroblastic proliferation with the concentric deposition of collagen and calcifications forming phleboliths are also seen (Fig. 4). Fatty elements are almost always present and frequently abundant.[1,9] The endothelium of vessels in IMVMs is immuno-reactive to vascular markers, such as CD31 (Fig. 5), CD34, and von Willebrand factor, but it is nonreactive to the glucose transporter protein (GLUT1), a marker associated with infantile hemangiomas, and D2-40, a marker associated with lymphatic vessels and lymphatic malformations.[1,17]

By definition, VMs should not have cellular proliferation or mitosis unless perturbed. However, VMs can exhibit cellular proliferation in the form of intravascular papillary endothelial hyperplasia (also known as Masson phenomenon), complicating the distinction between neoplasm and malformation. Masson phenomenon is a reactive condition to thrombosis or trauma that represents an exuberant organization and recanalization of a thrombus (Fig. 6A). Masson phenomenon is confined to the vascular spaces and is characterized by multiple papillary structures covered by a single layer of flattened endothelium around cores of fibrous connective tissue. Thrombi of various stages of organization are nearly always present (Fig. 6B). Masson phenomenon has a striking similarity to the very rare angiosarcoma histologically and could potentially prompt a biopsy to the unfamiliar eye. Masson phenomenon is exclusively intravascular, whereas angiosarcoma is rarely confined to a vascular lumen. Masson phenomenon can be seen as a reactive change inside a preexisting vascular lesion, most frequently in a venous malformation and especially if the location is intramuscular.[18–20]

Clinical Presentation

Most IMVMs are diagnosed in the first 3 decades, with most lesions discovered at birth.[1,9,21] A female predominance has been reported with a female:male ratio of 2:1.[1,7] IMVMs have a wide anatomic distribution throughout the body, potentially involving any muscle. The head and neck were found to be the most common locations in

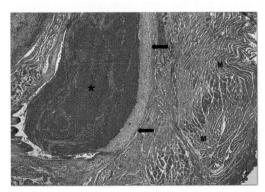

Fig. 3. Large early organizing thrombus (asterisk) within intramuscular vessel (arrows); (M) skeletal muscle (hematoxylin-eosin, original magnification ×40).

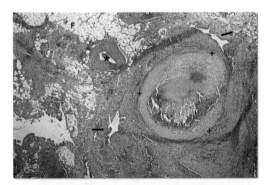

Fig. 4. Venous malformation with tortuous venous channels (arrows), small thick-walled artery (asterisk) and fibroblastic proliferation with concentric deposition of collagen and calcification forming a phlebolith (calipers). (F) Fat (hematoxylin-eosin, original magnification ×40).

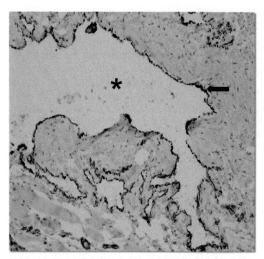

Fig. 5. Intramuscular venous malformation showing that the endothelium (*arrow*) of the abnormal vascular channels (*asterisk*) is immuno-reactive to the vascular marker CD31 (original magnification ×200).

the studies by Vogel and colleagues[7] and Hein and colleagues.[1] In the study by Hein and colleagues,[1] the orbicularis oris and masseter were the most frequently involved muscles. A lower-extremity predominance was found by Allen and Enzinger,[9] Wild and colleagues,[10] and Wu and colleagues,[11] with the most commonly involved muscle being the quadriceps. Based on the personal experience at our Vascular Anomaly Clinic, most IMVMs affect the lower extremities.

The most common symptoms associated with IMVMs are the presence of a mass (**Fig. 7**); pain due to thrombosis; or intermittent, localized swelling, or muscle hypoplasia. IMVMs are more likely to present as a mass because of the predominant spongiform morphology and are more likely to be painful and to interfere more with physical activity than the superficial counterparts do.[1,7,10,22]

A higher percentage of IMVMs are diagnosed later in life compared with the superficial

counterpart. This late diagnosis of IMVMs is probably multifactorial. IMVMs are confined to a muscle or muscle group, lacking the skin discoloration of their superficial counterpart and therefore are less apparent on physical examination at an early age (see **Fig. 7**).[7] In the study by Hein and colleagues,[1] only 68% of IMVMs were diagnosed at birth, with the average age at presentation being 13 years. In a later study, Vogel and colleagues[7] also found that when compared with VMs limited to the skin and subcutis, those restricted to the muscle compartment were less likely to present at birth (27% vs 53%) with a mean age of presentation of 6.7 ± 0.9 years. These results are echoed by the experience at our Vascular Anomaly Clinic. Furthermore, due to their location, IMVMs are subjected to additional compressive forces exerted by the surrounding muscle acting similarly to a compressive stocking, which may delay the development of symptoms.[7]

Another reason for a potential late diagnosis of IMVMs is the hormonal influence on these lesions during puberty. IMVMs, like any other vascular malformation, grow proportionate to the patient and never involute. The pubertal hormonal surge causes a temporary accelerated growth of these spongiform lesions, making them more apparent and causing potential confusion with a soft tissue sarcoma. Likewise, the pubertal surge in estrogens, due to a prothrombotic effect, may trigger pain, thus bringing attention to deeply seated lesions.[23,24]

IMVMs can also present with symptoms related to localized intravascular coagulopathy (LIC), such as thrombosis, hemorrhage, or thromboembolic events. The pathophysiology of LIC is explained by the stagnation of blood that occurs in these low-flow vascular malformations, causing the activation of the coagulation cascade, the consumption of coagulation factors, the generation of thrombin, and fibrin with the elevation of D-dimers

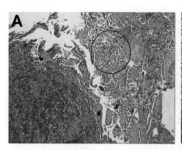
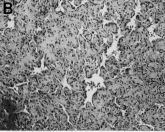

Fig. 6. (*A*) Large organizing thrombus with recanalization (*arrowheads*) and foci of intravascular papillary endothelial hyperplasia also known as Masson phenomenon (in *circle*) (hematoxylin-eosin, original magnification ×100). (*B*) At higher magnification, the exuberant fibroblastic and endothelial proliferation with the formation of papillary structures that fuse and form narrow interconnecting channels is better appreciated. This image shows the proliferative nature of Masson phenomenon resembling angiosarcoma (hematoxylin-eosin, original magnification ×200).

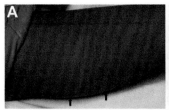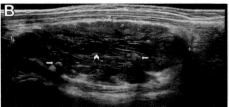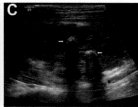

Fig. 7. A 5-year old boy with a lump in the proximal left thigh. (*A*) Clinical photograph shows a subtle bulge (*arrows*) in the proximal thigh medially with no skin discoloration. (*B*) Gray-scale ultrasound image shows the slightly bulging, lobulated, well-defined "masslike" lesion (*calipers*) with increased through transmission. The lesion is predominantly hyperechoic at the periphery with anechoic channels in the center (*arrowhead*) and echogenic shadowing foci representing phleboliths (*arrows*). (*C*) Color Doppler ultrasound image of the intramuscular venous malformation shows no internal vascularity confirming a low-flow vascular malformation. Two shadowing phleboliths (*arrows*) are present.

and hypofibrogenemia that may progress to disseminated intravascular coagulopathy. The spongiform IMVMs are more associated with LIC than the other morphologic types due to the greater lesion capacitance, slower flow, and more blood isolation due to the fewer or no systemic venous connections.[8,24,25] Therefore, spongiform VMs, especially in an intramuscular location, tend to develop painful intralesional thrombotic episodes that eventually lead to phlebolith formation.[8,24]

Imaging Approach

The 2 main imaging modalities used to evaluate IMVMs (as well as ICTH and FAVA) are ultrasound and MR imaging, which are complementary and therefore usually used in conjunction. Each has its own advantages; however, neither modality uses ionizing radiation.

As most IMVMs are of the spongiform type, they tend to present as masses for which ultrasound is usually the initial imaging modality for their evaluation in the pediatric population. Ultrasound confirms the presence of a mass and characterizes the location (superficial vs deep), the nature of the lesion (cystic vs solid), and the vascularity. On the other hand, MR imaging is helpful in evaluating the extension of the lesion, the pattern of enhancement, and the relationship with adjacent vital structures, such as the neurovascular bundle. The MR imaging protocol must include T1-weighted images without fat suppression, fluid-sensitive sequences, either short-T1 inversion recovery or T2-weighted images with fat suppression, and T1-weighted images with fat suppression before and after intravenous contrast. Early and delayed postcontrast images are critical for assessing the characteristic slow yet progressive enhancement of the lesion (**Table 1**). The initial MR imaging evaluation should

include a dynamic contrast-enhanced MR arteriogram to exclude arterial supply to the lesion commonly seen in neoplasms but absent in IMVMs. Different from malignant neoplasms, IMVMs enhance on the delayed venous phases rather than on the early arterial phases (see **Table 1**). In younger, less cooperative children, MR imaging usually requires sedation to avoid motion artifact.

Ultrasound features of intramuscular venous malformations

Considering their spongiform appearance, IMVMs on ultrasound are seen as well-defined, elliptical or oval-shaped masses with a lobulated contour, of variable echogenicity confined to a single muscle or muscle group. IMVMs are composed of blood-filled, tubular venous channels or cavernous spaces oriented along the long axis of the muscle fibers, hence their hypoechoic, multiseptated appearance with increased through transmission on ultrasound (**Fig. 8**). IMVMs may also appear hyperechoic and/or solid when composed of collapsed veins (see **Fig. 7**) or when thrombosed (**Fig. 9**).[26,27] Fatty elements secondary to muscle atrophy are seen as a peripheral echogenic rind simulating a capsule or scattered areas of increased echogenicity (**Fig. 10**).[10,11,28]

In cases of intralesional thrombosis, a more heterogeneous parenchyma can be seen with solid areas of varying echogenicity corresponding to thrombi at various stages (**Fig. 11**). Phleboliths are seen as small, echogenic, round foci with posterior acoustic shadowing (see **Fig. 7**). Because of the low flow in venous malformations, floating low-level echoes may fill the venous channels. Likewise, when color interrogation is applied, usually little or no color fills the venous channels (see **Figs. 7 and 8**).[29] Some lesions may display different degrees of internal and

Table 1 MR imaging protocol		
STIR	Coronal	• Best plane to evaluate lesions in extremities • Larger FOV includes the entire extremity to better evaluate the location and overall lesion extent
T1	Axial or coronal	• Best plane to evaluate relationship to anatomic landmarks, for example, neurovascular bundle • Best sequence and planes to evaluate muscle anatomy • Evaluates intralesional thrombi at different stages • Best sequence to evaluate fatty atrophy
STIR/T2 FS	Axial	• Smaller FOV for more detail. • Best sequence to evaluate lesion margins, size, and presence of fluid-fluid levels • Helpful sequence to evaluate intralesional thrombosis
Precontrast T1 FS	Axial	• Evaluates enhancement pattern • Helpful in evaluation of intralesional thrombi/phleboliths
Contrast enhaned MRA	Coronal	• Obtain several passes to include delayed venous phases • Early phases exclude arterial feeders, presence of a nidus or early draining vein
Early post contrast T1 FS	Axial	• Evaluates pattern of enhancement • Frequently there is mild or minimal patchy contrast enhancement
Delay post contrast T1 FS	Coronal or Sagittal	• Further evaluates enhancement pattern with increasing enhancement or more diffuse enhancement
Extra delayed postcontrast T1 FS	Axial	• Additional delays maybe needed to further evaluate late slow enhancement

Abbreviations: FOV, field of view; FS, fat suppression; MRA, magnetic resonance angiography; STIR, short-T1 inversion recovery.

peripheral vascularity with arterial waveforms in the solid elements and septum-like structures that histologically correspond to the fibrin-rich papillary endothelial proliferations and fibrovascular cores of Masson phenomenon (see **Fig. 9**; **Fig. 12**).[30–32]

MR imaging features of intramuscular venous malformations

On MR imaging, IMVMs are seen as well-defined, oval-shaped, intramuscular masses of different sizes that appear multiseptated, as they are composed of vascular channels longitudinally

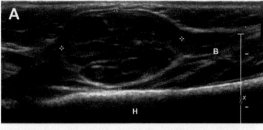
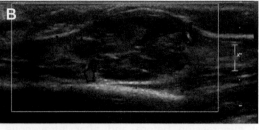

Fig. 8. Intramuscular venous malformation of the biceps in a 7-year old girl who presented with a mass. (*A*) Gray-scale ultrasound image shows a well-defined oval-shape mass (*calipers*) with increased through transmission containing anechoic tubular spaces embedded in the fibers of the biceps (B). Humerus (H). (*B*) Corresponding color Doppler ultrasound image shows the paucity of internal vascularity despite the vascular nature of the lesion, a common finding in venous malformations.

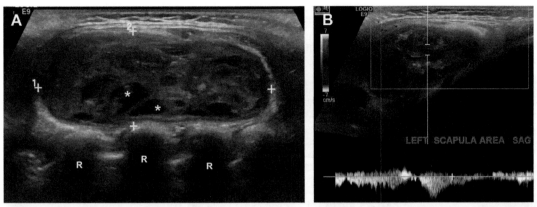

Fig. 9. A 6-year old boy with a venous malformation of the shoulder girdle muscles with Masson phenomenon. (A) Gray-scale ultrasound image shows a well-defined, round lesion (*calipers*) embedded in the fibers of the muscles overlying the rib cage. The lesion is echogenic and predominantly solid with scant cystic elements (*asterisks*). R, Rib. (B) Corresponding ultrasound image using color Doppler and spectral analysis shows internal arterial vascularity seen with Masson phenomenon.

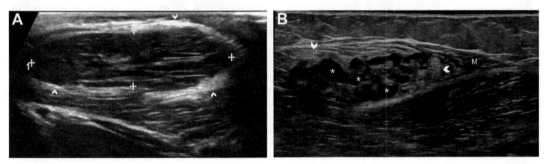

Fig. 10. (A) A 7-year old girl with an intramuscular venous malformation of a paraspinal muscle. Gray-scale ultrasound image shows an oval lesion (*calipers*) composed of anechoic vascular channels embedded in the muscle fibers with a peripheral echogenic rind corresponding to fat (*arrowheads*). (B) An 11-year old girl with an intramuscular venous malformation of the soleus muscle. Gray-scale ultrasound image shows an elliptical lesion (*arrowheads*) composed of anechoic vascular channels (*asterisks*) embedded in the muscle fibers (M) and interspersed echogenic elements corresponding to fat.

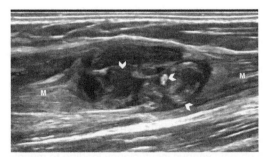

Fig. 11. Intramuscular venous malformation in the flexor compartment of the forearm. Gray-scale ultrasound image shows an oval-shaped lesion composed of venous channels with different echogenicities (*arrowheads*) corresponding to thrombi at different stages yielding a solid appearance. M, muscle.

oriented along the muscle fibers. IMVMs are isointense to slightly hyperintense to muscle on T1-weighted images and are markedly hyperintense on T2-weighted images (**Fig. 13**). The high signal on fluid-sensitive sequences is due to the cavernous, markedly dilated venous spaces filled with stagnant blood.[1,10,11] Stagnant intralesional flow leads to the separation of the blood elements into plasma and sediment, explaining the formation of fluid-fluid levels (**Fig. 14**) and thrombi.

IMVMs display different degrees of enhancement after the administration of intravenous gadolinium. On early phases, contrast enhancement tends to be less pronounced and markedly heterogeneous. On delayed phases, enhancement becomes more intense and homogeneous, an important clue to the diagnosis (see **Fig. 13**).[1] In

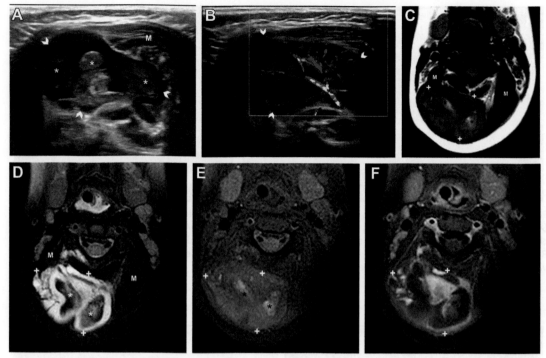

Fig. 12. Intramuscular venous malformation with secondary Masson phenomenon in a 1-month old girl who presented with a lump in the cervical region. (*A*) Gray-scale ultrasound image shows an oval-shaped lesion (*arrowheads*) embedded in the deep cervical muscles (*M*) with areas of different echogenicities (*asterisks*) representing thrombi at different stages. The lesion underwent biopsy with final diagnosis of venous malformation with Masson phenomenon. (*B*) Corresponding color Doppler ultrasound image shows substantially increased vascularity in the solid component and along the septa of the venous malformation (*arrowheads*). (*C*) Axial T1-weighted image shows an oval-shape lesion (*calipers*) isointense to muscle (*M*). The foci of increased signal intensity correspond to thrombi (*asterisks*). (*D*) Axial T2-weighted image with fat suppression shows an oval-shape lesion (*calipers*) markedly hyperintense to muscle (*M*). The foci of decreased signal intensity correspond to thrombi (*asterisks*). (*E*) Axial precontrast T1-weighted image with fat suppression shows foci of increased signal intensity corresponding to thrombi (*asterisks*) inside the lesion (*calipers*). (*F*) Axial postcontrast T1-weighted image with fat suppression shows patchy contrast enhancement by the lesion (*calipers*) around the intralesional thrombi (*asterisks*).The large size of the thrombi is better appreciated after contrast administration.

some cases, enhancement in early phases is scant and may not progress on delayed images (**Fig. 15**). This enhancement pattern is explained by the relative isolation from the systemic venous circulation, limiting the passage of contrast into these low-flow lesions. The presence of thrombi at various stages, including Masson phenomenon, also adds to the heterogeneous enhancement pattern of the lesion (see **Fig. 15C**). If the degree of intralesional thrombosis is extensive, the lesion may appear solid (see **Fig. 12**).[1,8,11,31–34]

When calcified, phleboliths are seen as round foci of drop signal (see **Fig. 13A**), which are an important clue to the diagnosis but are not to be confused with flow voids, which are typically absent due to the low-flow nature of VMs. Phleboliths are more commonly found in IMVMs compared with VMs in other locations.[1,7,8] Acute intralesional thrombosis may cause a mild degree of perilesional edema. On the 2-dimensional time of fly MR venogram, the lesion should not be seen due to the slow flow and the isolation from the peripheral circulation (see **Fig. 13F**). On a contrast-enhanced MR arteriogram (MRA), IMVMs typically display no arterial supply. On delayed (venous) phases of an MRA, a faint blush of contrast can be seen inside the lesion, but no arterial supply or nidus should be present on any phase (see **Fig. 13G**) except in cases of superimposed Masson phenomenon.

The presence of fatty elements, a common and important feature of IMVMs, has been attributed to chronic venous insufficiency leading to muscle atrophy, therefore is more common in older children and young adults[35] The presence of fat is best identified on T1-weighted images more frequently as a perilesional circumferential rind (see **Fig. 14B**) but also interspersed inside the

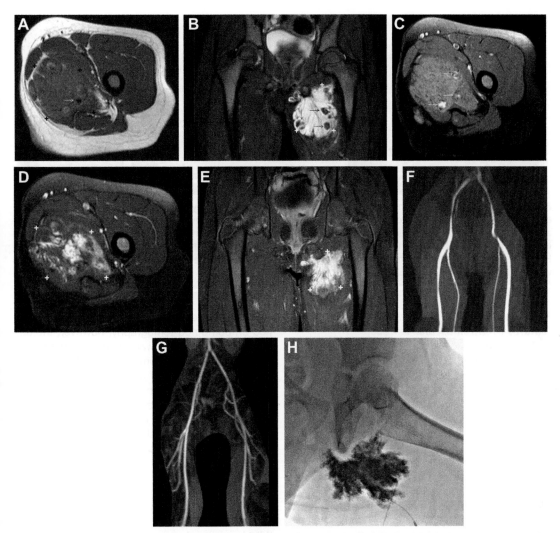

Fig. 13. A 6-year-old girl with an intramuscular venous malformation (IMVM) of the adductor compartment. (*A*) Axial T1-weighted image shows a lobulated mass (*calipers*) isointense to muscle. There are foci of increased signal intensity corresponding to acute thrombi (*black arrows*) as well as a focus of drop signal (*white arrow*) corresponding to a phlebolith. A peripheral hyperintense fatty halo is present indicating muscle atrophy. (*B*) Coronal T2-weighted image shows the IMVM as a hyperintense (fluid signal) lobulated mass (*calipers*). There are multiple foci or decreased signal intensity corresponding to thrombi (*black arrows*). (*C*) Axial precontrast T1-weighted image with fat suppression makes the foci of increased signal intensity corresponding to acute thrombi (*white arrows*) more conspicuous. (*D*) Axial early postcontrast T1-weighted image with fat suppression shows hyperintense areas of patchy enhancement throughout the IMVM (*calipers*). (*E*) Coronal delayed post-contrast T1-weighted image with fat suppression shows progressive and more homogeneous enhancement by the IMVM (*calipers*). (*F*) 2-D TOF MR venogram of both lower extremities shows normal and symmetric venous system to both thighs. No signal is seen in the area of the malformation. (*G*) Dynamic, contrast-enhanced MR arteriogram of both lower extremities shows normal and symmetric arterial system to both thighs. No arterial supply or nidus is seen in the area of the malformation. (*H*) Spot image of a conventional venogram using image intensifier at the time of the sclerotherapy shows a spongiform type IMVM with no connections with the peripheral circulation.

lesion (**Fig. 16**).[10,11,28] The "split fat" sign frequently associated with peripheral nerve tumors can be present at the cephalad and caudal edges of IMVMs, as these lesions are oriented along the long axis of the muscle (see **Fig. 14**C).

As a general rule, the presence of fatty elements in soft tissue masses (especially in childhood when liposarcoma is exceedingly rare) should support the diagnosis of a benign type of pathology.[28]

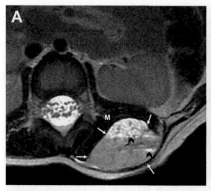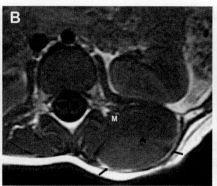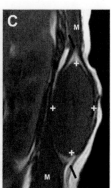

Fig. 14. Intramuscular venous malformation of a paraspinal muscle in a 5-year-old girl. (*A*) Axial T2-weighed image shows the oval-shaped hyperintense lesion (*arrows*) with fluid-fluid levels (*arrowheads*). The nondependent area is more hyperintense corresponding to the plasma and the dependent area is less hyperintense corresponding to the sediment. M, muscle. (*B*) On the Axial T1-weighted image, the F-F level (*arrowhead*) is less conspicuous. However, a fatty rind around the periphery (*arrows*) of the lesion is more apparent. M, muscle. (*C*) Sagittal T1-weighted image shows the "split fat" sign (*arrows*) at the superior and inferior edge of the lesion (*calipers*). (M) muscle.

Radiographic and computed tomography features of intramuscular venous malformations

Radiographs are not routinely used to diagnose IMVM; however, in patients presenting with pain, radiographs are frequently the first type of imaging obtained. Depending on the lesion size, soft tissue fullness can be present in the area of the malformation. Intralesional thrombosis may lead to phlebolith formation, which on radiographs are seen as single or multiple round, lamellated, calcified foci with a lucent center. Focal linear lucent streaks over the muscle involved represent fatty atrophy. When the malformation is juxta-cortical, hyperostosis with periosteal scalloping and cortical wavy margins as well as nonaggressive periosteal

reaction can be seen.[11,36,37] IMVMs can be identified on computed tomography; however, the use of radiation and the lower contrast resolution are clear disadvantages compared with MR imaging. In addition, because of the slow and progressive enhancement pattern inherent to IMVMs, several exposure events would be required to properly characterize the lesion. Phleboliths and fatty muscle atrophy can be easily detected on computed tomography and should raise the possibility of an IMVM.[37]

Treatment

Not only the diagnosis but also the treatment of IMVMs can be challenging. To minimize morbidity,

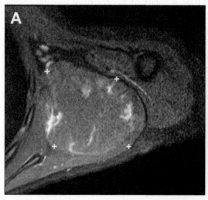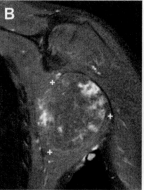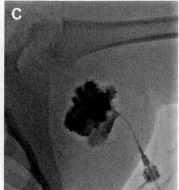

Fig. 15. A 10-year old girl with a large intramuscular venous malformation (IMVM) of the latissimus dorsi muscle. (*A*) Axial early postcontrast T1-weighted image with fat suppression shows a few small hyperintense areas of patchy enhancement throughout the IMVM (*calipers*). (*B*) Coronal delayed postcontrast T1-weighted image with fat suppression shows only minimal progression of the enhancement by the IMVM (*calipers*). (*C*) Spot image of a conventional venogram using image intensifier at the time of the sclerotherapy shows a spongiform type IMVM with no connections with the peripheral circulation.

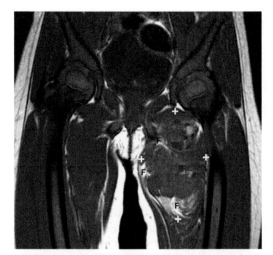

Fig. 16. A 3-year old girl with an intramuscular venous malformation of the adductor compartment. Coronal T1-weighted image shows a lobulated mass (*calipers*) isointense to muscle with areas of increased signal intensity corresponding to fat (F) indicating muscle atrophy.

the approach should be multidisciplinary and ideally by a vascular anomaly team.[38,39] Observation is advocated for asymptomatic lesions. For symptomatic lesions, medical treatment can be the first line of approach, especially if the symptoms are mild. Medical treatment includes compression garment, nonsteroidal anti-inflammatory drugs, prophylactic aspirin, or low molecular weight heparin if thrombosis is present.

Sclerotherapy, surgery, or a combination is usually reserved for the more symptomatic lesions.[1,7,22,40] In the study by Wieck and colleagues,[22] sclerotherapy was found to be more effective for pain-related symptoms, whereas surgery was more effective for muscle contractures. If sclerotherapy, surgery, or even biopsy is contemplated, the possibility of LIC-related complications must be considered. A baseline preprocedural complete blood count as well as a coagulation profile that includes partial thromboplastin time, prothrombin time, international normalized ratio, fibrinogen, and D-dimer levels must be obtained. In cases of LIC in which the level of D-dimers is elevated and fibrinogen is low, the patient must be placed on a prophylactic regimen of low-molecular-weight heparin (Lovenox) for several days before and after the procedure.[8,24]

At our institution, we routinely administer Lovenox subcutaneously for a total of 20 days: 10 days before and after the procedure in patients with evidence of LIC. Because these lesions are confined to the muscle, we have found that the inflammatory reaction after sclerotherapy is a source of substantial pain with daily activities. Usually in combination with acetaminophen, a short course of opioids that do not interfere with or halt the expected inflammation after sclerotherapy can be prescribed. The risk of skin necrosis related to sclerotherapy is substantially lower than that of the superficial VMs because these lesions are confined to muscle.

INTRAMUSCULAR CAPILLARY-TYPE HEMANGIOMA

Hein and colleagues[1] in 2002 were the first to hypothesize that small vessel hemangioma described by Allen and Enzinger in 1972 represented a benign vascular neoplasm with a capillary structure. In 2014, Yilmaz and colleagues[12] formally proposed that this lesion was indeed a benign neoplasm, and they named it ICTH. In the last revised ISSVA classification,[2] intramuscular hemangioma remains in the provisionally, unclassified category, although it is recognized as a separate entity distinct from infantile hemangioma, IMVM, and fibroadipose vascular anomaly.

Histologic Appearance

Intramuscular capillary-type hemangioma, being a true neoplasm, is histologically composed of lobules or sheets of multiple thin-wall capillaries embedded in collagen and surrounded by fat (**Fig. 17A**). The lesions appear very cellular with large endothelial cells, causing the obliteration of the lumen of the small vessels yielding a solid appearance (**Fig. 17B**). The presence of plump nuclei, mitotic activity, and intraluminal papillary projections can convey a malignant appearance. Various amounts of adipose tissue separating individual or groups of skeletal muscle fibers is a constant feature. Intravascular thrombosis is not a prominent feature, and calcifications (ie, phleboliths) are not seen.[1,9,12] Small-size arteries and thin-wall draining veins with variable smooth muscle but no arteriovenous shunting are also present. Being a vascular lesion, ICTH is reactive to CD31, CD34, and von Willebrand factor and similar to IMVMs is nonreactive to glucose transporter protein (GLUT1).[1,12]

Clinical Presentation

In the largest and only pediatric series published by Yilmaz and colleagues,[12] which included 18 children with ICTHs, 10 were boys with a mean age of 8.1 years and a median age of 6.8 years. The third decade predominance reported in the seminal article by Allen and Enzinger was probably

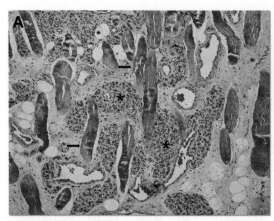 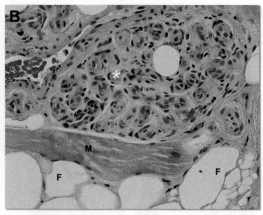

Fig. 17. (A) Intramuscular capillary-type hemangioma (ICTH) is characterized by lobules of capillaries (GLUT-1 negative) with plump endothelium (*asterisk*) containing variable amount of adipose tissue and infiltrating skeletal muscle (*arrows*) (hematoxylin-eosin, original magnification X100). (B) Higher magnification of ICTH shows a proliferation of small capillaries with plump endothelium (*asterisk*) in between skeletal muscle fibers (M) and fat (F). (hematoxylin-eosin, original magnification ×400).

a selection bias, as almost half of the patients were from military hospitals[9] The lesions were present in the head and neck, trunk, and extremities with a lower-limb predominance,[12] which is in contradistinction from the head and neck predominance found in the seminal article.[9]

The clinical presentation of ICTH is similar to that of IMVMs with a palpable, soft tissue mass; however, they are less painful, which is in accordance with the symptomatology originally described by Allen and Enzinger. Due to the intramuscular location, skin discoloration is not present.[9]

Imaging Approach

Because ICTHs and IMVMs present as a mass, they have a similar imaging approach, which should include ultrasound followed by MR imaging as discussed in the IMVMs section (see **Table 1**).

On ultrasound and MR imaging, ICTH is seen as a predominantly well-defined, solid soft tissue mass confined to a single or to multiple muscles. Mild extension into the subcutis is occasionally present. No calcifications in the form of phleboliths are identified on ultrasound or MR imaging. On ultrasound, the lesions have a heterogeneous echogenicity with hyperechoic fatty elements. Intralesional fast flow vessels with arterial waveforms and no evidence of arteriovenous shunting are identified.[12,41] On MR imaging, the lesions are heterogeneously hyperintense on T2-weighted images, isointense to muscle on T1-weighted images with the presence of flow voids and intralesional and perilesional fatty elements. The lesions display a rather homogeneous contrast enhancement indicating a hypervascular nature (**Fig. 18**). Diffuse involvement and

expansion of the involved muscle with relative preservation of the shape is a distinct imaging feature of ICTH (see **Fig. 18**A).[42]

The presence of an intramuscular enhancing mass with arterial and venous components and fatty elements causing muscle expansion is suggestive of ICTHs. The presence of a mass and the lack of arteriovenous shunting are features that are helpful for differentiating ICTHs from arteriovenous malformations. A late age at presentation, the lack of involution, and an intramuscular location are differentiating features from infantile hemangiomas. Fatty elements in a soft tissue mass almost always heralds a benign pathology (except for the exceedingly rare liposarcoma in children) and speak against a malignant neoplasm.[28] An ICTH is less defined and can be more infiltrative within the muscle compared with IMVMs.[10,11] Some lesions may require a biopsy to reach a final diagnosis.

Treatment

These lesions can be observed but when symptomatic, complete resection to include the surrounding muscle fibers is advocated.

FIBROADIPOSE VASCULAR ANOMALY

Since its original description in the series of 18 patients by Alomari and colleagues[13] in 2014, little has been written about FAVA with only a few additional articles written in the English literature.[43–45] Currently, FAVA, along with ICTH, is considered a separate entity in the still unclassified category by ISSVA.[2] However, recent genetic studies of FAVA specimens have identified mutations in

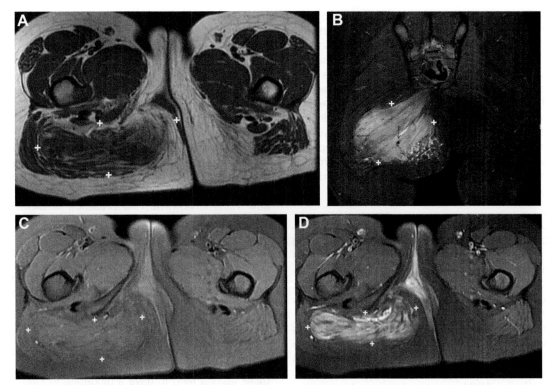

Fig. 18. A 14-year old girl with an intramuscular capillary-type hemangioma (ICTH) of the right gluteus maximus. (A) Axial T1-weighted image shows a heterogeneous and expanded appearance of the right gluteus maximus (*asterisks*) which is infiltrated by fat. (B) Coronal T2-weighted image with fat suppression shows the increased signal intensity (less than fluid) of the right gluteal lesion (*calipers*). Several flow voids (*arrows*) representing arteries are seen. (C) Axial precontrast T1-weighted image with fat suppression shows the lesion (*calipers*) before contrast. (D) Axial postcontrast T1-weighted image with fat suppression shows fairly homogeneous and vivid enhancement by the right gluteal lesion (*calipers*).

phosphoinositide 3-kinase, the same mutations found in overgrowth syndromes (PROS: PIK3CA-related overgrowth spectrum).[46,47] These often symptomatic lesions require a precise diagnosis as correct treatment is critical.

Histologic Appearance

FAVA consists of 2 predominant components: prominent fibrofatty tissue infiltrating skeletal muscle and slow flow vascular malformations of the venous and lymphatic type (**Fig. 19**). The

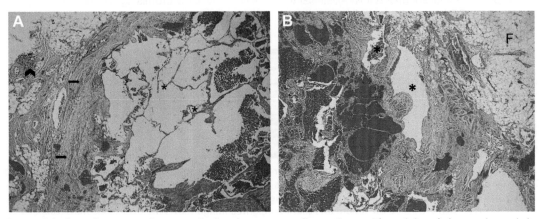

Fig. 19. (A) Fibroadipose vascular anomaly showing mature adipose tissue with nodules of abnormal vessels (*arrows*) with numerous diverticula that simulate pulmonary alveoli (*asterisks*), surrounded by fibrous tissue and with lymphoid aggregates scattered throughout (*arrowhead*). H&E, 40X. (B) The muscularized abnormal venous channels (*asterisks*) within mature fatty overgrowth (F) is seen. H&E, 40X.

venous component has small and large, irregular, muscularized venous channels with occasional thrombi and rare phleboliths as well as smaller clusters of vascular channels resembling pulmonary alveoli. The abnormal lymphatics are clustered and thin-walled with little or no muscle in the walls. Lymphoplasmatic aggregates are usually seen scattered throughout the lesion. Having a lymphatic component, this lesion is immune-positive to D2-40 a marker for lymphatic endothelium. Entrapment of nerves by surrounding fibrous tissue may explain the localized pain typical of this lesion.[13,43]

Clinical Presentation

Like intramuscular venous malformations and hemangiomas, FAVA usually presents as a palpable mass. Differing from IMVM, FAVAs are hard and noncompressible. These lesions have a female predominance and more commonly involve the calf musculature, particularly the gastrocnemius. Other locations have been reported, such as the forearm and thigh, but in our practice, we have also found them involving the chest and abdominal wall musculature (**Fig. 20**). Both, FAVA and IMVM are painful and tend to present during puberty. Unlike IMVM, FAVA typically has constant and severe pain leading to limb atrophy, a result of muscle fibrosis. Limb contracture and limited range of motion is unique to FAVA and, even if absent at the time of initial diagnosis, they eventually develop in due course. Due to its intramuscular location, skin discoloration is not characteristically present but superficial phlebectasia of the overlying tissues can be seen.[13,43–45,47]

Imaging Approach

Fibroadipose vascular anomalies (FAVA), similar to IMVM and ICTH, should be imaged with ultrasound and MR imaging. All 3 entities are seen as an intramuscular mass that can involve a single muscle, a muscle group either focally or diffusely, or involve multiple compartments. FAVA surrounds or displaces neurovascular structures and may extend across and distort fascial planes. On ultrasound, FAVA is seen as a solid mass (differing from the rather cystic IMVM) replacing the muscle fibers with indistinct borders and a heterogeneous but predominantly increased echogenicity attributable to fatty elements. The mass is not particularly hypervascular on color Doppler ultrasound because is composed of low-flow vessels, however, the presence of dilated veins with thrombi and even the occasional phlebolith are characteristic and helpful in differentiating them from ICTH (see **Fig. 20**A). MR imaging has a higher diagnostic value than ultrasound for this entity, and FAVA is seen as a heterogeneously hyperintense mass on T2-weighted images but with less hyperintensity than the blood-filled venous malformations. On T1-weighted images, the affected muscle has also a heterogeneous signal with hyperintense areas corresponding to fatty elements. After gadolinium administration, these lesions tend to have a moderate to strong enhancement different than IMVM at least on the early phase (see **Fig. 20**B–E).[13,44]

Treatment

The treatment of FAVA is variable. Symptomatic patients may require surgical resection, whereas asymptomatic patients may simply be observed. Physical therapy and sclerotherapy can help alleviate symptoms, but these tend to be only temporary measures.[13] More recently, image-guided thermal ablation (cryoablation) and sirolimus have been used as a promising alternative with good results.[48–50]

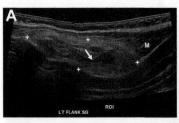
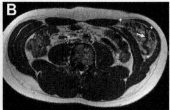
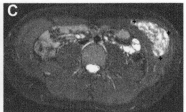

Fig. 20. An 18-year old man with a fibroadipose vascular anomaly of the abdominal wall (same as on **Fig. 19**). (*A*) Gray-scale ultrasound image shows an oval-shape mass (*calipers*) with poorly defined borders and a predominantly increased echogenicity replacing part of the left external oblique muscle (M). Hypoechoic, dilated, tortuous veins (*arrow*) are inside the lesion. (*B*) Axial T1-weighted image shows the oval-shape mass (*calipers*) replacing the external oblique muscle. The mass (*calipers*) has interspersed predominantly hyperintense fatty elements and dilated and tortuous veins (*arrow*). (*C*) Axial T2-weighted image with fat suppression shows the mass (*calipers*) as predominantly hyperintense with suppression of the fatty elements. (*D*) Axial postcontrast T1-weighted image with fat suppression shows substantial heterogeneous enhancement by the mass (*calipers*).

SUMMARY

The unification and proper use of terminology of vascular anomalies is essential to attain a correct diagnosis and treatment for general radiologists. It is now recognized that IMVMs, ICTH, and FAVA are 3 distinct pathologies with unique clinical, histologic and imaging features. Histologically, IMVMs correspond to the large vessel–type lesion originally described by Allen and Enzinger, whereas ICTHs, which are neoplasms, correspond to the small-vessel type. All 3 pathologies tend to present beyond the neonatal period because of their confinement to muscle and can potentially be confused with a malignancy. These potentially confusing lesions are best evaluated with ultrasound and MR imaging, which are complementary modalities. Familiarity with the clinical presentation as well as the histologic and imaging appearance can increase diagnostic confidence. However, dubious cases may still require a biopsy. The presence of LIC may support the diagnosis of IMVMs and should be considered when biopsy, surgery, or sclerotherapy are contemplated to avoid potentially life-threatening complications.

REFERENCES

1. Hein KD, Mulliken JB, Kozakewich HPW, et al. Venous malformations of skeletal muscle. Plast Reconstr Surg 2002;110(7):1625–35.

2. Classification | International Society for the study of vascular anomalies. Available at: http://www.issva.org/classification. Accessed August 16, 2018.

3. Hassanein AH, Mulliken JB, Fishman SJ, et al. Evaluation of terminology for vascular anomalies in current literature. Plast Reconstr Surg 2011;127(1):347.

4. Dubois J, Soulez G, Oliva VL, et al. Soft tissue venous malformations in adult patients: imaging and therapeutic issues. Radiographics 2001;21(6): 1519–31.

5. Puig S, Casati B, Staudenherz A, et al. Vascular low-flow malformations in children: current concepts for classification, diagnosis and therapy. Eur J Radiol 2005;53(1):35–45.

6. Puig S, Aref H, Chigot V, et al. Classification of venous malformations in children and implications for sclerotherapy. Pediatr Radiol 2003;33(2): 99–103.

7. Vogel SA, Hess CP, Dowd CF, et al. Early versus later presentations of venous malformations: where and why? Pediatr Dermatol 2013;30(5):534–40.

8. Koo KSH, Dowd CF, Mathes EF, et al. MRI phenotypes of localized intravascular coagulopathy in venous malformations. Pediatr Radiol 2015;45(11): 1690–5.

9. Allen PW, Enzinger FM. Hemangioma of skeletal muscle. An analysis of 89 cases. Cancer 1972; 29(1):8–22.

10. Wild AT, Raab P, Krauspe R. Hemangioma of skeletal muscle. Arch Orthop Trauma Surg 2000;120(3–4): 139–43.

11. Wu J-L, Wu C-C, Wang S-J, et al. Imaging strategies in intramuscular haemangiomas: an analysis of 20 cases. Int Orthop 2007;31(4):569–75.

12. Yilmaz S, Kozakewich HP, Alomari AI, et al. Intramuscular capillary-type hemangioma: radiologic–pathologic correlation. Pediatr Radiol 2014;44(5):558–65.

13. Alomari AI, Spencer SA, Arnold RW, et al. Fibro-adipose vascular anomaly: clinical-radiologic-pathologic features of a newly delineated disorder of the extremity. J Pediatr Orthop 2014;34(1):109.

14. Ahlawat S, Fayad LM, Durand DJ, et al. International Society for the Study of Vascular Anomalies classification of soft tissue vascular anomalies: survey-based assessment of musculoskeletal radiologists' use in clinical practice. Curr Probl Diagn Radiol 2017;48(1): 10–6. Available at: http://www.sciencedirect.com/science/article/pii/S0363018817300993. Accessed August 16, 2018.

15. Mulliken JB, Glowacki J. Hemangiomas and vascular malformations in infants and children: a classification based on endothelial characteristics. Plast Reconstr Surg 1982;69(3):412–22.

16. Hand JL, Frieden IJ. Vascular birthmarks of infancy: resolving nosologic confusion. Am J Med Genet 2002;108(4):257–64.

17. Bruder E, Alaggio R, Kozakewich HPW, et al. Vascular and perivascular lesions of skin and soft tissues in children and adolescents. Pediatr Dev Pathol 2012;15(1_suppl):26–61.

18. Hashimoto H, Daimaru Y, Enjoji M. Intravascular papillary endothelial hyperplasia. A clinicopathologic study of 91 cases. Am J Dermatopathol 1983;5(6):539–46.

19. Guledgud MV, Patil K, Saikrishna D, et al. Intravascular papillary endothelial hyperplasia: diagnostic sequence and literature review of an orofacial lesion. Case Rep Dent 2014;2014:934593. Available at: https://www.ncbi.nlm.nih.gov/pmc/articles/PMC4033548/. Accessed August 18, 2018.

20. Beutler BD, Cohen PR. Intravascular papillary endothelial hyperplasia of the vulva: report of a patient with Masson tumor of the vulva and literature review. Dermatol Online J 2016;22(5). Available at: https://escholarship.org/uc/item/0ss9x4vf. Accessed August 18, 2018.

21. Shallow TA, Eger SA, Wagner FB. Primary hemangiomatous tumors of skeletal muscle. Ann Surg 1944;119(5):700–40.

22. Wieck MM, Nowicki D, Schall KA, et al. Management of pediatric intramuscular venous malformations. J Pediatr Surg 2017;52(4):598–601.

618   Restrepo et al

23. Hassanein AH, Mulliken JB, Fishman SJ, et al. Venous malformation: risk of progression during childhood and adolescence. Ann Plast Surg 2012; 68(2):198.

24. Mazoyer E, Enjolras O, Bisdorff A, et al. Coagulation disorders in patients with venous malformation of the limbs and trunk: a case series of 118 patients. Arch Dermatol 2008;144(7):861–7.

25. Dompmartin A, Ballieux F, Thibon P, et al. Elevated D-dimer level in the differential diagnosis of venous malformations. Arch Dermatol 2009;145(11):1239–44.

26. Paltiel HJ, Burrows PE, Kozakewich HPW, et al. Soft-tissue vascular anomalies: utility of US for diagnosis. Radiology 2000;214(3):747–54.

27. Trop I, Dubois J, Guibaud L, et al. Soft-tissue venous malformations in pediatric and young adult patients: diagnosis with doppler US. Radiology 1999;212(3): 841–5.

28. Sung J, Kim J-Y. Fatty rind of intramuscular soft-tissue tumors of the extremity: is it different from the split fat sign? Skeletal Radiol 2017;46(5):665–73.

29. Greenspan A, McGahan JP, Vogelsang P, et al. Imaging strategies in the evaluation of soft-tissue hemangiomas of the extremities: correlation of the findings of plain radiography, angiography, CT, MRI, and ultrasonography in 12 histologically proven cases. Skeletal Radiol 1992;21(1):11–8.

30. Kim OH, Kim YM, Choo HJ, et al. Subcutaneous intravascular papillary endothelial hyperplasia: ultrasound features and pathological correlation. Skeletal Radiol 2016;45(2):227–33.

31. Craig KA, Escobar E, Inwards CY, et al. Imaging characteristics of intravascular papillary endothelial hyperplasia. Skeletal Radiol 2016;45(11):1467–72.

32. Lee SJ, Choo HJ, Park JS, et al. Imaging findings of intravascular papillary endothelial hyperplasia presenting in extremities: correlation with pathological findings. Skeletal Radiol 2010;39(8):783–9.

33. Juan Y-H, Huang G-S, Chiu Y-C, et al. Intravascular papillary endothelial hyperplasia of the calf in an infant: MR features with histological correlation. Pediatr Radiol 2009;39(3):282–5.

34. Corti R, Osende JI, Fayad ZA, et al. In vivo noninvasive detection and age definition of arterial thrombus by MRI. J Am Coll Cardiol 2002;39(8):1366–73.

35. Olsen KI, Stacy GS, Montag A. Soft-tissue cavernous hemangioma. Radiographics 2004; 24(3):849–54.

36. Ly JQ, Sanders TG, Mulloy JP, et al. Osseous change adjacent to soft-tissue hemangiomas of the extremities: correlation with lesion size and proximity to bone. Am J Roentgenol 2003;180(6):1695–700.

37. Kudawara I, Yoshikawa H, Araki N, et al. Intramuscular haemangioma adjacent to the bone surface with periosteal reaction. Report of three cases and review of the literature. J Bone Joint Surg Br 2001; 83(5):659–62.

38. Greene AK, Liu AS, Mulliken JB, et al. Vascular anomalies in 5621 patients: guidelines for referral. J Pediatr Surg 2011;46(9):1784–9.

39. Rochon PJ. Importance of multidisciplinary approach to vascular malformation management. Semin Intervent Radiol 2017;34(3):301–2. Available at: https:// eurekamag.com/research/059/842/059842270.php. Accessed August 20, 2018.

40. Jayaraman V, Austin RD, Kannan S. Nonsurgical management of vascular malformation of masseter. Indian J Dent Res 2015;26(1):96.

41. Johnson CM, Navarro OM. Clinical and sonographic features of pediatric soft-tissue vascular anomalies part 1: classification, sonographic approach and vascular tumors. Pediatr Radiol 2017;47(9): 1184–95.

42. Merrow AC, Gupta A, Adams DM. Additional imaging features of intramuscular capillary-type hemangioma: the importance of ultrasound. Pediatr Radiol 2014;44(11):1472–4.

43. Fernandez-Pineda I, Marcilla D, Downey-Carmona FJ, et al. Lower extremity Fibro-Adipose Vascular Anomaly (FAVA): a new case of a newly delineated disorder. Ann Vasc Dis 2014;7(3):316–9.

44. Cheung K, Taghinia AH, Sood RF, et al. Fibroadipose vascular anomaly in the upper extremity: a distinct entity with characteristic clinical, radiological, and histopathological findings. J Hand Surg 2019;45(1): 68.e1-13. Available at: https://www.jhandsurg.org/ article/S0363-5023(19)30028-0/abstract. Accessed September 8, 2019.

45. Wang KK, Glenn RL, Adams DM, et al. Surgical management of fibroadipose vascular anomaly of the lower extremities. J Pediatr Orthop 2020;40(3): e227–36.

46. Luks VL, Kamitaki N, Vivero MP, et al. Lymphatic and other vascular malformative/overgrowth disorders are caused by somatic mutations in PIK3CA. J Pediatr 2015;166(4):1048–54.e1-5.

47. Bertino F, Braithwaite KA, Hawkins CM, et al. Congenital limb overgrowth syndromes associated with vascular anomalies. Radiographics 2019; 39(2):491–515.

48. Shaikh R, Alomari AI, Kerr CL, et al. Cryoablation in fibro-adipose vascular anomaly (FAVA): a minimally invasive treatment option. Pediatr Radiol 2016; 46(8):1179–86.

49. Adams DM, Trenor CC, Hammill AM, et al. Efficacy and safety of sirolimus in the treatment of complicated vascular anomalies. Pediatrics 2016;137(2): e20153257. Available at: https://www.ncbi.nlm.nih. gov/pmc/articles/PMC4732362/. Accessed September 8, 2019.

50. Erickson J, McAuliffe W, Blennerhassett L, et al. Fibroadipose vascular anomaly treated with sirolimus: Successful outcome in two patients. Pediatr Dermatol 2017;34(6):e317–20.

Genetic Syndromes Affecting Both Children and Adults
A Practical Guide to Imaging-based Diagnosis, Management, and Screening Recommendations for General Radiologists

Bradford Hastings, MD, MPH[a], Koenraad Mortele, MD[b],
Edward Y. Lee, MD, MPH[c],*

KEYWORDS

- Pediatric • Adult • Genetic syndrome • Neurofibromatosis • Von Hippel-Lindau syndrome (VHL)
- Tuberous sclerosis • Multiple endocrine neoplasia • Li-Fraumeni syndrome (LFS)

KEY POINTS

- Genetic syndromes are infrequently encountered but challenging group of conditions for both pediatric and adult radiologists.
- Both pediatric and adult radiologists should be familiar with characteristic syndromic imaging features and common complications. Such knowledge can assist in image interpretation, guide management, and guide appropriate surveillance.

INTRODUCTION

Although genetic syndromes are often thought of as entities falling under the scope of pediatrics and pediatric radiology, the sequelae of these conditions frequently extend into adulthood and are often associated with significant morbidity and mortality. Therefore, both pediatric and adult radiologists should be familiar with characteristic syndromic features and the most common complications, including malignant transformation of benign neoplasms. Such knowledge can assist in image interpretation and help guide management and appropriate surveillance.

Although a complete discussion of every aspect of the included genetic syndromes is beyond the scope of this review article, the overarching goal is to provide an up-to-date review of characteristic imaging findings, management, and screening recommendations for a select group of clinically important genetic syndromes that are encountered in daily clinical practice by general radiologists (Table 1).

SPECTRUM OF GENETIC SYNDROMES AFFECTING BOTH CHILDREN AND ADULTS
Neurofibromatosis Type 1

Neurofibromatosis type 1 (NF 1) is a multisystemic neurocutaneous disorder with a broad range of clinical manifestations predominantly involving the skin, orbits, nervous system, and musculoskeletal

a Department of Radiology, Beth Israel Deaconess Medical Center, Harvard Medical School, 330 Brookline Avenue, Boston, MA 02215, USA; b 24 Walpole Street, Dover, MA 02030, USA; c Division of Thoracic Imaging, Department of Radiology, Boston Children's Hospital, Harvard Medical School, 300 Longwood Avenue, Boston, MA 02115, USA
* Corresponding author.
E-mail address: Edward.Lee@childrens.harvard.edu

Radiol Clin N Am 58 (2020) 619–638
https://doi.org/10.1016/j.rcl.2020.01.003
0033-8389/20/© 2020 Elsevier Inc. All rights reserved.

Table 1
Key imaging features and current selected imaging screening recommendations

Genetic Syndromes	Key Imaging Features	Current Selected Imaging Screening Recommendations
NF 1[2,10]	Neurofibromas, CNS gliomas, skeletal involvement (eg, scoliosis, pseudarthrosis), malignant peripheral nerve sheath tumors, neuroendocrine tumors (eg, pheochromocytoma), embryonal rhabdomyosarcoma, breast malignancy	• Consider full body MR imaging in young adults to establish baseline • NCCN guidelines recommend an annual mammogram starting at age 30 y and consideration of contrast-enhanced breast MR imaging for female patients with NF 1 • Screening imaging is otherwise not recommended in asymptomatic patients
NF 2[15]	Schwannomas (eg, bilateral schwannomas involving the vestibulocochlear nerve), meningiomas, spinal lesions (eg, low-grade ependymoma)	• Screening for neoplasms is recommended in patients with family history of NF 2 or those presenting with a unilateral vestibular schwannoma or other type of schwannoma, meningioma, or retinal hamartoma • Annual or biannual brain MR imaging starting at 10 y using high-resolution technique (1–3 mm slice thickness) with coverage of the internal acoustic meatus in at least 2 planes (enhanced study preferred) • Imaging of the spine should be obtained starting at 10 y and repeated at intervals of 24–36 mo, preferably with contrast • If NF 2–associated lesions are detected on either brain or spinal imaging, the next repeat examination should occur 6 mo later to assess rate of growth • As patients enter adulthood, annual MR imaging of the brain is still recommended; however, the interval of spinal imaging can be extended to 3–5 y
VHL[22]	CNS and retinal hemangioblastomas, pheochromocytomas, renal cysts and RCCs, pancreatic cysts and cystadenomas, pancreatic neuroendocrine tumors, endolymphatic tumors	• In patients age 16 y and older, annual abdominal US (with MR imaging of the abdomen at least every other year) is recommended as well as annual imaging of the brain, petrous temporal bone, and total spine with and without contrast • In younger patients, decision regarding screening for abdominal or CNS disease can be made from the clinical assessment and history
TS[34]	Subcortical tubers, subependymal ependymomas, subependymal giant cell astrocytoma, renal angiomyolipoma, RCCs, cardiac rhabdomyomas, pulmonary lymphangioleiomyomatosis	• MR imaging of the brain and abdomen every 1–3 y for symptom-free patients with TS <25 y old • CNS screening can stop after age 25 y for patients without subependymal astrocytoma. More frequent

(continued on next page)

Table 1
(continued)

Genetic Syndromes	Key Imaging Features	Current Selected Imaging Screening Recommendations
		imaging is recommended for patients with known lesions • Continued surveillance is recommended to assess for renal complications (interval not specified) • In asymptomatic women at risk for LAM, HRCT should be performed at intervals of 5–10 y. If cysts are detected, the interval should be reduced to 2–3 y
Multiple endocrine neoplasia syndrome type 1[44,45]	Parathyroid adenomas, pituitary adenomas, pancreatic neuroendocrine tumors, adrenal lesions, carcinoid tumors	• Endocrine Society guidelines published in 2012 recommend annual imaging surveillance for pancreatic neuroendocrine tumors and adrenal lesions with MR imaging, CT, or US before the age of 10 y • Starting at age 5 y, patients should undergo MR imaging every 3 y for pituitary lesions surveillance • The guidelines recommend CT or MR imaging screening every 1–2 y for thymic and bronchial carcinoid lesions starting at age 15 y
Multiple endocrine neoplasia type 2[36]	Medullary thyroid carcinoma, pheochromocytoma, parathyroid lesions	• Variability in screening recommendations with some investigators recommending imaging only in the setting of biochemical abnormalities and others recommending organ-specific screening, such as MR imaging of the abdomen every 3 y to evaluate for pheochromocytoma with optional scintigraphy
LFS[49,56–58]	Osteosarcoma, soft tissue sarcomas (eg rhabdomyosarcomas), brain tumors (eg astrocytoma, choroid plexus carcinoma), adrenal cortical tumors, breast cancer	• Mai and colleagues[49] described an LFS surveillance protocol including abdominal sonography every 4 mo, annual brain MR imaging, and annual rapid whole-body MR imaging for children aged 3–16 y • For patients older than 16 y, the surveillance protocol included annual brain MR imaging and annual rapid whole-body MR imaging • In addition, for female patients 20–40 y old, annual breast MR imaging was recommended and for patients >40 y old annual breast MR imaging and mammography was recommended

(continued on next page)

Table 1
(continued)

Genetic Syndromes	Key Imaging Features	Current Selected Imaging Screening Recommendations
DICER 1 syndrome[61]	Pleuropulmonary blastoma, renal lesions (eg cystic nephroma, Wilms tumor), ovarian sex cord-stromal tumors, genitourinary rhabdomyosarcomas, and pituitary blastoma. Patients also may develop other lesions, such as multinodular goiter	• Shultz and colleagues[61] recommend a comprehensive imaging surveillance for patients with DICER 1. • Pelvic and abdominal US every 6–12 mo for female patients beginning at 8–10 y until age 40 y • For evaluation of renal abnormalities, abdominal US is recommended every 6 mo until age 8 y, then annually until 12 y • Baseline thyroid US by 8 y of age, then once per 3 y in asymptomatic patients • CXR every 4–6 mo from birth until age 8 y, then annually until age 12 y with consideration of chest CT

Abbreviations: CNS, central nervous system; CT, computed tomography; CXR, chest radiography; HRCT, high-resolution computed tomography; LAM, lymphangioleiomyomatosis; LFS, Li-Fraumeni syndrome; MR, magnetic resonance; NCCN, national comprehensive cancer network; NF 1, neurofibromatosis type 1; NF 2, neurofibromatosis type 2; RCC, renal cell carcinoma; TS, tuberous sclerosis; US, ultrasonography; VHL, von Hippel-Lindau syndrome.

system. NF 1 is the most common neurocutaneous disorder and one of the most common genetic disorders overall, affecting 1 in 2500 to 3000.[1] There is variable expression of the most common systemic abnormalities in NF 1; however, most patients are diagnosed using major or minor criteria by 1 year of age. The condition is associated with an reduction in life expectancy of 8 to 15 years secondary to associated neoplasms and cardiovascular causes.[2] The NF 1 gene is located on chromosome 17 and produces neurofibromin, a tumor suppressor of the Ras/mitogen-activated protein kinase (MAPK) pathway that, when mutated, predisposes to tumor development in both pediatric and adult populations.[3] The inheritance pattern is considered autosomal dominant; however, the condition occurs sporadically in up to 50% of cases.

Neurofibromas are benign peripheral nerve sheath tumors classified as plexiform neurofibromas, localized neurofibromas, and diffuse cutaneous neurofibromas. Localized neurofibromas are not specific to NF 1, and diffuse cutaneous neurofibromas are not typically a radiologic diagnosis. Plexiform neurofibromas are frequently seen in patients with NF 1, involve long segments of nerves typically extending into adjacent soft tissues, and present clinically as a so-called bag-of-worms subcutaneous mass. On plain radiography, these lesions are seen as a nonspecific soft tissue mass without calcification. If the lesions are large enough, bony remodeling can be seen secondary to mass

effect. On computed tomography (CT), the lesions are typically low density. Magnetic resonance (MR) imaging is the recommended modality for more comprehensive evaluation, and lesions are typically T1 hypointense, T2 hyperintense, and show variable postgadolinium enhancement patterns. On T2-weighted images, these lesions may show the target sign characterized by peripheral hyperintensity and central hypointensity.[4] Of particular concern is the potential for plexiform neurofibromas to undergo malignant degeneration into malignant peripheral nerve sheath tumors (MPNSTs). MPNSTs are aggressive lesions that frequently metastasize. Malignant degeneration occurs in approximately 5% of patients with NF 1. Although differentiation of benign plexiform neurofibromas and MPNSTs is difficult from imaging alone, lesions that are symptomatic show substantial interval growth, show cystic degeneration/necrosis, or have infiltrative margins should alert the reader of the possibility of malignant degeneration (**Fig. 1**).[4,5] 18F-fluorodeoxyglucose (FDG) PET can be helpful because MPNST typically shows increased FDG avidity.

NF 1 is associated with several central nervous system (CNS) neoplasms, such as optic pathway gliomas and brain stem gliomas.[6] Optic glioma affects 15% to 20% of patients with NF 1 and represents one of the diagnostic criteria of NF 1 (**Fig. 2**). These lesions are typically considered low-grade lesions (World Health Organization grade I). A

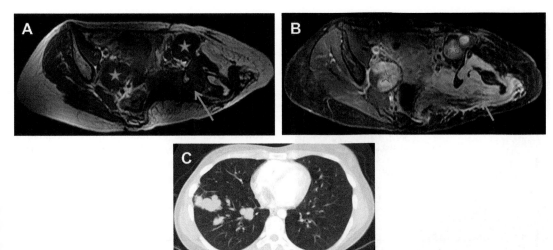

Fig. 1. Neurofibromatosis type 1 in a 28-year-old woman. (*A, B*) Axial T1-weighted and T1-weighted postcontrast MR images show an enhancing and infiltrative soft tissue mass (*arrows*) extending from the left hemipelvis into and around the left acetabular region and upper thigh consistent with malignant peripheral nerve sheath tumor. Multiple additional enhancing soft tissue masses (*asterisks*) are seen in the pelvis consistent with neurofibromas. (*C*) Axial lung window CT image shows multiple pulmonary masses consistent with metastatic disease.

common diagnostic dilemma in patients with NF 1 is the classically described unidentified neurofibromatosis objects (UNOs), which are T2 hyperintense and T1 isointense and are most commonly seen in the globi pallidi. Depending on location, these lesions may or may not resolve with age. Persistent UNO lesions may mimic CNS neoplasms associated with NF 1, such as a brainstem glioma. In such situations, MR spectroscopy may assist the reader in making such a distinction.[7]

Skeletal abnormalities in patients with NF 1 can often be described using plain radiography and include characteristic findings of sphenoid wing

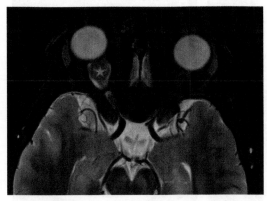

Fig. 2. Neurofibromatosis type 1 in a 12-year-old girl. Axial T2-weighted MR image with fat suppression shows an optic glioma (*asterisk*) of the intraconal portion of the right optic nerve with associated mild exophthalmos.

dysplasia, scoliosis, neuroforaminal widening, pseudoarthrosis of the tibia, and rib notching (**Fig. 3**).[8,9] Because these changes progress over time, skeletal involvement of NF 1 may cause substantial morbidity in adulthood. Patients are also at risk for vertebral degenerative changes, dural ectasia, and spinal compression as well as osteoporosis, which typically occurs at an earlier age.[10]

NF 1 is associated with increased incidence of several neoplasms outside of the CNS, including embryonal rhabdomyosarcoma, juvenile myelomonocytic leukemia, and neuroendocrine tumors. Despite their increased incidence relative to the general population, the overall incidence remains low. For example, the incidence of embryonal rhabdomyosarcoma is approximately 1% in patients with NF 1. As such, routine asymptomatic imaging of pediatric patients with NF 1 is not currently recommended. However, clinicians may consider whole-body MR imaging between the ages of 16 and 20 years to assess internal tumor burden and assist with long-term care planning.[10]

Adult patients with NF 1 are at risk for malignancies related to NF 1. For example, NF-associated pheochromocytomas are more commonly diagnosed in adult patients with NF 1, with a median age at diagnosis of 43 years.[2] Adult women with NF 1 are at increased risk of breast cancer, especially before the age of 40 years, and show significantly poorer 5-year survival. The National Comprehensive Cancer Network guidelines recommend an annual mammogram starting at age 30 years and consideration of

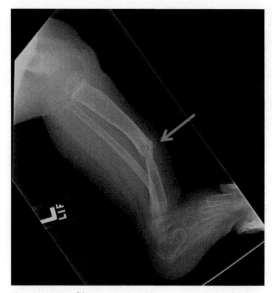

Fig. 3. Neurofibromatosis 1 in a 15-month-old boy. Radiograph of the left lower extremity shows pseudarthrosis (*arrow*) of the left tibial shaft and substantial anterolateral bowing of the left tibia and fibula.

contrast-enhanced breast MR imaging for female patients with NF 1.[2]

Neurofibromatosis Type 2

Neurofibromatosis type 2 (NF 2) is an autosomal dominant neurocutaneous disorder unrelated to NF 1 or neurofibromas. NF 2 is characterized by the development of multiple CNS lesions, including intracranial schwannomas, meningiomas, and spinal lesions such as low-grade ependymomas. NF 2 typically presents in young

adults aged 18 to 24 years with an incidence of 1 in 50,000.[11] The NF 2 gene is located on chromosome 22 and encodes the merlin protein, which plays a role in tumor suppression in neuronal cells, Schwann cells, and meningeal cells.

NF 2 presents differently in pediatric and adult populations. The Manchester diagnostic criteria are one of several diagnostic tools that have evolved over time to become more sensitive in diagnosing NF2 in typical pediatric and adult population presentations.[12] The classic adult presentation of NF 2 consists of bilateral schwannomas involving the vestibulocochlear nerve with clinical presentations of hearing difficulties, tinnitus, and balance issues (**Fig. 4**). Schwannomas also frequently involve spinal and peripheral nerves. Meningiomas may occur throughout the CNS, and intracranial meningiomas are associated with increased mortality in patients with NF 2.[4] Intraspinal ependymomas are typically low grade and indolent. MR imaging is the imaging modality of choice in the evaluation of NF 2–related CNS lesions. In the evaluation of vestibular schwannomas, readers should turn their attention to the internal auditory canal/cerebellar pontine angle, where lesions are typically T1 hypointense to isointense, T2 hyperintense, and avidly and homogeneously enhancing on postcontrast MR images. Meningiomas are typically T1 isointense or hypointense and diffusely enhancing with a dural tail. T2 bright perilesional edema and calcification seen as blooming on T2* gradient recalled echo may be encountered. Indistinct and infiltrating margins with restricted diffusion can signal atypical and malignant meningiomas. Ependymoma presents as an expansile cord lesion that is T1 isointense

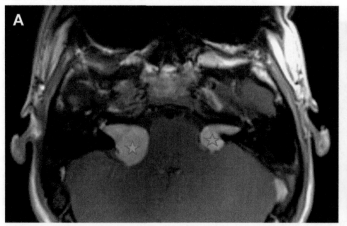
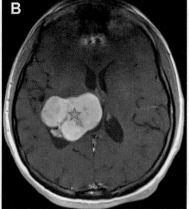

Fig. 4. Neurofibromatosis type 2 in a 12-year-old boy. (*A*) Axial T1-weighted postcontrast MR image of the brain shows bilateral avidly enhancing cerebellopontine angle lesions (*asterisks*) consistent with cranial nerve 8 schwannomas. (*B*) Axial T1-weighted postcontrast MR image shows a large right atrial meningioma (*asterisk*) with peripheral calcification.

or hypointense, T2 bright, and avidly enhancing. A T2 dark peripheral rim represents associated hemorrhage and is seen in up to 33% of cases (the cap sign).[13]

Pediatric patients with NF 2 often do not present with bilateral cranial nerve 8 schwannomas but with symptoms related to a nonspecific neuropathy, an apparently isolated meningioma, an extracranial schwannoma, or ocular symptoms. Pediatric patients with NF 2 initially presenting with nonclassic lesions may harbor severe multitumor disease. Baser and colleagues[14] showed that the risk of mortality increases with younger age at diagnosis.

Evans and colleagues[15] recommend MR screening for neoplasms in patients with family history of NF 2 or those presenting with a unilateral vestibular schwannoma or other type of schwannoma, meningioma, or retinal hamartoma. For those patients in whom the diagnosis of NF2 is established, the investigators recommend annual or biannual brain MR imaging starting at 10 years using a high-resolution technique (slice thickness 1–3 mm) with coverage of the internal acoustic meatus in at least 2 planes. Because CNS lesions associated with NF2 are avidly enhancing, gadolinium administration is recommended if clinically appropriate. Imaging of the spine should be obtained starting at 10 years and repeated at intervals of 24 to 36 months, preferably with contrast. If NF 2–associated lesions are detected on either brain or spinal imaging, the next repeat examination should occur 6 months later to assess rate of growth. As patients enter into adulthood, annual MR imaging of the brain is still recommended; however, the interval of spinal imaging can be extended to 3 to 5 years.

Von Hippel-Lindau Syndrome

Von Hippel-Lindau syndrome (VHL) is a rare, autosomal dominant syndrome with incidence of 1 in 35,000 to 50,000. VHL is characterized by a germline mutation resulting in inactivation of the VHL tumor suppressor gene on chromosome 3. This mutation has variable expression and can result in dozens of both benign and malignantneoplasms affecting more than 10 organs.[16] The most common lesions include CNS and retinal hemangioblastomas (HBs), pheochromocytomas, renal cysts and renal cell carcinoma (RCC), pancreatic cysts, pancreatic cystadenomas, pancreatic neuroendocrine tumors, endolymphatic sac tumors, and epididymal cystadenomas (Figs. 5 and 6). Although most of the lesions associated with VHL are treatable, affected patients experience increased morbidity and mortality. The most common causes of death in patients

with VHL are RCC and complications resulting from cerebellar hemangioblastomas.[17] VHL shows high penetrance, with 90% of patients diagnosed with a tumor by age 65 years and a mean age of 26 years at first tumor detection.[18]

The most characteristic tumor in VHL is the CNS hemangioblastoma, which can occur in the cerebellum, brainstem, spinal cord, and less frequently in the supratentorial brain (Fig. 7). Of all locations, spinal cord HBs are most specific to VHL.[17] CNS HBs are reported in 60% to 80% of patients with VHL, with 44% to 72% of these lesions found in the cerebellum. The mean age at diagnosis is 33 years, with symptoms including headaches and ataxia. HBs are often multifocal and, if a cerebellar HB is detected, imaging of the spinal cord is recommended because coexisting lesions are commonly seen.[19] HBs are typically characterized on imaging as having both solid nodular and cystic components, although cystic components are not always seen. CT shows a low-density cyst and an isodense/hyperdense nodule that enhances avidly after contrast administration. MR imaging findings are similar, with the nodule isointense to brain on T1-weighted images and avidly enhancing after gadolinium administration with both the nodule and cyst hyperintense on T2-weighted images. Development of new cystic components or enlargement of existing cystic components of an HB often correlate with worsening symptoms, especially when seen with peritumoral edema, and may redirect from expectant management to surgical resection.

Particular attention must be made to renal imaging in patients with VHL because RCC is responsible for the death of 50% of patients with VHL. Complicating evaluation is the fact that approximately 60% of patients with VHL have renal cysts that can be simple or complex and atypical. These renal cysts are usually multiple and bilateral. RCCs in VHL have a mean age of 35 to 40 years at presentation. They are most commonly multifocal and bilateral, with morphology ranging from solid hyperenhancing lesions to complex cystic masses with thick septations and nodularity. The underlying histology is the clear cell subtype, which is known to have the worst prognosis of all RCCs and frequently metastasizes to liver, lung, and bone. Ultrasonography can be used to distinguish cystic and solid renal lesions and has an advantage given its lack of ionizing radiation; this is an important feature in this group of patients who need lifelong surveillance imaging. However, CT and MR imaging are increasingly preferred in both surveillance and evaluation of suspicious renal lesions. CT evaluation should include unenhanced, corticomedullary, nephrogenic, and

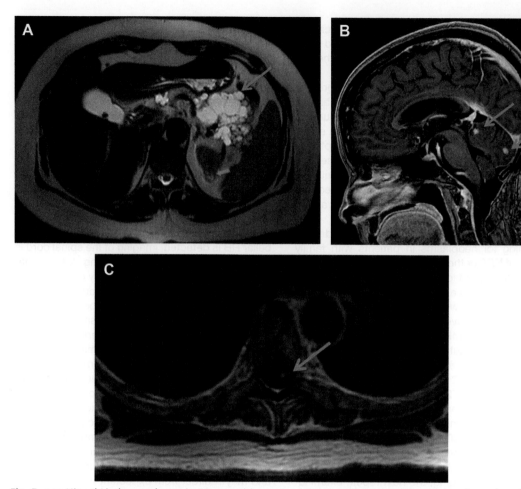

Fig. 5. von Hippel-Lindau syndrome in 52-year-old woman. (*A*) Axial T2-weighted single-shot fast spin-echo MR image shows numerous epithelial cysts (*long arrow*) in the pancreatic parenchyma. A centrally T2 bright, exophytic lesion extending from the interpolar region of the left kidney represents a renal cell carcinoma (*short arrow*). (*B*) Sagittal magnetization-prepared rapid gradient-echo brain MR image shows multiple cerebellar hyperintensities consistent with hemangioblastomas (*arrows*). (*C*) Axial T1-weighted postcontrast MR image of the thoracic spine shows a punctate focal area of enhancement consistent with a hemangioblastoma (*arrow*).

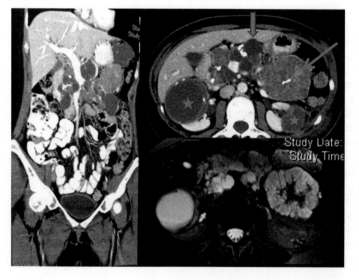

Fig. 6. von Hippel-Lindau syndrome in a 20-year-old woman. Coronal and axial contrast-enhanced CT images of the abdomen and pelvis and axial T2-weighted half-fourier acquisition single-shot turbo spin-echo (HASTE) MR image show pancreatic serious cystadenoma (*thin arrow*), upper abdominal epithelial cysts (*wide arrow*), and bilateral cystic renal cell carcinomas (*asterisks*).

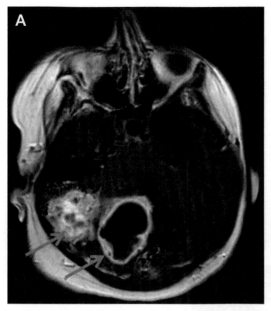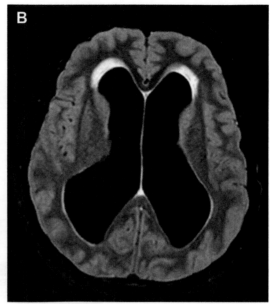

Fig. 7. von Hippel-Lindau syndrome in a 17-year-old girl. (A) Axial postcontrast T1-weighted MR image of the brain shows multiple hyperenhancing lesions (arrows) within the posterior fossa consistent with hemangioblastomas. (B) Axial T1-weighted MR image with fat suppression shows the posterior fossa lesions, which are associated with mass effect effacing the fourth ventricle with hydrocephalus of the lateral and third ventricles.

excretory phases to optimize sensitivity. For example, cortically based clear cell RCCs can be missed on the corticomedullary phase because their degree of enhancement is typically similar to the adjacent cortex. However, on the nephrogenic phase, these lesions are hypoenhancing relative to the normal parenchyma and thus more easily detected.[20] MR imaging is increasingly used for surveillance and lesion characterization given its lack of ionizing radiation. On MR imaging, clear cell RCC may present as T1-hypointense and T2-hyperintense lesions with heterogeneous enhancement or may show cystic components with thickened and nodular septations and enhancing solid components. There may be a decrease in signal on out-of-phase imaging because a portion of clear cell RCCs may contain intralesional fat. These MR imaging findings are in juxtaposition to simple renal cysts, which are homogeneously T1 hypointense and T2 hyperintense, and complex cysts, which should not show postcontrast internal enhancement.

Imaging and screening protocols for both adult and pediatric patients with VHL have shown benefits in reducing mortality.[21] Numerous surveillance protocols exist, including a commonly followed protocol in United States centers authored by the VHL Alliance Surveillance, which includes recommended imaging surveillance. For example, in patients aged 16 years and older, annual abdominal ultrasonography (with MR imaging of the abdomen at least every other year) is recommended as well as annual imaging of the brain, petrous temporal bone, and total spine with and without contrast.[22]

Tuberous Sclerosis

Tuberous sclerosis is a rare autosomal dominant neurocutaneous disorder characterized by a broad spectrum of abnormalities, including hamartomatous tumors involving multiple organs such as the brain, kidneys, lung, and heart (Fig. 8). Tuberous sclerosis occurs secondary to a familial or spontaneous mutation in either the TSC1 or TSC2 genes (on chromosomes 9 and 16, respectively) resulting in errors in tumor suppression along the mammalian target of rapamycin (mTOR) pathway.[23] Tuberous sclerosis has an incidence of approximately 1 in 6000 and is classically described as the triad of epilepsy, mental retardation, and facial angiofibromas, although this presentation is infrequent. Diagnosis of tuberous sclerosis can be made from combinations of both major and minor criteria with imaging playing a critical role in diagnosis, determining extent of disease, and monitoring for complication.[24] Tuberous sclerosis is associated with increased mortality, with 40% of patients dying by age 40 years. Younger patients typically experience increased mortality secondary to complications from CNS involvement, and older patients from complications related to renal disease.[25–27]

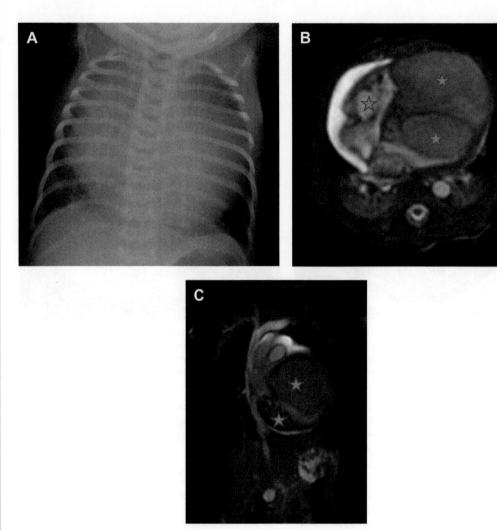

Fig. 8. Cardiac rhabdomyoma in a 5-year-old boy with tuberous sclerosis. (*A*) Chest radiograph shows marked cardiomegaly without pulmonary edema. (*B, C*) Subsequently obtained axial and coronal cardiac MR images show multiple large tumors (*asterisks*) in both ventricles and causing complete obliteration of the right ventricle. These lesions are compatible with cardiac rhabdomyomas in pediatric patients with tuberous sclerosis.

Common neurologic findings in tuberous sclerosis include subcortical tubers, subependymal ependymomas (less commonly subependymal giant cell astrocytomas), and white matter abnormalities such as radial migration lines. Subcortical tubers represent developmental abnormalities of the cortex, and the extent of cortical tubers has been shown to relate to the degree of underlying neurologic symptoms (eg, seizures, intellectual disability).[28] Best visualized on MR imaging, 90% of subcortical tubers are located in the frontal lobes, typically show subcortical or cortical T1 hypointensity and T2 hyperintensity, and rarely enhance. The T2 sequences can be less helpful in neonates and infants because the lesion signal characteristics can be similar to unmyelinated brain.[25] Subependymal ependymomas represent small hamartomatous nodules typically lining the walls of the lateral ventricles and are usually apparent on nonenhanced CT given their propensity to calcify. Subependymal ependymomas can degenerate into subependymal giant cell astrocytomas, which are seen in 10% to 15% of patients (**Fig. 9**).[23] These enhancing, pathologically benign tumors of astrocytes and giant cells are typically located at the foramen of Monro and can slowly grow over time, resulting in ventricular obstruction and hydrocephalus.[29] MR spectroscopy may be useful in distinguishing subependymal ependymomas from an subependymal giant cell astrocytoma at the foramen of Monro in challenging cases. Enlarging or symptomatic lesions may be managed surgically with mTOR pathway inhibitors in nonsurgical patients.[23,30]

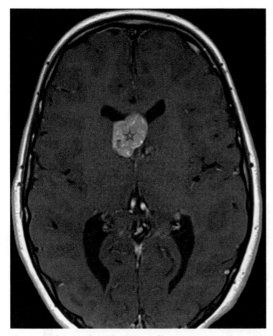

Fig. 9. Subependymal giant cell astrocytoma in a 10-year-old boy with tuberous sclerosis. Axial T1-weighted postcontrast MR image of the brain shows an enhancing lesion (*asterisk*) arising from the foramen of Monro consistent with a subependymal giant cell astrocytoma.

Renal involvement of tuberous sclerosis includes renal angiomyolipomas, renal cysts, and early development of RCC (**Fig. 10**). Angiomyolipomas are composed of blood vessels, fat, and smooth muscle cells. They are seen in up to 80% of patients with tuberous sclerosis, in whom angiomyolipomas are often multiple, bilateral, and seen at younger ages than in nontuberous sclerosis–associated acute myeloid leukemias (AMLs).[31] An important complication of AMLs is the propensity to hemorrhage, particularly when lesions grow larger than 4 cm or contain an associated aneurysm greater than 5 mm.[32] In the presence of a hemorrhagic AML, it is important to evaluate for the presence of an underlying lesion. Angiomyolipomas are frequently homogeneously hyperechoic on ultrasonography but can become more heterogeneous with increasing size. Because a small portion of RCCs may also present as hyperechoic lesions on ultrasonography, CT and MR imaging are often used for further diagnostic evaluation. On noncontrast CT, AMLs typically show macroscopic fat and measure less than −20 Hounsfield units (HU).[25] On MR imaging, AMLs typically lose signal on T1-weighted fat-suppression sequences and show India ink etching artifact on out-of-phase imaging. However, some AMLs are fat poor and not easily distinguished from RCC (**Fig. 11**). Park[33] reports several imaging

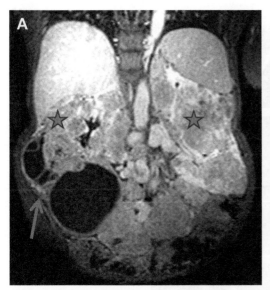
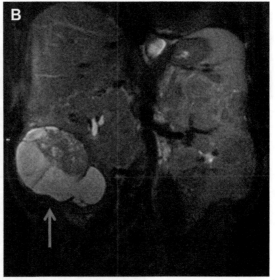

Fig. 10. Renal angiomyolipoma and renal cell carcinoma in a 41-year-old man with tuberous sclerosis. (*A*) Coronal T1-weighted postcontrast MR image shows marked enlargement of both kidneys with multiple enhancing masses (*asterisks*) consistent with angiomyolipomatosis. A complex cystic and solid mass (*arrow*) arising from the mid to lower pole of the right kidney is noted. The lesion was resected with pathology consistent with RCC. (*B*) Coronal T2-weighted MR image with fat suppression shows the cystic and solid components of the suspicious right renal lesion (*arrow*).

criteria to assist in the distinction between fat-poor AML and clear cell RCC. For example, fat-poor AMLs tend to be hyperattenuating on nonenhanced CT, T2 hypointense and relatively hyperintense on diffusion-weighted imaging, and hypointense on apparent diffusion coefficient (ADC) compared with clear cell RCC. However, the necessity of biopsy to distinguish these conditions remains controversial. In contrast, fat-invisible AMLs and non–clear cell RCCs are not readily distinguishable on imaging, and biopsy is necessary for differentiation.[33] Although the

incidence of RCC in patients with tuberous sclerosis is similar to that of the general population, lesions tend to occur at an average age of 28 years, approximately 25 years younger than in the general population.[25] Clear cell carcinoma is the most common subtype of renal tumors seen.

Several types of thoracic involvement can occur in tuberous sclerosis. For example, cardiac rhabdomyomas are striated muscle tumors seen in approximately 50% of patients with tuberous sclerosis, typically before 1 year of age. These lesions are typically found on the interventricular septum

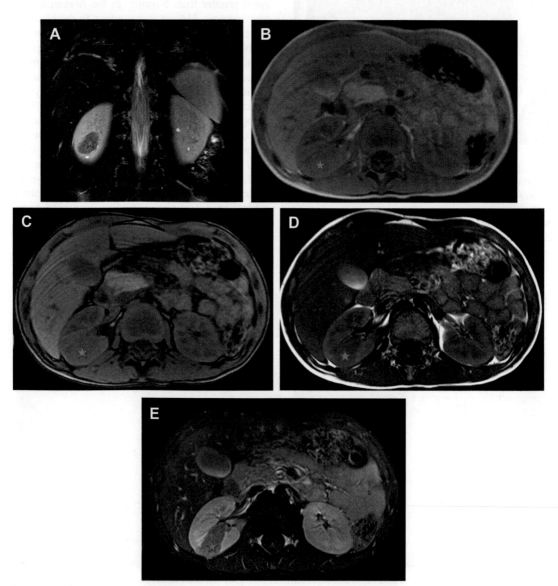

Fig. 11. Lipid-poor angiomyolipoma versus renal cell carcinoma in a 4-year-old boy with tuberous sclerosis. Coronal HASTE (*A*), axial in-phase T1-weighted (*B*), out-of-phase T1-weighted (*C*), T1-weighted precontrast (*D*), and T1-weighted postcontrast fat-suppressed (*E*) MR images show a T1 and T2 hypointense right interpolar lesion (*asterisks*) without signal drop on out-of-phase imaging. Differential considerations include lipid-poor angiomyolipoma with renal cell carcinoma and oncocytoma not excluded.

and when large can be associated with arrhythmia or hemodynamic compromise. These lesions often regress spontaneously but may require intervention if symptomatic. Echocardiography is the modality of choice in evaluating these lesions, but MR imaging is helpful in describing the size and extent of these lesions.[25,29] Another important thoracic association with tuberous sclerosis is pulmonary lymphangioleiomyomatosis (LAM). LAM affects approximately 40% of women and 15% of men with tuberous sclerosis and is characterized by diffuse interstitial smooth muscle proliferation with cystic changes developing throughout the pulmonary parenchyma resulting in progressive dyspnea on exertion and eventual respiratory failure in young adults. Complications include pneumothorax, pulmonary hemorrhage, and chylous effusions or ascites. The characteristic appearance of LAM on thin-section CT is round, thin-walled (<3 mm), cystic lesions of varying sizes and contours typically symmetrically distributed throughout the lungs.[29] Patients with LAM frequently encounter complications after lung transplant, including disease recurrence.[30]

Krueger and Northrup[34] formulated a set of clinical and imaging surveillance recommendations as part of a 2012 consensus conference and included recommendation for MR imaging of the brain and abdomen every 1 to 3 years for symptom-free patients less than 25 years old. More frequent imaging was recommended for patients with known lesions to evaluate for interval growth or development of suspicious features. In asymptomatic women at risk for LAM, high-resolution CT should be performed at intervals of 5 to 10 years. If cysts are detected, the interval should be reduced to 2 to 3 years.

Multiple Endocrine Neoplasia Syndrome Type 1

Multiple endocrine neoplasia type 1 (MEN-1) is an autosomal dominant disorder occurring secondary to a mutation of the MEN-1 tumor suppressor gene on chromosome 11, with a prevalence of 2 to 3 per 100,000.[35] MEN-1 is predominantly characterized by parathyroid adenomas, pancreatic neuroendocrine tumors, and pituitary adenomas. Additional features are also frequently seen, such as adrenal lesions, carcinoid tumors, and multiple facial angiofibromas.[35]

Primary hyperparathyroidism secondary to a parathyroid adenoma is frequently the presenting symptom in MEN-1 and occurs in 95% of patients, usually by the third decade.[36] Decreased bone mineral density and nephrolithiasis are common sequelae.[37] Evaluation for a parathyroid adenoma can be performed with ultrasonography, which shows an oval, usually hypoechoic lesion best appreciated when greater than 1 cm.[38] Limitations of ultrasonography include operator dependence and potential for ectopic adenomas, which cannot be visualized. Contrast-enhanced CT can identify ectopic adenomas within the mediastinum or adjacent to the trachea. On MR imaging, parathyroid adenomas are typically T1 dark and T2/short tau inversion recovery bright. Nuclear medicine studies with 99m Tc-methoxyisobutylisonitrile and single-photon emission computed tomography are frequently used for adenoma evaluation. Early images can show asymmetric radiotracer uptake, with delayed sequences (usually 2 hours) showing increased radiotracer activity, which is particularly helpful in cases of recurrent disease.[38]

Pancreatic neuroendocrine (islet cell) tumors are the second most common lesions in MEN-1 and occur in 40% of affected patients. The most common lesions are nonhyperfunctioning tumors, followed by gastrinomas (40%) and insulinomas (30%), and are typically indolent and functional but can be aggressive malignancies with a propensity for metastatic disease[39] (**Fig. 12**). A variety of imaging modalities are used in the evaluation of primitive neuroectodermal tumors (pNETs). Transabdominal ultrasonography has limited sensitivity for these lesions. However, endoscopic ultrasonography (EUS) may be the most sensitive imaging modality available, although the technique is invasive and operator dependent.[40] CT with a dedicated pancreatic protocol and narrow window settings is a sensitive modality for detection of pNETs and evaluation of metastatic disease. Most lesions are less than 2 cm in size and isointense to the pancreatic parenchyma on the unenhanced and portal venous phases but avidly enhancing on the late arterial phase. In detecting pNETs, MR imaging is more sensitive compared with CT (65%–85% and 70%–80%, respectively[39]). Lesions are T1 hypointense and moderately T2 hyperintense compared with the adjacent parenchyma and show homogeneous arterial enhancement in small lesions and heterogeneous enhancement if necrosis is present. Theoni and colleagues[41] report that MR imaging sensitivity can approach that of EUS, with appropriate sequence selection with T1 fat-suppression sequences being particularly helpful.

Pituitary adenomas are seen in 30% of patients with MEN-1, more commonly female, and may present as a hyperfunctioning lesion or secondary to associated mass effect. MR imaging is the imaging modality of choice in the detection of these lesions, with thin-slice (≤3 mm), small field of view, spin-echo T1 images with coronal and sagittal reformations the modality of choice. Pituitary adenomas are typically hypointense on both

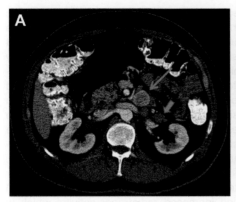 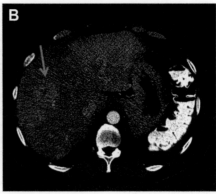 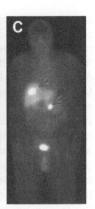

Fig. 12. Pancreatic neuroendocrine tumor in a 39-year-old man with history of multiple endocrine neoplasia type 1. (*A*) Axial enhanced CT image shows a 3-cm enhancing lesion (*long arrow*) in the pancreatic body/tail concerning for neuroendocrine tumor. Note is made of multifocal adenomas in the left adrenal gland (*short arrow*). (*B*) Axial enhanced CT image shows a low-density enhancing lesion (*arrow*) in the liver corresponding with the findings on the octreotide study and consistent with metastases. (*C*) Octreotide study shows increased radiotracer uptake (*arrows*) in the region of the pancreas and liver.

precontrast and postcontrast imaging. Adenomas larger than 10 mm are classified as macroadenomas and may compress adjacent structures. Although small microadenomas may not be readily visible, secondary features may be present, such as erosion of the sellar floor.[39]

Approximately 40% of patients with MEN-1 develop an adrenal cortical tumor, most typically a benign adenoma. Adrenal cortical adenomas are typically characterized using cross-sectional imaging, including CT, on which they measure less than 10 HU on noncontrast phases or show a relative washout greater than 40% or an absolute washout of greater than 60% on a dedicated adrenal protocol CT. These lesions are most reliably characterized on MR imaging, with a decrease in signal intensity of greater than 20% on out-of-phase imaging being diagnostic of a benign adenoma.[42] Rarely (<5%), patients with MEN-1 can present with adrenal cortical carcinoma, which typically presents as large tumors with necrosis, hemorrhage, and calcification. Evidence of local invasion and metastatic disease is frequently identified.[39]

A small percentage of patients with MEN-1 develop carcinoid tumors of the foregut, including the thymus, respiratory tract, and upper gastrointestinal tract.[39] Of particular interest is thymic carcinoid tumor, which, although rare (0%–8% of patients), has been found to be the second most common cause of MEN-1–related deaths.[43] This lesion typically presents on contrast-enhanced CT as a large, enhancing, prevascular mediastinal mass that can be difficult to distinguish from a thymoma and that may be locally invasive at the time of diagnosis.

Metastatic disease is most frequently seen in regional nodes, adrenal glands, and bones.

Endocrine Society guidelines published in 2012 recommend annual imaging surveillance for pancreatic neuroendocrine tumors and adrenal lesions with MR imaging, CT, or ultrasonography before the age of 10 years. Starting at age 5 years, patients should undergo MR imaging every 3 years for pituitary lesions surveillance. The guidelines recommend CT or MR imaging screening every 1 to 2 years for thymic and bronchial carcinoid lesions starting at age 15 years.[44,45]

Multiple Endocrine Neoplasia Type 2

Multiple endocrine neoplasia type 2 (MEN-2) is an autosomal dominant condition occurring secondary to a mutation of the MEN-1 tumor suppressor gene on chromosome 10 with an incidence of 1 in 200,000 births.[35] There are 3 distinct subtypes: MEN-2A, familial medullary thyroid carcinoma (MTC), and MEN-2B. The most common of these is MEN-2A, which accounts for 60% to 90% of cases and is characterized by MTC, pheochromocytoma, and parathyroid tumors. Familial MTC is characterized by medullary thyroid cancer whereas MEN-2B is characterized by MTC, pheochromocytomas, and additional abnormalities such as a marfanoid habitus.[35]

MTC shows 100% penetrance in patients with MEN-2 by the age of 70 years, is typically diagnosed between 20 and 30 years, and is the largest contributor to MEN-2–related mortality.[35] The earliest and most aggressive disease is seen in MEN-2B disease. MTC is often multicentric and bilateral in patients with MEN-2 and presents with increased calcitonin and carcinoembryonic antigen levels. Ultrasonography is often the first-line imaging technique in patients presenting with a thyroid mass and allows the performance of fine-needle aspiration if a suspicious lesion is identified. Cross-sectional imaging with CT with intravenous contrast can show a hypodense, heterogeneous thyroid mass that may be calcified. Extension beyond the thyroid and nodal metastatic disease should also be carefully assessed. Common sites of metastatic disease include liver, lung, and bone. Given the aggressive nature of this malignancy and complete penetrance in patients with MEN-2, prophylactic thyroidectomy is currently recommended between the ages of 5 and 10 years in MEN-2A and familial MTC and by 6 months in MEN-2B if a RET oncogene is present.[35,46]

Pheochromocytomas develop in about half of patients with MEN-2A and MEN-2B, with a mean age of 36 years at the time of diagnosis. These lesions are typically diagnosed after MTC and are often bilateral. Excluding the presence of a pheochromocytoma is critical in patients with MEN-2A/MEN-2B before any interventional procedures given the risk of pheochromocytoma crisis, a catecholamine-induced hemodynamic disturbance.[47] Contrast-enhanced CT and MR imaging have similar sensitivities in the detection of pheochromocytomas. CT should be performed with nonionic contrast media and can show an avidly enhancing adrenal mass (>110 HU on arterial phase) with regions of cystic necrosis, hemorrhage, and calcification sometimes seen. On MR imaging, the classic appearance is a markedly T2 bright adrenal mass (eg, so-called light-bulb sign) that has a heterogeneous enhancement pattern on postcontrast T1-weighted imaging.

Diffusion-weighted imaging can be helpful in distinguishing benign and malignant lesions, with lower ADC values in malignant lesions.[48] 123-I-MIBG (metaiodobenzylguanidine) scintigraphy can be used for whole-body localization of pheochromocytomas and metastatic disease. Further, it is more sensitive than CT and MR imaging in the detection of adrenal medullary hyperplasia, a precursor lesion to pheochromocytoma.[36] There is some variability in screening recommendations for patients with MEN-2, with some investigators recommending imaging only in the setting of biochemical abnormalities and others recommending MR imaging of the abdomen every 3 years to evaluate for pheochromocytoma with optional scintigraphy.[36]

Li-Fraumeni Syndrome

Li-Fraumeni syndrome (LFS) is a rare, autosomal dominant cancer predisposition syndrome of unknown prevalence most often related to a loss-of-function mutation in the TP53 gene, which encodes the p53 tumor suppressor protein.[49,50] Patients with Li-Fraumeni are at increased risk for numerous tumors, including osteosarcomas, soft tissue sarcomas (**Fig. 13**), leukemia, breast cancer, brain tumors (astrocytoma, choroid plexus carcinoma), adrenal cortical tumors, and melanoma.[49] Although breast cancer is the most common malignancy seen in these patients, childhood adrenocortical carcinoma, choroid plexus carcinoma, rhabdomyosarcoma, and multiple childhood cancers are most associated with germline TP53 gene mutations.[51] Patients with LFS have an approximately 50% chance of developing cancer by the age of 40 years and a 90% risk by age 60 years. The lifetime risk of malignancy is up to

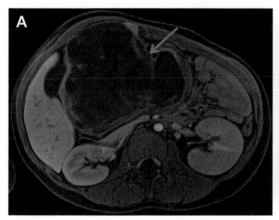
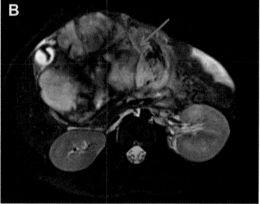

Fig. 13. Hepatic embryonal sarcoma in a 6-year-old girl with LFS. Axial T1-weighted (*A*) and T2-weighted (*B*) MR images show a large and heterogeneously enhancing mass (*arrows*) arising from the liver. Pathology showed undifferentiated embryonal sarcoma of the liver.

90% by age 60 years, with women having a higher lifetime risk largely related to breast cancer.[49]

Adrenal cortical carcinoma (ACC) typically presents as a large adrenal mass. On CT, ACC typically shows a well-defined mass with heterogeneous enhancement, a nonenhancing central stellate hypodense area, and calcifications. On MR imaging, ACC is typically T1 isointense, with a T2 bright central stellate region and showing heterogeneous postcontrast enhancement. Findings of hemorrhage and necrosis are frequently encountered.[52] In pediatric patients, ultrasonography is often the first imaging modality used for evaluation and can show a suprarenal, hyperechoic lesion that may contain calcification and potentially invade or compress the inferior vena cava and may invade the renal vein. Metastases to the lungs, liver, and nodes are common. Of particular interest in pediatric patients is the differentiation of ACC from neuroblastoma. Although differentiation by imaging alone is difficult, Ribiero and colleagues[52] report that the presence of a central stellate zone may assist in favoring ACC rather than neuroblastoma. Choroid plexus carcinoma is a rare intraventricular malignancy associated with LFS most often arising from the lateral ventricles in young children and that often caries a poor prognosis secondary to large size at presentation and propensity for spread along cerebrospinal fluid pathways.[53] These lesions are isoattenuating to hyperattenuating on noncontrast CT with avid postcontrast enhancement. Necrosis, lesion hemorrhage, and brain invasion are common. On MR imaging, periventricular T2/fluid-attenuated inversion recovery white matter hyperintensity is suggestive of brain invasion. Hydrocephalus is common secondary to mechanical obstruction.

Rhabdomyosarcoma is a highly malignant tumor seen in patients with LFS and is the most common soft tissue sarcoma in children (Fig. 14). In up to 79% of patients, the diagnosis is established in the first decade of life.[54] Rhabdomyosarcoma can occur virtually anywhere in the body but typically arises within the head and neck (35%), genitourinary system (26%), and extremities (19%).[55] Metastases are common at presentation, with liver, lung, and bone the most common sites. For example, rhabdomyosarcoma of the head and neck are typically T1 isointense, T2 bright, enhancing with possible necrosis and restricted diffusion.

Kim and colleagues[56] reported a series of patients with treated rhabdomyosarcoma who underwent surveillance for disease recurrence and who presented with distant metastatic disease without locoregional recurrence. As such, whole-body imaging, such as MR imaging, is of particular

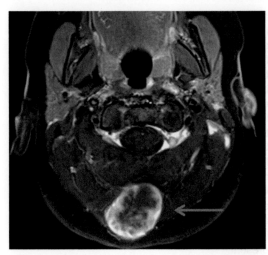

Fig. 14. Rhabdomyosarcoma in a 4-year-old girl with history of Li-Fraumeni syndrome. Axial T1-weighted postcontrast fat-suppressed MR image of the neck shows an enhancing mass (*arrow*) with necrosis consistent with rhabdomyosarcoma.

interest in surveillance of patients with LFS. Several recent studies have shown the efficacy and feasibility of using whole-body MR imaging in the early detection of malignancy in patients with LFS (Fig. 15).[57,58] Mai and colleagues[49] described an LFS surveillance protocol including abdominal sonography every 4 months, annual brain MR imaging, and annual rapid whole-body MR imaging for children aged 3 to 16 years. For patients older than 16 years, the surveillance protocol included annual brain MR imaging and annual rapid whole-body MR imaging. In addition, for female patients 20 to 40 years old, annual breast MR imaging was performed and, for patients older than 40 years, annual breast MR imaging and mammography were performed.

DICER 1 Syndrome

DICER 1 syndrome is a rare genetic cancer predisposition syndrome placing patients at increased risk of several malignant and benign tumors. The DICER 1 gene is located on chromosome 14 and contributes to the production of microRNA, which is essential in cell growth, division, differentiation, and maturation.[59] DICER 1 has moderate penetrance and most mutation carriers are phenotypically normal throughout life.[60] Typical lesions associated with DICER 1 syndrome include pleuropulmonary blastoma, cystic nephroma, ovarian sex cord-stromal tumors, genitourinary rhabdomyosarcomas, and pituitary blastoma. Affected patients also may develop other lesions, such as pineoblastoma, Wilms tumor, and multinodular goiter.[61]

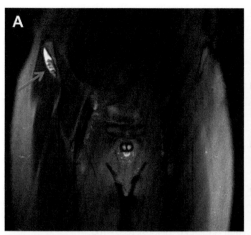
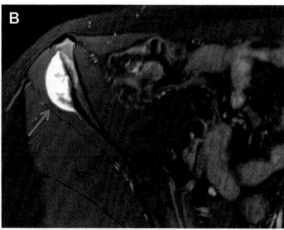

Fig. 15. Osteosarcoma in a 14-year-old boy with history of LFS who presented for whole-body screening MR imaging. (*A*) Coronal T2-weighted MR image with fat suppression shows a T2 bright 4.5-cm lenticular-shaped lesion (*arrow*) along the outer cortex of the right iliac bone. (*B*) Axial T2-weighted MR image with fat suppression shows an enhancing mass (*arrow*) causing underlying bony remodeling. Biopsy was consistent with osteosarcoma.

Pleuropulmonary blastoma (PPB) is the most common primary lung malignancy in children and is typically diagnosed in young children before the age of 7 years (**Fig. 16**). PPB is thought to progress from type I (cystic) to type II (cystic and solid) to type III (solid) with progressively older age at diagnosis and worse prognosis.[60] On plain radiography, the appearance of PPB may range from a large, cystic-appearing mass in type I to a complete opacification of the hemithorax with mass effect on the mediastinum in type III disease. On CT, type I lesions may show a single cyst or a multifocal cystic lesion without solid components or thickened septa. Type II disease can show air-filled or fluid-filled cystic cavities with solid nodular components and possible solid nodules. Type III

neoplasms are principally solid and may show homogeneous or heterogeneous postcontrast enhancement. Type III lesions are classically heterogeneously enhancing on MR imaging with regions of hemorrhage and may restrict diffusion. Associated pleural effusion and pneumothorax are common.[62] Metastatic disease can be seen to the CNS, bone, and liver.[59]

Cystic renal nephroma is an uncommon benign renal neoplasm that most typically presents as an abdominal mass. These lesions may be visible as soft tissue masses on plain radiography but they are frequently first evaluated on ultrasonography in pediatric patients. Ultrasonography may show a cystic mass without solid components. On CT, cystic nephroma typically appears as a

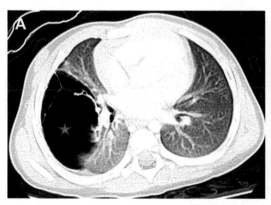
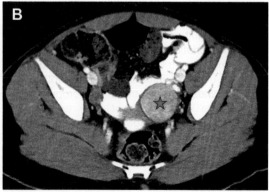

Fig. 16. Type 1 pleuropulmonary blastoma and ovarian Sertoli-Leydig cell tumor in a 19-month-old girl with DICER 1 syndrome. (*A*) Axial noncontrast CT image shows a large cystic lesion (*asterisk*) in the right upper lobe with internal septations and nodular components. Pathology was consistent with pleuropulmonary blastoma type 1. (*B*) Axial enhanced CT image obtained 16 years later shows a 4-cm enhancing left adnexal lesion (*asterisk*) with pathology consistent with Sertoli-Leydig cell tumor.

well-circumscribed, encapsulated mass with variably enhancing septations. On MR imaging, cystic nephroma is T2 bright with variable T1 signal and possible enhancement of intralocular septa. Of note, these lesions are typically resected because of an inability to distinguish them from cystic partially differentiated nephroblastoma (Wilms tumor).[63,64]

Sex cord-stromal tumors are also associated with DICER 1.[65] Sertoli-Leydig cell tumors (SLCTs) are usually unilateral and restricted to the ovary. On ultrasonography, these lesions have a nonspecific appearance and may appear as a distinct hypoechoic mass or a heterogeneous solid mass with cystic spaces. On CT, SLCT may appear as a soft tissue attenuation adnexal lesion with avid contrast enhancement in the solid portions of the tumor. On MR imaging, these lesions are typically T1 hypointense with varying degrees of T2 hyperintensity depending on the extent of fibrous content. The lesions show homogeneous or heterogeneous avid contrast enhancement on postgadolinium sequences.[66]

Shultz and colleagues[61] recommend a comprehensive imaging surveillance for patients with DICER 1. For example, a chest radiograph is recommended every 4 to 6 months from birth until age 8 years, and then annually until age 12 years, with consideration of chest CT in the surveillance for pleuropulmonary blastoma. Surveillance for gynecologic lesions is recommended with pelvic and abdominal ultrasonography performed every 6 to 12 months beginning at age 8 to 10 years until at least age 40 years.

SUMMARY

Genetic syndromes are a challenging group of conditions for both pediatric and adult general radiologists given the multitude of syndromic findings and associated complications. Both pediatric and adult radiologists should be familiar with characteristic syndromic imaging features and the most common complications, including malignant transformation of benign neoplasms. Such knowledge can allow radiologists to suggest the possibility of an underlying syndrome, assist in image interpretation, help guide management, and direct appropriate surveillance.

REFERENCES

1. Levy AD, Patel N, Dow N, et al. Abdominal neoplasms in patients with neurofibromatosis type 1: radiologic-pathologic correlations. Radiographics 2005;25(2):455–80.

2. Stewart DR, Korf BR, Nathanson KL, et al. Care of adults with neurofibromatosis type 1: a clinical practice resource of the American College of Medical Genetics and Genomics (ACMG). Genet Med 2018;20(7):671–82.

3. Tidyman WE, Rauen KA. The RASopathies: developmental syndromes of Ras/MAPK pathway dysregulation. Curr Opin Genet Dev 2009;19(3):230–6.

4. Wilkinson LM, Manson D, Smith CR. Best cases from the AFIP: Plexiform Neurofibroma of the bladder. Radiographics 2004;24(suppl_1):S237–42.

5. Broski SM, Johnson GB, Howe BM, et al. Evaluation of (18)F-FDG PET and MRI in differentiating benign and malignant peripheral nerve sheath tumors. Skeletal Radiol 2016;45(8):1097–105.

6. Campian J, Gutmann DH. CNS tumors in neurofibromatosis. J Clin Oncol 2017;35(21):2378–85.

7. Bekiesinksa-Figatowska M. A mini review on neurofibromatosis type 1 from the radiologic point of view. J Rare Dis Treat 2017;2(6):45–9.

8. Patel NB, Stacy GS. Musculoskeletal manifestations of neurofibromatosis type 1. AJR Am J Roentgenol 2012;199(1):W99–106.

9. Shah H, Rousset M, Canavese F. Congenital pseudarthrosis of the tibia: management and complications. Indian J Orthop 2012;46(6):616–26.

10. Evans DGR, Salvador H, Chang VY, et al. Cancer and central nervous system tumor surveillance in pediatric neurofibromatosis 1. Clin Cancer Res 2017;23(12):e46–53.

11. Borofsky S, Levy LM. Neurofibromatosis: types 1 and 2. AJNR Am J Neuroradiol 2013;34(12):2250–1.

12. Smith MJ, Bowers NL, Bulman M, et al. Revisiting neurofibromatosis type 2 diagnostic criteria to exclude LZTR1-related schwannomatosis. Neurology 2017;88(1):87–92.

13. Koeller KK, Rosenblum RS, Morrison AL, et al. Neoplasms of the spinal cord and Filum Terminale: radiologic-pathologic correlation. Radiographics 2001;20(6):1721–49.

14. Baser ME, Friedman JM, Aeschliman D, et al. Predictors of the risk of mortality in neurofibromatosis 2. Am J Hum Genet 2002;71(4):715–23.

15. Evans DGR, Salvador H, Chang VY, et al. Cancer and central nervous system tumor surveillance in pediatric neurofibromatosis 2 and related disorders. Clin Cancer Res 2017;23(12):e54–61.

16. Karsdorp N, Elderson A, Wittebol-Post D, et al. Von hippel-lindau disease: new strategies in early detection and treatment. Am J Med 1994;97(2):158–68.

17. Leung RS, Biswas SV, Duncan M, et al. Imaging features of von Hippel-Lindau disease. Radiographics 2008;28(1):65–79.

18. NORD (National Organization for Rare Disorders). Von Hippel-Lindau disease - NORD (National Organization for Rare Disorders). 2019. Available at:

https://rarediseases.org/rare-diseases/von-hippel-lindau-disease/. Accessed July 26, 2019.

19. Rankin D, Menias CO, Pickhardt PJ, et al. Tumors in von Hippel-Lindau syndrome: from head to toe – comprehensive state-of-the-art review. Radiographics 2018;38(3):849–66.

20. Dyer R, DiSantis DJ, McClennan BL, et al. Simplified imaging approach for evaluation of the solid renal mass in adults. Radiology 2008;247(2):331–43.

21. Hes FJ, Feldberg MA. Von Hippel-Lindau disease: strategies in Early Detection (renal-, adrenal-, pancreatic masses). Eur Radiol 1998;9(4): 598–610.

22. VHLA Suggested Active Surveillance Guidelines. (2017). Boston: VHL Family Alliance. Available at: https://www.vhl.org/wp-content/uploads/2017/07/Active-Surveillance-Guidelines.pdf. Accessed July 16, 2019.

23. Manoukian SB, Kowal DJ. Comprehensive imaging manifestations of tuberous sclerosis. AJR Am J Roentgenol 2015;204(5):933–43.

24. Northrup H, Krueger DA, International Tuberous Sclerosis Complex Consensus Group. Tuberous sclerosis complex diagnostic criteria update: recommendations of the 2012 International Tuberous Sclerosis Complex Consensus Conference. Pediatr Neurol 2013;49(4):243–54.

25. Umeoka S, Koyama T, Miki Y, et al. Pictorial review of tuberous sclerosis in various organs. Radiographics 2008;28(7):e32.

26. Amin S, Lux A, Calder N, et al. Causes of mortality in individuals with tuberous sclerosis complex. Dev Med Child Neurol 2017;59(6):612–7.

27. Shepard CW, Gomez MR, Lie JT, et al. Causes of death in patients with tuberous sclerosis. Mayo Clin Proc 1991;66(8):792–6.

28. Klantari BN, Salamon N. Neuroimaging of tuberous sclerosis: spectrum of pathologic findings and frontiers in imaging. AJR Am J Roentgenol 2008;190: W304–9.

29. Radhakrishnan R, Verma S. Clinically relevant imaging in tuberous sclerosis. J Clin Imaging Sci 2011;1: 39.

30. Pallisa E, Sanz P, Roman A, et al. Lymphangioleiomyomatosis: pulmonary and abdominal findings with pathologic correlation. Radiographics 2002; 22(suppl_1):S185–98.

31. Redkar N, Patil MA, Dhakate T, et al. Tuberous sclerosis complex presenting as bilateral large renal angiomyolipomas. BMJ Case Rep 2012;2012. bcr2012006412.

32. Yamakado K, Tanaka N, Nakagawa T, et al. Renal angiomyolipoma: relationships between tumor size, aneurysm formation, and rupture. Radiology 2002; 225(1):78–82.

33. Park BK. Renal angiomyolipoma based on new classification: how to differentiate it from renal cell carcinoma. AJR Am J Roentgenol 2019;212(3):582–8.

34. Krueger DA, Northrup H, International Tuberous Sclerosis Complex Consensus Group. Tuberous sclerosis complex surveillance and management: recommendations of the 2012 international tuberous sclerosis complex consensus conference. Pediatr Neurol 2013;49(4):255–65.

35. Norton JA, Krampitz G, Krampitz RT. Multiple endocrine neoplasia: genetics and clinical management. Surg Oncol Clin N Am 2015;24(4):795–832.

36. Scarsbrook AF, Thakker RV, Wass JA, et al. Multiple endocrine neoplasia. spectrum of radiologic appearances and discussion of a multitechnique imaging approach. Radiographics 2006;26(2): 433–51.

37. Giusti F, Tonelli F, Brandi M. Primary hyperparathyroidism in multiple endocrine neoplasia type 1: when to perform surgery? Clinics (Sao Paulo) 2012;67(S1):141–4.

38. Johnson NA, Tublin ME, Ogilvie JB. Parathyroid imaging technique and role in the preoperative. Evaluation of primary hyperparathyroidism. AJR Am J Roentgenol 2007;188(6):1706–15.

39. Grajo JR, Paspulati RM, Sahani DV, et al. Multiple endocrine neoplasia syndromes: a comprehensive imaging review. Radiol Clin North Am 2016;54(3): 441–51.

40. Langer P, Kann PH, Fendrich V, et al. Prospective evaluation of imaging procedures for the detection of pancreaticoduodenal endocrine tumors in patients with multiple endocrine neoplasia type 1. World J Surg 2004;28(12):1317–22.

41. Thoeni RF, Mueller-Lisse UG, Chan R, et al. Detection of small, functional islet cell tumors in the pancreas: selection of MR imaging sequences for optimal sensitivity. Radiology 2000;214(2): 483–90.

42. Elsayes KM, Mukundan G, Narra VR, et al. Adrenal masses: MR imaging features with pathologic correlation. Radiographics 2004;24(suppl_1). S73–86.

43. Ito T, Igarashi H, Uehara H, et al. Causes of death and prognostic factors in multiple endocrine neoplasia type 1: a prospective study: comparison of 106 MEN1/Zollinger-Ellison syndrome patients with 1613 literature MEN1 patients with or without pancreatic endocrine tumors. Medicine (Baltimore) 2013;92(3):135–81.

44. Kamilaris CDC, Stratakis CA. Multiple Endocrine Neoplasia Type 1 (MEN1): an update and the significance of early genetic and clinical diagnosis. Front Endocrinol (Lausanne) 2019;10:339.

45. Thakker RV, Newey PJ, Walls GV, et al. Clinical practice guidelines for Multiple Endocrine Neoplasia Type 1 (MEN1). J Clin Endocrinol Metab 2012; 97(9):2990–3011.

46. Wells SA, Asa SL, Dralle H, et al. Revised American Thyroid Association Guidelines for the management

of medullary thyroid carcincoma. Thyroid 2015; 25(6):567–610.

47. James MF, Cronjé L. Pheochromocytoma crisis: the use of magnesium sulfate. Anesth Analg 2004; 99(3):680–6.

48. Dong Y, Liu Q. Differentiation of malignant from benign pheochromocytomas with diffusion-weighted and dynamic contrast-enhanced magnetic resonance at 3.0 T. J Comput Assist Tomogr 2012; 36(4):361–6.

49. Mai PL, Khincha PP, Loud JT, et al. Prevalence of cancer at baseline screening in the national cancer institute Li-Fraumeni syndrome cohort. JAMA Oncol 2017;3(12):1640–5.

50. U.S. National Library of Medicine, Genetics Home Reference. Li-Fraumeni Syndrome. Available at: https://ghr.nlm.nih.gov/condition/li-fraumeni-syndrome#statistics. Accessed July 22, 2019.

51. Monsalve J, Kapur D, Babyn PS. Imaging of cancer predisposition syndromes in children. Radio-graphics 2011;31(1):263–80.

52. Ribeiro J, Ribeiro RC, Fletcher BD. Imaging findings in pediatric adrenocortical carcinoma. Pediatr Radiol 2000;30(1):45–51.

53. Meyers SP, Khademian ZP, Chuang SH, et al. Choroid plexus carcinomas in children: MRI features and patient outcomes. Neuroradiology 2004;46(9):770–80.

54. Chung EM, Biko DM, Arzamendi AM, et al. Solid tumors of the peritoneum, omentum, and mesentery in children: radiologic-pathologic correlation: from the radiologic pathology archives. Radiographics 2015;35(2):521–46.

55. McHugh K, Boothroyd AE. The role of radiology in childhood rhabdomyosarcoma. Clin Radiol 1999; 54(1):2–10.

56. Kim JR, Yoon HM, Koh K-N, et al. Rhabdomyosarcoma in children and adolescents: patterns and risk factors of distant metastasis. AJR Am J Roentgenol 2017;209(2):409–16.

57. Ballinger ML, Best A, Mai PL, et al. Baseline surveillance in Li-Fraumeni syndrome using whole-body magnetic resonance imaging: a meta-analysis. JAMA Oncol 2017;3(12):1634–9.

58. Anupindi SA, Bedoya MA, Lindell RB, et al. Diagnostic performance of whole-body MRI as a tool for cancer screening in children with genetic cancer-predisposing conditions. AJR Am J Roentgenol 2015;205(2):400–8.

59. Bartley et al. The imaging findings of DICER 1 syndrome – a pictorial review. European Society of Radiology Educational Exhibit. Congress ECR 2014, Poster C-2331.

60. Bueno MT, Martínez-Ríos C, la Puente Gregorio AD, et al. Pediatric imaging in DICER1 syndrome. Pediatr Radiol 2017;47(10):1292–301.

61. Schultz KAP, Williams GM, Kamihara J, et al. DICER1 and associated conditions: identification of at-risk individuals and recommended surveillance strategies. Clin Cancer Res 2018;24(10):2251–61.

62. Lichtenberger JP, Biko DM, Carter BW, et al. Primary lung tumors in children: radiologic-pathologic correlation from the radiologic pathology archives. Radiographics 2018;38(7):2151–72.

63. Granja MF, O'Brien AT, Trujillo S, et al. Multilocular cystic nephroma: a systematic literature review of the radiologic and clinical findings. AJR Am J Roentgenol 2015;205(6):1188–93.

64. Silver IMF, Boag AH, Soboleski DA. Best cases from the AFIP: multilocular cystic renal tumor: cystic nephroma. Radiographics 2008;28(4):1221–5.

65. Witkowski L, Mattina J, Schönberger S, et al. DICER1 hotspot mutations in non-epithelial gonadal tumours. Br J Cancer 2013;109(10):2744–50.

66. Horta M, Cunha TM. Sex cord-stromal tumors of the ovary: a comprehensive review and update for radiologists. Diagn Interv Radiol 2015;21(4):277–86.

Congenital Incidental Findings in Children that Can Be Mistaken as True Pathologies in Adults
Pearls and Pittfalls of Imaging Diagnosis

Gary R. Schooler, MD[a], Ricardo Restrepo, MD[b], Robert P. Mas, BAS[b],
Edward Y. Lee, MD, MPH[c],*

KEYWORDS

- Congenital • Incidental • Developmental variant • Disease mimic • Pediatric • Adult

KEY POINTS

- Congenital incidental findings are not uncommonly encountered in adults.
- Radiographic analysis of the incidental finding frequently provides an inconclusive assessment.
- Careful evaluation of ultrasound, computed tomography, and/or MR imaging can help distinguish the incidental congenital process from a true pathologic process.
- Radiologists should be familiar with common congenital entities and variants of development that may simulate disease in the adult.

INTRODUCTION

Congenital entities and variants of development occasionally are discovered incidentally in adult patients. Many of these incidental findings share similar imaging characteristics with and may mimic true pathologic entities. Persistence of developmental structures, accessory structures from development, and incomplete maturation all may result in an appearance that simulates true pathologic processes, such as infection and neoplasia. Although these congenital incidental findings share similar imaging features with true pathologic processes, up-to-date knowledge and careful assessment with the most appropriate imaging modalities generally can allow a distinction between congenital entities that may be safely dismissed and those pathologic processes requiring further assessment and treatment.

The overarching aim of this article is to review several of the most common congenital processes that may present incidentally in the adult patient mimicking disease. An emphasis is placed on imaging findings that can be used to distinguish the congenital process from disease processes in need of additional evaluation and treatment.

SPECTRUM OF CONGENITAL INCIDENTAL FINDINGS
Neck

Ectopic thymus
The thymus begins development during weeks 4 to 6 of gestation, arising from the third branchial pouch.[1] By the end of the eighth to ninth weeks, the primordial thymus descends caudally into the anterior mediastinum and fuses in the midline.[2]

[a] Department of Radiology, Duke University Medical Center, 2301 Erwin Road, Durham, NC 27005, USA; [b] Ross University School of Medicine, Two Mile Hill, St. Michael BB11093, Barbados, West Indies; [c] Division of Thoracic Imaging, Department of Radiology, Boston Children's Hospital, Harvard Medical School, 300 Longwood Avenue, Boston, MA 20115, USA
* Corresponding author.
E-mail address: Edward.Lee@childrens.harvard.edu

Radiol Clin N Am 58 (2020) 639–652
https://doi.org/10.1016/j.rcl.2020.01.006
0033-8389/20/© 2020 Elsevier Inc. All rights reserved.

Ectopic thymus may be found anywhere along the path of descent from the cervical region to the mediastinum owing to failure or incomplete descent, sequestration, or persistence of a remnant and failure of involution within the thymo-pharyngeal duct.[1,3]

Thymic tissue is instrumental in development of B cells and T cells and is disproportionally larger in infants, with a gradual involution and replacement by fat with maturation.[4] Cervical ectopic tissue may present as a painless lump or mass in child-hood or be discovered incidentally in childhood, adolescence, or adulthood. Ectopic tissue may be positioned laterally or midline in the neck, simulating many other pathologic processes, including lymphadenopathy and primary neck neoplasia (Fig. 1). Ectopic thymic tissue also may be located in the thyroid and is found in approximately 1% of the pediatric and adult pop-ulation,[5] potentially mimicking malignant thyroid nodules, especially those with microcalcification (Fig. 2).[6]

The key to making a diagnosis of ectopic cervi-cal thymus, both within and outside the thyroid, is to recognize the potential for its presence and the characteristic imaging appearance. Normal thy-roid tissue has multiple linear hyperechoic septa and discrete homogeneously distributed hypere-choic foci, resulting in a speckled appearance on ultrasound.[1,7] On MR imaging, ectopic thymic tissue is homogenous, isointense, or slightly hyperintense to skeletal muscle on T1-weighted images and hyperintense on T2-weighted images and typically has angulated margins that mold to adjacent structures rather than displacing them.[8] In adolescents and adults, the thymic tissue ma-tures, showing progressive involution and an increasingly fatty appearance (after orthotopic, normal thymus maturation), resulting in an in-crease in echogenicity on ultrasound.[9] Obser-vance of the typical appearance on imaging may obviate biopsy or removal of a significant amount of thymic tissue, which may have detrimental ef-fects on immune system development in younger patients.

Branchial cleft cyst

The branchial apparatus develops between the fourth and seventh weeks of gestation and forms the precursors of the ear, blood vessels, bones, cartilage, and mucosal lining of the face, neck, and pharynx.[10] Branchial apparatus anomalies result from incomplete obliteration of the associ-ated cleft or pouch during development and are the second most common congenital neck lesion, behind thyroglossal duct cysts.[11]

Second branchial cleft anomalies are the most common of all of the branchial apparatus anoma-lies to develop.[12,13] Cysts are the most likely anomaly to be seen.[14] Second branchial cleft

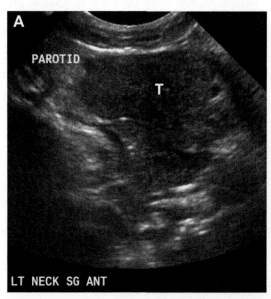
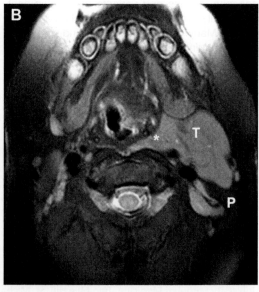

Fig. 1. A 3-year-old girl with ectopic cervical thymus presenting as a painless mass in the left side of the neck. (A) Longitudinal ultrasound image shows ectopic thymus (T) presenting as a solid soft tissue mass with a speckled appearance in the left side of the neck adjacent to the parotid gland. (B) Axial T2-weighted, fat-suppressed MR image shows the ectopic cervical thymus (T) as a solid soft tissue structure with characteristic homogenous hyperintense T2 signal on the left side of the neck overlying the vessels and adjacent to the parotid gland (P). The thymus is insinuating in between structures with a deep extension (asterisk) into the retropharyngeal space.

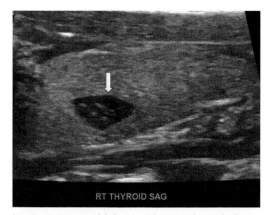

Fig. 2. A 3-year-old boy with intrathyroid thymus discovered incidentally on ultrasound of the neck. Sagittal ultrasound image of the right thyroid lobe shows a well-defined, oval-shaped hypoechoic nodule (*arrow*) in the right lobe of the thyroid with a speckled appearance internally characteristic of normal thymic tissue ectopically positioned in the thyroid.

anomalies are encountered lateral to the midline, along the developmental tract, extending from the tonsillar fossa inferior-laterally between the internal and external carotid arteries to the level of the skin anterior to the sternocleidomastoid (SCM) muscle.

On imaging, the second branchial cleft cysts are seen most commonly anterior to the SCM muscle, resulting in posterior displacement of the SCM, medial displacement of the carotid sheath structures, and anterior displacement of the submandibular gland (**Fig. 3**).[15] Ultrasound typically shows a well-circumscribed round or oval hypoechoic or anechoic cyst with posterior acoustic enhancement. Occasionally, the internal fluid may be complex and the wall thickened in the setting of infection.[1] Computed tomography (CT) and MR imaging may better elucidate the precise location of the cyst, with attenuation and internal signal characteristics reflecting the complexity of the fluid.

Although many second branchial cleft cysts are diagnosed in the pediatric population, branchial cleft cysts that are small and/or asymptomatic may remain undetected into adulthood. The branchial cleft cyst may mimic other pathologies within the neck, including necrotic lymph nodes and primary head/neck malignancies. One key to differentiation is recognition of their characteristic anatomic positioning, although surgical resection may be required for definitive diagnosis in questionable cases.

Chest

Lung agenesis

Lung agenesis is a rare congenital anomaly.[16] Embryonic development of the lung begins early in gestation, with the development of 2 lung buds that grow to form the left and right mainstem bronchi during the embryonic phase. With

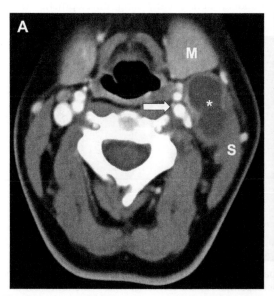
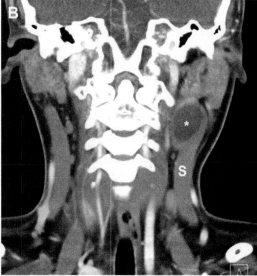

Fig. 3. A 1-year-old boy with a type II branchial cleft cyst who presented with a palpable neck mass. (*A*) Axial contrast-enhanced CT image of the neck reveals a hypodense cystic structure (*asterisk*) that is displacing the carotid sheath medially (*arrow*), displacing the submandibular gland (M) anteriorly, and anteriorly positioned to the SCM muscle (S). (*B*) Coronal contrast-enhanced CT image of the neck shows the hypodense cystic structure (*asterisk*) along the superior and deep margin of the sternocleidomastoid muscle (S).

pulmonary agenesis, there is complete absence of all normal pulmonary structures on the affected side.[17] The cause of pulmonary agenesis is not definitively known, although it may be related to abnormal blood flow in the dorsal aortic arch during the fourth week of gestation, mechanical or genetic causes, or teratogenic effects.[18,19] Approximately 50% of patients with lung agenesis have concomitant congenital anomalies involving the cardiovascular, central nervous, gastrointestinal, and genitourinary systems.[20,21] Those with unilateral lung agenesis, however, may reach adulthood and remain asymptomatic.[16,22]

Unilateral lung agenesis results in mediastinal shift toward the hemithorax with absent lung and compensatory hypertrophy and hyperexpansion of the contralateral lung, which herniates across midline. Chest radiography typically shows opacification of the affected hemithorax and ipsilateral mediastinal shift that can mimic complete lung atelectasis and those findings seen postpneumonectomy (**Fig. 4**).[23] The differential diagnosis for patients with unilateral lung atelectasis is broad but includes obstructing bronchial entities, such as primary lung cancer in adults. CT can help distinguish between an acquired disease process and congenital absence of the lung, revealing the absence of the lung parenchyma, bronchus, and ipsilateral pulmonary artery.[24]

Pulmonary arteriovenous malformation

A pulmonary arteriovenous malformation (PAVM) is an abnormal communication between the pulmonary artery and pulmonary vein, bypassing the normal pulmonary capillary network. PAVMs are relatively uncommon in the general population, although they occur more commonly in patients with hereditary hemorrhagic telangiectasia.[25,26] PAVMs usually are discovered incidentally in asymptomatic patients, but when large or multiple may result in right-to-left shunting and embolic phenomena.[27]

On chest radiography, PAVMs appear as pulmonary nodules (**Fig. 5**). When the feeding vessels are large enough to be radiographically conspicuous, they help establish a diagnosis. Smaller lesions, however, may have inconspicuous vasculature, resulting in a pulmonary nodule that has a broad differential diagnosis, including other vascular etiologies, such as pulmonary artery aneurysms, infectious entities, and neoplastic entities, including primary lung cancer—especially in adult patients. CT angiography may be necessary to help distinguish the incidentally discovered asymptomatic PAVM from other entities requiring further investigation and treatment. On CT, PAVMs most commonly appear as well-defined peripheral nodules that may be lobulated, into which a feeding pulmonary artery and at least 1 draining pulmonary vein can be identified (see **Fig. 5**).[28,29]

Bronchogenic cyst

Bronchogenic cysts arise from defective foregut budding during early lung development. They

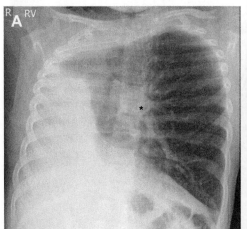
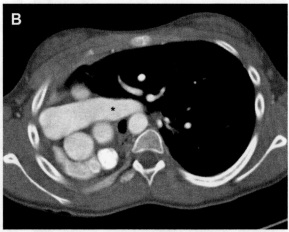

Fig. 4. A 30-year-old woman who presented with chest pain and was incidentally discovered to have right lung agenesis. (*A*) Frontal radiograph of the chest shows hyperexpansion of the left lung, which extends across the midline into the right hemithorax. The mediastinal structures are deviated into the right hemithorax. Note the prominent left pulmonary artery (*asterisk*). (*B*) Axial contrast-enhanced CT image of the chest demonstrates the complete absence of the right lung, compensatory enlargement and hyperexpansion of the left lung, and deviation of the mediastinal cardiovascular structures into the posterior right hemithorax. Left pulmonary artery crossing midline (*asterisk*).

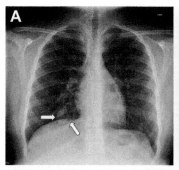
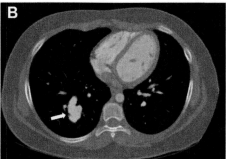
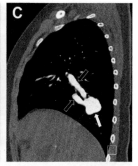

Fig. 5. An 18-year-old man with an incidentally discovered right lower lobe pulmonary arteriovenous malformation (AVM). (*A*) Frontal chest radiograph shows a round opacity (*arrows*) in the right lung base. (*B*) Axial contrast-enhanced CT image demonstrates the avidly enhancing structure (*white arrow*) in the right lower lobe is a vascular structure compatible with a PAVM. (*C*) Sagittal contrast-enhanced CT image demonstrates to better advantage the feeding and draining pulmonary artery and vein (*black arrows*) of the PAVM (*white arrow*).

may arise in the paratracheal, hilar, or most commonly the subcarinal regions.[30,31] More rarely, bronchogenic cysts can be found within the lung parenchyma or in the cervical region.[32,33] When the bronchogenic cysts are intrapulmonary, they usually are solitary with thin walls and are seen most commonly in the lower lobes.[23] Affected patients generally present within the first 4 decades of life, although approximately half of patients are asymptomatic with the bronchogenic cyst detected incidentally on an imaging study performed for alternate indications.[31]

Bronchogenic cysts generally appear as a round or oval-shaped opacity on radiographs. CT provides better characterization, especially of internal fluid attenuation, which may have density similar to that of water or soft tissue.[18,31] On MR imaging, those bronchogenic cysts with simple internal fluid exhibit high signal intensity on T2-weighted images and low signal intensity on T1-weighted images. Those bronchogenic cysts with internal fluid that is not simple typically display variable signal intensity on T1-weighted and T2-weighted images, reflecting the internal composition of the fluid. The cysts do not have central enhancement on postcontrast MR images.

When found incidentally, bronchogenic cysts may mimic other pathologies found in the mediastinum or hilum. Specifically, a bronchogenic cyst identified on CT with low internal attenuation may mimic a necrotic lymph node from an infectious or neoplastic source.[34,35] When solid-appearing on CT, bronchogenic cysts may mimic solid lymph nodes or neoplasms. MR imaging may provide additional helpful information on the characteristics of the fluid and, when contrast is given, reveal the uniformly enhancing thin wall of the cyst and lack of central enhancement (**Fig. 6**).[31] In distinction, solid masses and lymph nodes typically show central enhancement and those masses with central necrosis are less likely to have a uniformly thin wall rather than a thick or irregular wall.

Pulmonary sequestration

Pulmonary sequestrations are the second most common congenital pulmonary anomaly (behind congenital pulmonary airway malformations).[18] They are characterized by a portion of dysplastic lung not in connection with the tracheobronchial tree that have a systemic arterial supply, generally from the thoracic or abdominal aorta, and either pulmonary or systemic venous drainage.[17,18,36–38] Two types of pulmonary sequestrations have been described based on venous drainage pattern and pleural investment: the intralobar types do not have their own pleural investment and generally drain via the pulmonary venous system and the extralobar types have their own pleural investment and drain via the systemic venous system. Intralobar pulmonary sequestrations are more common than extralobar pulmonary sequestrations and although some investigators suggest intralobar pulmonary sequestrations may be acquired after birth, at least some of these pulmonary sequestrations are congenital because they are identified on prenatal imaging.[17,39,40]

Although extralobar pulmonary sequestrations are diagnosed in the prenatal-neonatal period, intralobar pulmonary sequestrations are found more commonly incidentally in childhood or adulthood at chest radiography.[18,23,41] Pulmonary sequestrations tend to appear as an area of increased opacity, usually in the lower lobes, that may mimic other pathologic processes, such as pneumonia. With recurrent infection, the pulmonary sequestration may develop intralesional necrosis, generating a more cystic appearance, occasionally with air-fluid levels. The necrotic

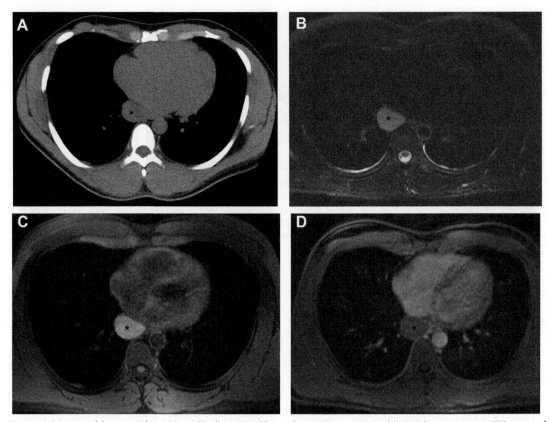

Fig. 6. A 30-year-old man with incidentally discovered bronchogenic cyst on CT. (*A*) Axial noncontrast CT image of the chest shows a mass (*asterisk*) posterior to the atria along the right posterior mediastinum that has intermediate internal attenuation (30 Hounsfield units). (*B*) Axial T2-weighted, fat-suppressed MR image reveals the internal contents of the structure (*asterisk*) are moderately hyperintense but not as intense as cerebrospinal fluid. (*C*) Axial T1-weighted, fat-suppressed MR image shows the internal contents of the structure (*asterisk*) are moderately hyperintense, suggesting the internal fluid is proteinaceous and correlating with the density seen on CT. (*D*) Axial T1-weighted, fat-suppressed MR image reveals a lack of enhancement of the structure (*asterisk*), confirming the cystic nature.

appearance can further mimic cavitary variants of pneumonia or a neoplastic process. CT with intravenous contrast generally is needed for diagnosis. The use of intravenous contrast and angiographic technique can highlight the systemic feeding artery(s) and the draining veins, confirming the diagnosis of pulmonary sequestration (**Fig. 7**).

Abdomen and Pelvis

Persistent fetal lobation of the kidneys

The adult kidney is composed of 14 lobes, or reniculi, which, during early fetal development, are made up of numerous lobules. Each reniculus is like a small kidney with cortex and medullary tissues, blood supply, and collecting system. During normal renal development, the lobes coalesce to form the kidney. When the lobation normally found in the fetal kidney persists into adulthood, it is referred to as persistent *fetal lobation*. The term,

fetal lobulation, also has been used to describe the undulating contour referring to fetal lobation, although fetal lobation is the more precise and preferred term.[42–44]

Persistent fetal lobation is usually identified on ultrasound. It is characterized by undulations of the renal contour corresponding to the bulge of the renal lobule with normal thickness cortex overlying a renal pyramid, such that each indentation is between the renal lobes (**Fig. 8**). Fetal lobation may mimic renal scarring. On careful observation, however, scarring is observed over the middle of the bulge of the renal lobule (ie, over a pyramid) rather than between the renal lobules and always coincides with thinning of the associated cortex. A prominent renal bulge generated by the indentions also may mimic a renal cortical tumor—so-called renal pseudotumor.[45] Careful evaluation of the regions on ultrasound can reveal the presence of the renal pyramid. On CT or MR imaging, a

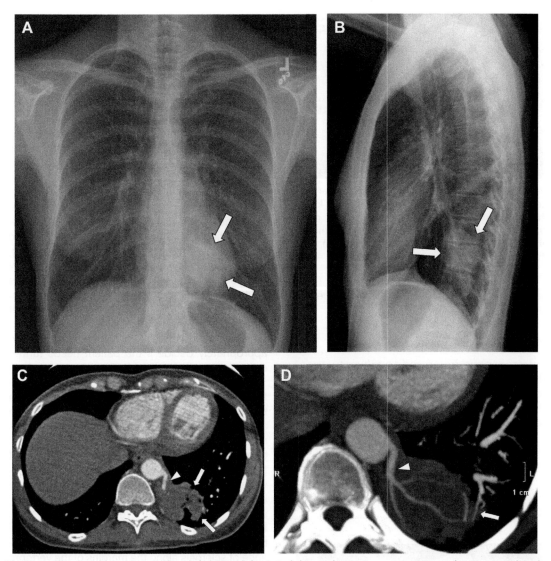

Fig. 7. A 35-year-old woman with a left lower lobe intralobar pulmonary sequestration who presented with recurrent pneumonia. (*A*) Frontal chest radiograph shows a retrocardiac opacity (*arrows*), residing in the left lower lobe. (*B*) Lateral chest radiograph confirms the presence of the opacity (*arrows*) in the left lower lobe and was suspicious for pneumonia. (*C*) Axial CT image from contrast-enhanced angiogram of the chest shows the left lower lobe consolidation is a mass (*arrows*) with arterial blood supply (*arrowhead*) arising from the descending thoracic aorta. (*D*) Axial MIP image from CT angiography shows the full extent of the feeding artery (*arrowhead*) and the pulmonary venous drainage (*arrow*).

pseudotumor remains isodense or isointense to the normal renal parenchyma on all sequences and phases of contrast enhancement.[45–47]

Dromedary hump
The renal dromedary hump is a description given to the focal contour bulge of the lateral interpolar region of the left kidney. The term, *dromedary*, comes from the Arabian 1-hump dromedary camel. This renal contour bulge is caused by molding of the normal renal parenchyma by the adjacent spleen and originally was described on excretory urography.[48] The dromedary hump also is evident on ultrasound, CT, and MR imaging. The bulge can mimic a renal mass. Differentiation usually can be made, however, by recognizing the parenchyma within the dromedary hump is equivalent to that of normal renal parenchyma on ultrasound, CT, and MR imaging (**Fig. 9**). Additionally, the perfusion and contrast enhancement of the parenchyma within the dromedary hump typically match that of surrounding normal renal

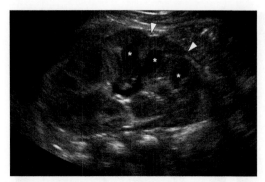

Fig. 8. A 6-month-old boy with persistent fetal lobation. Sagittal ultrasound image of the left kidney shows the undulating contour of the renal cortex with the indentions (*arrowheads*) overlying the columns between the renal pyramids (*asterisks*). Note the normal, uniform renal cortical thickness.

parenchyma, rather than the altered enhancement identified within a renal mass.[49]

Musculoskeletal System

Accessory ossicles/unfused apophyses
The growing and developing pediatric skeleton can pose diagnostic challenges for those evaluating radiologic studies where variants of ossification are found. Numerous anatomic variants exist in the development of the pediatric skeleton, many of which may simulate a disease process, either during development or after development is complete and the skeleton reaches maturity.[50,51] Select variants of musculoskeletal development are discussed.

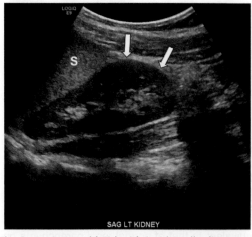

Fig. 9. A 10-year-old girl with incidentally discovered dromedary hump. Sagittal ultrasound image of the left kidney shows the characteristic parenchymal bulge (*arrows*) along the lower kidney due to the impression by the spleen (S).

Os odontoideum Os odontoideum refers to an independent osseous structure lying cephalad to the axis body in the location of the odontoid process.[52] Although originally believed to be a congenital variant,[53] there are many investigators who consider the finding an acquired abnormality and a result of traumatic injury.[54–56] Both etiologies may play a role in development of this finding. Os odontoideum may be identified during childhood or adulthood and may be asymptomatic or result in instability in the upper cervical spine with substantial narrowing of the spinal canal and compression of the spinal cord.[57,58]

On radiographic imaging, the os may mimic the presence of an odontoid fracture. CT can be helpful to distinguish between acute injury and chronic abnormality, when radiographs are confusing, because chronic variants/abnormalities typically show sclerosis around the ossific bodies whereas acute fractures do not (**Fig. 10**). Although an os odontoideum may be discovered incidentally, it generally is recommend that patients be evaluated by a provider familiar with the entity who can appropriately decide if the patient needs further evaluation and/or treatment.[56]

Limbus vertebra The limbus vertebra is a defect in the margin of the vertebral body that may be seen at either anterior or posterior and superior or inferior endplate that results in a detached triangular bony fragment and sclerosis at the interface of the bone defect.[59] The defect arises from the intravertebral herniation of the intervertebral disk[60] and is seen most commonly along the anterosuperior aspect of the lumbar vertebral body.[59] The triangular-shaped fragment can mimic a vertebral body fracture at radiography or CT.[61] The presence of sclerosis along the margins of the vertebra and adjacent triangular bony fragment help identify the process as chronic rather than sequalae of acute traumatic injury (**Fig. 11**).

Os acromiale The acromion develops from multiple ossification centers that fuse to form the mature acromion between the ages of 15 years and 25 years.[62] When the ossification centers fail to completely fuse in individuals older than 25 years, the term os acromiale is applied to the finding.[63] Two types of os acromiale have been described: (1) large relatively triangular mesoacromion that forms an interface with the acromion in proximity to the acromioclavicular joint and (2) the smaller preacromion that is noted at the distal tip of the acromion.[64] Os acromiale is found in approximately 3% to 4% of the population, more frequently in the right shoulder, with the mesoacromion variant identified most commonly.[65,66]

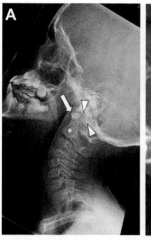
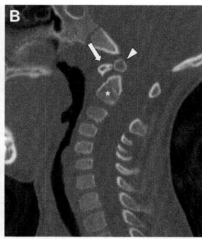

Fig. 10. A 15-year-old boy with an incidentally discovered os odontoideum. (*A*) Lateral radiograph of the cervical spine shows a round and well-corticated ossific body (*arrowheads*) adjacent to the superior aspect of the C2 vertebra (*asterisk*) and posterior to the anterior arch of C1 (*arrow*). (*B*) Sagittal reconstructed CT image from a noncontrast cervical spine CT demonstrates a well-corticated ossicle (*arrowhead*) adjacent to the superior aspect of the CT vertebra (*asterisk*) and immediately superior to the anterior arch of C1 (*arrow*). Note the well-corticated nature of the ossicle indicative of a chronic process rather than acute fracture.

The os may be identified incidentally on radiographic, CT, or MR imaging and can mimic a fracture, especially on radiography when the indication for the examination is related to traumatic injury.[67] The os can be identified, however, as having sclerotic margins indicative of the chronic nature of its presence. In some patients, this variant may be symptomatic, with MR imaging

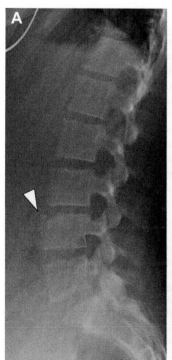
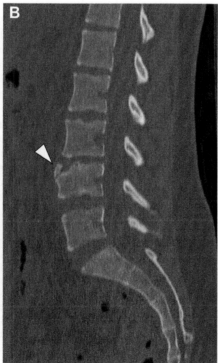
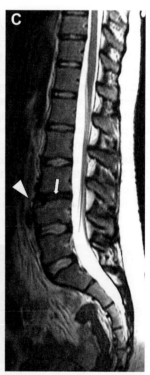

Fig. 11. An 18-year-old man status post–motor vehicle collision with an incidentally discovered limbus vertebra. (*A*) Lateral radiograph of the lumbar spine shows a bony fragment (*arrowhead*) along the anterosuperior corner of the L4 vertebral body. Note the irregular sclerosis of the adjacent vertebral body at the interface. (*B*) Sagittal reconstructed CT image from a noncontrast CT of the lumbar spine shows the ossific fragment is well corticated with a thin sclerotic margin of the bony fragment and adjacent vertebral body, compatible with a limbus vertebra (*arrowhead*). (*C*) Sagittal T2-weighted MR image reveals the bony fragment (*arrowhead*) along the anterosuperior aspect of the L2 vertebral body has no abnormal edema-like bone marrow signal, nor does the adjacent vertebral body, indicating this process is not acute. Note the relative hypointensity of the L3-L4 disk (*arrow*) compatible with early degenerative change.

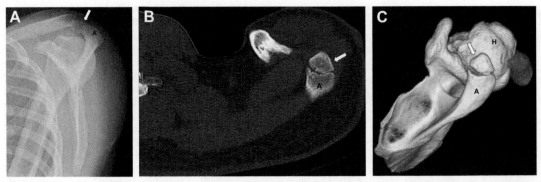

Fig. 12. A 26-year-old man with an os acromiale. (*A*) Radiograph of the left shoulder (scapular Y view) shows a well-corticated ossicle (*arrow*) adjacent to the acromion (A). (*B*) Axial noncontrast CT image of the left shoulder shows the os acromiale (*arrow*) closely opposed to the acromion (A). Note the sclerotic borders where at the interface of the os acromiale and acromion. (*C*) Three-dimensional, volume-rendered CT image of the left shoulder shows the os acromiale (*arrow*) and its relationship to the adjacent acromion (A) lying superior to humeral head (H).

demonstrating edema at the opposing bone surfaces and/or clinical signs of painful impingement (**Fig. 12**).[63,68,69]

Multipartite patella Patellar ossification begins at 4 years to 6 years of age with multiple ossification centers coalescing to form 1 ossification center. When secondary ossification centers develop and fail to fuse, a multipartite patella forms, most commonly a bipartite or tripartite patella. A multipartite patella is found in approximately 2% of the population and is bilateral in approximately 40% of patients.[69,70] The accessory ossification center is characteristically located superolaterally and has cartilaginous continuity with the rest of the patella. The multipartite patella can mimic a patellar fracture, although the characteristic location and round contour of the ossicles distinguish the multipartite patella from fractures (**Fig. 13**).

Accessory muscles

Accessory muscles are anatomic variants representing distinct muscles that are found in addition to the normal complement of muscles. Accessory muscles can be found in the upper and lower extremities and within the trunk. Examples of accessory muscles include (1) the anconeus epitrochlearis muscle that attaches at the medial cortex of the olecranon and the inferior surface of the medial epicondyle in the upper extremity (**Fig. 14**); (2) the accessory extensor carpi radialis brevis muscle that arises from the medial aspect of the normal extensor carpi radialis brevis muscle,

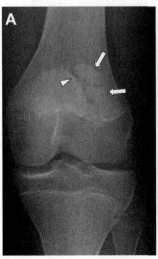

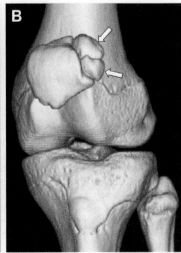

Fig. 13. A 14-year-old boy with incidentally discovered multipartite patella. (*A*) Frontal radiograph of the knee demonstrates 2 well-corticated ossicles (*arrows*) along the superolateral margin of the patella. Note the sclerotic nature of the bone at the interface with the adjacent major patellar ossification center (*arrowhead*) indicative of a chronic or developmental process. (*B*) Three-dimensional, volume-rendered CT image from a CT scan of the knee without contrast shows to better advantage the rounded nature of the ossicles (*arrows*) along the superolateral patella, a classic appearance and location for a multipartite patella.

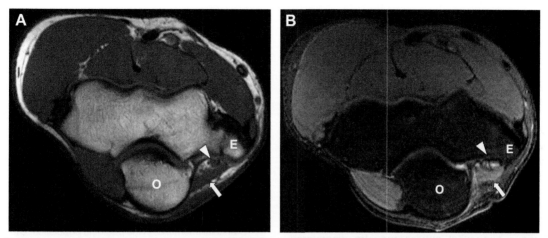

Fig. 14. A 15-year-old boy with an anconeus epitrochlearis. (*A*) Axial T1-weighted MR image shows the anconeus epitrochlearis (*arrow*) extending from the medial surface of the olecranon (O) to the inferior surface of the medial epicondyle (E) that shares signal characteristics with the other muscles in the field of view. Note the ulnar nerve's (*arrowhead*) close approximation to the anconeus epitrochlearis. (*B*) Proton-density MR image with fat suppression reveals the anconeus epitrochlearis (*arrow*) shares identical signal characteristics with the other regional muscles. Arrowhead, ulnar nerve; E, medial epicondyle; O, olecranon.

with the tendon passing deep to the main tendon and entering the second extensor tunnel of the wrist (**Fig. 15**); and (3) the accessory soleus muscle in the lower extremity that arises proximally from multiple sites including the posterior aspect of the proximal fibula, the soleal line of the tibia, the middle third of the medial tibia, and a fibrous band bridging its fibular and tibial origins, joining the deep surface of the Achilles tendon distally.[71]

Most accessory muscles are incidental findings. They may, however, mimic a soft tissue tumor as well as result in impingement on neurovascular structures. Accessory muscles may cause obliteration of fat planes on radiography, but these

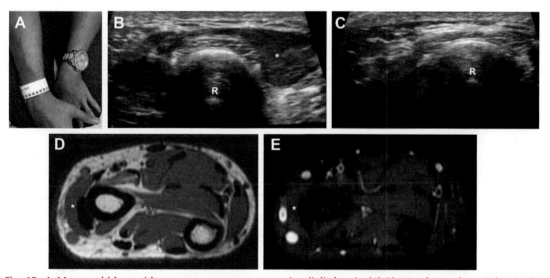

Fig. 15. A 14-year-old boy with an accessory extensor carpi radialis brevis. (*A*) Picture shows the painless in the distal right forearm (*encircled by the dashed line*). (*B*) Transverse ultrasound image of the right forearm shows the accessory extensor carpi radialis brevis (*asterisk*) along the dorsal aspect of the superficial compartment of the distal right forearm. (*C*) Comparison transverse ultrasound image from the same location in the left upper extremity demonstrates absence of the accessory muscle seen in the left upper extremity. (*D, E*) Axial T1-weighted MR image (*D*) and T2-weighted MR image with fat suppression (*E*) show the accessory extensor carpi radialis brevis (*asterisk*) has similar signal to other normal forearm musculature on both sequences. (R), radius.

studies rarely are diagnostic. Assessment with ultrasound can be helpful, with dynamic assessment demonstrating muscular contraction and echogenicity and architecture similar to adjacent muscles.[72] Evaluation with CT or MR imaging can reveal the accessory muscle, which shares similar attenuation/signal intensity and enhancement characteristics with normal muscles. When using MR imaging for assessment, T1-weighted images without fat suppression are most helpful in identifying accessory muscles due to the intrinsic contrast with adjacent fat.[73]

SUMMARY

Various congenital entities may be discovered incidentally for the first time in adults and occasionally mimic a true pathologic process. These congenital entities may be found in the neck, chest, abdomen/pelvis, and musculoskeletal system. Radiologists should be familiar with the most commonly encountered congenital entities and their characteristic imaging features described in this article, so the chance of misdiagnosis is minimized.

REFERENCES

1. Bansal AG, Oudsema R, Masseaux JA, et al. US of pediatric superficial masses of the head and neck. Radiographics 2018;38(4):1239–63.
2. Yildiz AE, Elhan AH, Fitoz S. Prevalence and sonographic features of ectopic thyroidal thymus in children: a retrospective analysis. J Clin Ultrasound 2018;46(6):375–9.
3. Bach AM, Hilfer CL, Holgersen LO. Left-sided posterior mediastinal thymus–MRI findings. Pediatr Radiol 1991;21(6):440–1.
4. Nasseri F, Eftekhari F. Clinical and radiologic review of the normal and abnormal thymus: pearls and pitfalls. Radiographics 2010;30(2):413–28.
5. Fukushima T, Suzuki S, Ohira T, et al. Prevalence of ectopic intrathyroidal thymus in Japan: the Fukushima health management survey. Thyroid 2015; 25(5):534–7.
6. Frates MC, Benson CB, Dorfman DM, et al. Ectopic intrathyroidal thymic tissue mimicking thyroid nodules in children. J Ultrasound Med 2018;37(3): 783–91.
7. Han BK, Yoon HK, Suh YL. Thymic ultrasound. II. Diagnosis of aberrant cervical thymus. Pediatr Radiol 2001;31(7):480–7.
8. Zielke AM, Swischuk LE, Hernandez JA. Ectopic cervical thymic tissue: can imaging obviate biopsy and surgical removal? Pediatr Radiol 2007;37(11): 1174–7.
9. Ota H, Hirokawa M, Suzuki A, et al. Phantom nodules detected by ultrasound examination of the neck: the possibility of ectopic cervical thymic tissue in adults. Ultrasound Int Open 2018;4(4): E119–23.
10. Waldhausen JH. Branchial cleft and arch anomalies in children. Semin Pediatr Surg 2006;15(2):64–9.
11. Adams A, Mankad K, Offiah C, et al. Branchial cleft anomalies: a pictorial review of embryological development and spectrum of imaging findings. Insights Imaging 2016;7(1):69–76.
12. Prosser JD, Myer CM 3rd. Branchial cleft anomalies and thymic cysts. Otolaryngol Clin North Am 2015; 48(1):1–14.
13. Schroeder JW Jr, Mohyuddin N, Maddalozzo J. Branchial anomalies in the pediatric population. Otolaryngol Head Neck Surg 2007;137(2):289–95.
14. Telander RL, Filston HC. Review of head and neck lesions in infancy and childhood. Surg Clin North Am 1992;72(6):1429–47.
15. Koch BL. Cystic malformations of the neck in children. Pediatr Radiol 2005;35(5):463–77.
16. Kaya O, Gulek B, Yilmaz C, et al. Adult presentation of symptomatic left lung agenesis. Radiol Case Rep 2017;12(1):25–8.
17. Thacker PG, Schooler GR, Caplan MJ, et al. Developmental lung malformations in children recent advances in imaging techniques, classification system, and imaging findings. J Thorac Imaging 2015;30(1):29–45.
18. Biyyam DR, Chapman T, Ferguson MR, et al. Congenital lung abnormalities: embryologic features, prenatal diagnosis, and postnatal radiologic-pathologic correlation. Radiographics 2010;30(6): 1721–38.
19. Berrocal T, Madrid C, Novo S, et al. Congenital anomalies of the tracheobronchial tree, lung, and mediastinum: embryology, radiology, and pathology. Radiographics 2004;24(1):e17.
20. Cooney TP, Thurlbeck WM. Lung growth and development in anencephaly and hydranencephaly. Am Rev Respir Dis 1985;132(3):596–601.
21. Robertson N, Miller N, Rankin J, et al. Congenital lung agenesis: incidence and outcome in the North of England. Birth Defects Res 2017;109(11):857–9.
22. El-Badrawy A, El-Badrawy MK. Adult presentation of asymptomatic right lung agenesis: a rare anatomical variation. Surg Radiol Anat 2019;41(2):247–9.
23. Zylak CJ, Eyler WR, Spizarny DL, et al. Developmental lung anomalies in the adult: radiologic-pathologic correlation. Radiographics 2002;22(Spec No):S25–43.
24. Sadiqi J, Hamidi H. CT features of lung agenesis - a case series (6 cases). BMC Med Imaging 2018; 18(1):37.
25. Nakayama M, Nawa T, Chonan T, et al. Prevalence of pulmonary arteriovenous malformations as

estimated by low-dose thoracic CT screening. Intern Med 2012;51(13):1677–81.

26. Gossage JR, Kanj G. Pulmonary arteriovenous malformations. A state of the art review. Am J Respir Crit Care Med 1998;158(2):643–61.

27. Tellapuri S, Park HS, Kalva SP. Pulmonary arteriovenous malformations. Int J Cardiovasc Imaging 2019; 35(8):1421–8.

28. Gill SS, Roddie ME, Shovlin CL, et al. Pulmonary arteriovenous malformations and their mimics. Clin Radiol 2015;70(1):96–110.

29. Tokunaga K, Kubo T, Yamaoka T, et al. Can the "pine-needle sign" on computed tomography be used to differentiate pulmonary arteriovenous malformation from its mimics? Analysis based on dynamic contrast-enhanced chest computed tomography in adults. Eur J Radiol 2017;95:314–8.

30. Lee EY, Boiselle PM, Cleveland RH. Multidetector CT evaluation of congenital lung anomalies. Radiology 2008;247(3):632–48.

31. McAdams HP, Kirejczyk WM, Rosado-de-Christenson ML, et al. Bronchogenic cyst: imaging features with clinical and histopathologic correlation. Radiology 2000;217(2):441–6.

32. Suen HC, Mathisen DJ, Grillo HC, et al. Surgical management and radiological characteristics of bronchogenic cysts. Ann Thorac Surg 1993;55(2): 476–81.

33. Jiang JH, Yen SL, Lee SY, et al. Differences in the distribution and presentation of bronchogenic cysts between adults and children. J Pediatr Surg 2015; 50(3):399–401.

34. Homewood R, Darby M, Medford AR. Bronchogenic cyst mimicking an isolated paratracheal lymph node. Br J Hosp Med (Lond) 2017;78(1):52–3.

35. Jun HH, Kim SM, Lee YS, et al. Cervical bronchogenic cysts mimic metastatic lymph nodes during thyroid cancer surgery. Ann Surg Treat Res 2014; 86(5):227–31.

36. Lee EY, Dorkin H, Vargas SO. Congenital pulmonary malformations in pediatric patients: review and update on etiology, classification, and imaging findings. Radiol Clin North Am 2011;49(5): 921–48.

37. Thacker PG, Rao AG, Hill JG, et al. Congenital lung anomalies in children and adults: current concepts and imaging findings. Radiol Clin North Am 2014; 52(1):155–81.

38. Panicek DM, Heitzman ER, Randall PA, et al. The continuum of pulmonary developmental anomalies. Radiographics 1987;7(4):747–72.

39. Eustace S, Valentine S, Murray J. Acquired intralobar bronchopulmonary sequestration secondary to occluding endobronchial carcinoid tumor. Clin Imaging 1996;20(3):178–80.

40. Stocker JT. Sequestrations of the lung. Semin Diagn Pathol 1986;3(2):106–21.

41. Sun X, Xiao Y. Pulmonary sequestration in adult patients: a retrospective study. Eur J Cardiothorac Surg 2015;48(2):279–82.

42. Hodson J. The lobar structure of the kidney. Br J Urol 1972;44(2):246–61.

43. Patriquin H, Lefaivre JF, Lafortune M, et al. Fetal lobation. An anatomo-ultrasonographic correlation. J Ultrasound Med 1990;9(4):191–7.

44. Yeh HC. Some misconceptions and pitfalls in ultrasonography. Ultrasound Q 2001;17(3):129–55.

45. Nazim SM, Bangash M, Salam B. Persistent fetal lobulation of kidney mimicking renal tumour. BMJ Case Rep 2017;2017 [pii:bcr-2017-219856].

46. Tynski Z, MacLennan GT. Renal pseudotumors. J Urol 2005;173(2):600.

47. Millet I, Doyon FC, Hoa D, et al. Characterization of small solid renal lesions: can benign and malignant tumors be differentiated with CT? AJR Am J Roentgenol 2011;197(4):887–96.

48. Stine VE, Wolfman NT, Dyer RB. The "dromedary hump" appearance. Abdom Imaging 2015;40(8): 3346–7.

49. Bhatt S, MacLennan G, Dogra V. Renal pseudotumors. AJR Am J Roentgenol 2007;188(5):1380–7.

50. Keats TE, Anderson MW. Atlas of normal roentgen variants that may simulate disease. 7th edition. St Louis (MO): Mosby; 2001.

51. Kellenberger CJ. Pitfalls in paediatric musculoskeletal imaging. Pediatr Radiol 2009;39(Suppl 3): 372–81.

52. Smoker WR. Craniovertebral junction: normal anatomy, craniometry, and congenital anomalies. Radiographics 1994;14(2):255–77.

53. Fielding JW, Hensinger RN, Hawkins RJ. Os odontoideum. J Bone Joint Surg Am 1980;62(3):376–83.

54. Fielding JW, Griffin PP. Os odontoideum: an acquired lesion. J Bone Joint Surg Am 1974;56(1): 187–90.

55. Brecknell JE, Malham GM. Os odontoideum: report of three cases. J Clin Neurosci 2008;15(3):295–301.

56. Arvin B, Fournier-Gosselin MP, Fehlings MG. Os odontoideum: etiology and surgical management. Neurosurgery 2010;66(3 Suppl):22–31.

57. Choit RL, Jamieson DH, Reilly CW. Os odontoideum: a significant radiographic finding. Pediatr Radiol 2005;35(8):803–7.

58. White D, Al-Mahfoudh R. The role of conservative management in incidental Os Odontoideum. World Neurosurg 2016;88:695.e15-17.

59. Henales V, Hervas JA, Lopez P, et al. Intervertebral disc herniations (limbus vertebrae) in pediatric patients: report of 15 cases. Pediatr Radiol 1993; 23(8):608–10.

60. Ghelman B, Freiberger RH. The limbus vertebra: an anterior disc herniation demonstrated by discography. AJR Am J Roentgenol 1976;127(5): 854–5.

61. Yagan R. CT diagnosis of limbus vertebra. J Comput Assist Tomogr 1984;8(1):149–51.

62. Macalister A. Notes on Acromion. J Anat Physiol 1893;27(Pt 2):244.1-251.

63. Roedl JB, Morrison WB, Ciccotti MG, et al. Acromial apophysiolysis: superior shoulder pain and acromial nonfusion in the young throwing athlete. Radiology 2015;274(1):201–9.

64. Zember JS, Rosenberg ZS, Kwong S, et al. Normal skeletal maturation and imaging pitfalls in the pediatric shoulder. Radiographics 2015;35(4):1108–22.

65. Rockwood CA. The shoulder. 4th edition. Philadelphia: Saunders/Elsevier; 2009.

66. Rovesta C, Marongiu MC, Corradini A, et al. Os acromiale: frequency and a review of 726 shoulder MRI. Musculoskelet Surg 2017;101(3):201–5.

67. Berko NS, Kurian J, Taragin BH, et al. Imaging appearances of musculoskeletal developmental variants in the pediatric population. Curr Probl Diagn Radiol 2015;44(1):88–104.

68. Baheti AD, Iyer RS, Parisi MT, et al. "Children are not small adults": avoiding common pitfalls of normal developmental variants in pediatric imaging. Clin Imaging 2016;40(6):1182–90.

69. Lawson JP. International Skeletal Society Lecture in honor of Howard D. Dorfman. Clinically significant radiologic anatomic variants of the skeleton. AJR Am J Roentgenol 1994;163(2):249–55.

70. Lawson JP. Not-so-normal variants. Orthop Clin North Am 1990;21(3):483–95.

71. Sookur PA, Naraghi AM, Bleakney RR, et al. Accessory muscles: anatomy, symptoms, and radiologic evaluation. Radiographics 2008;28(2):481–99.

72. Martinoli C, Perez MM, Padua L, et al. Muscle variants of the upper and lower limb (with anatomical correlation). Semin Musculoskelet Radiol 2010; 14(2):106–21.

73. Vanhoenacker FM, Desimpel J, Mespreuve M, et al. Accessory muscles of the extremities. Semin Musculoskelet Radiol 2018;22(3):275–85.

Moving?

Make sure your subscription moves with you!

To notify us of your new address, find your **Clinics Account Number** (located on your mailing label above your name), and contact customer service at:

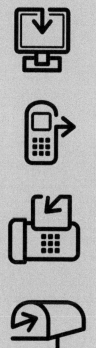

Email: journalscustomerservice-usa@elsevier.com

800-654-2452 (subscribers in the U.S. & Canada)
314-447-8871 (subscribers outside of the U.S. & Canada)

Fax number: 314-447-8029

Elsevier Health Sciences Division
Subscription Customer Service
3251 Riverport Lane
Maryland Heights, MO 63043

*To ensure uninterrupted delivery of your subscription, please notify us at least 4 weeks in advance of move.

Printed and bound by CPI Group (UK) Ltd, Croydon, CR0 4YY

08/05/2025

01864691-0019

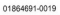